Pharmacology for the Surgical Technologist

evolve
learning system

ELSEVIER

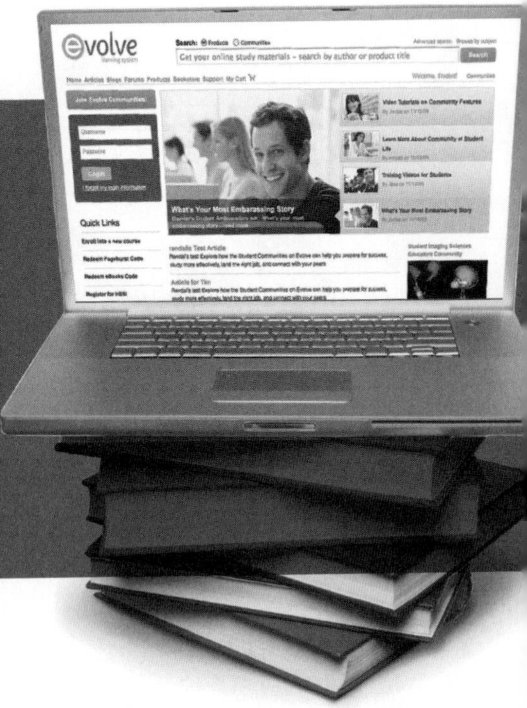

YOU'VE JUST PURCHASED MORE THAN A TEXTBOOK

ACTIVATE THE COMPLETE LEARNING EXPERIENCE THAT COMES WITH YOUR BOOK BY REGISTERING AT

http://evolve.elsevier.com/Snyder/pharmacologyST/

Once you register, you will have access to your

FREE STUDY TOOLS:

Evolve Resources for Pharmacology for the Surgical Technologist, Third Edition, offer the following features:
Instructor Resources:

- TEACH Lesson Plans
- TEACH Lecture Outlines
- TEACH PowerPoint Slides
- Image Collection
- Test Bank
- Unit Exams

Student and Instructor Resources

- Drag and Drop Exercises
- Drug Flash Card
- Key Term Flash Cards
- Medication Information Worksheet
- Visual Exercises
- Internet Exercises
- Utilizing Pharmacology Resources
- Weblinks

http://evolve.elsevier.com/Snyder/pharmacologyST/

REGISTER TODAY!

Pharmacology for the Surgical Technologist

THIRD EDITION

Katherine C. Snyder, CST, FAST, BS
Surgical Technology Program Director and Instructor
Laramie County Community College
Cheyenne, Wyoming

Chris Keegan, CST, FAST, MS
Professor and Chair
Surgical Technology Program
Vincennes University
Vincennes, Indiana

ELSEVIER

ELSEVIER
SAUNDERS

3251 Riverport Lane
St. Louis, Missouri 63043

PHARMACOLOGY FOR THE SURGICAL TECHNOLOGIST,
THIRD EDITION

ISBN: 978-1-4377-1002-1

Notices

Knowledge and best practice in this field are constantly changing. As new research and experience broaden our understanding, changes in research methods, professional practices, or medical treatment may become necessary.

Practitioners and researchers must always rely on their own experience and knowledge in evaluating and using any information, methods, compounds, or experiments described herein. In using such information or methods they should be mindful of their own safety and the safety of others, including parties for whom they have a professional responsibility.

With respect to any drug or pharmaceutical products identified, readers are advised to check the most current information provided (i) on procedures featured or (ii) by the manufacturer of each product to be administered, to verify the recommended dose or formula, the method and duration of administration, and contraindications. It is the responsibility of practitioners, relying on their own experience and knowledge of their patients, to make diagnoses, to determine dosages and the best treatment for each individual patient, and to take all appropriate safety precautions.

To the fullest extent of the law, neither the Publisher nor the authors, contributors, or editors, assume any liability for any injury and/or damage to persons or property as a matter of products liability, negligence or otherwise, or from any use or operation of any methods, products, instructions, or ideas contained in the material herein.

ISBN: 978-1-4377-1002-1

Managing Editor: Jennifer Janson
Developmental Editor: Kristen Mandava
Editorial Assistant: Anne Simon
Publishing Services Manager: Julie Eddy, Hemamalini Rajendrababu
Project Manager: Marquita Parker, Priya Dauntess
Designer: Amy Buxton

Printed in the United States of America

Last digit is the print number: 9 8 7 6 5 4 3 2

This textbook is dedicated to
the students and the instructors of surgical technology and surgical first assisting—
and to the patients we serve.

Kathy and Chris

Reviewers

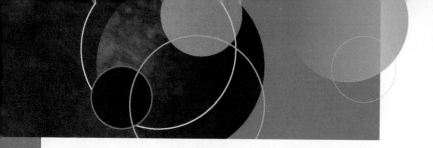

Tom McKibban, CRNA, MS
Mid-America Anesthesia Professionals, LLC
Susan B. Allen Memorial Hospital
El Dorado, Kansas

Renee Nemitz, CST, RN, AAS
Surgical Technology Program Director and Instructor
Western Iowa Tech Community College
Sioux City, Iowa

Stephen M. Setter, PharmD, CDE, CGP, FASCP
Associate Professor of Pharmacotherapy
Washington State University
Elder Services/Visiting Nurses Association
Spokane, WA

Clifford W. Smith, MSN, RN, ONC, CRNFA
Burke & Bradley Orthopedics
Pittsburg, PA

Erin Sullivan, MD
Associate Professor of Anesthesiology
Director of Cardiothoracic Anesthesiology
University of Pittsburgh Physicians
Department of Anesthesiology
Associate Chief Anesthesiologist
University of Pittsburgh Medical Center Presbyterian Hospital
Pittsburg, PA

Terry C. Wicks, CRNA, MHS, BSN
Staff Nurse Anesthetist
Obstetric Anesthesia Service
Catawba Valley Medical Center
Hickory, North Carolina

Preface

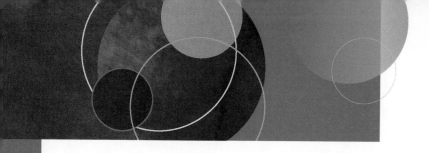

More than 15 years ago, a committee of instructors met to work on revisions to the *Core Curriculum for Surgical Technology.* During the meeting, the topic of textbooks surfaced—in particular pharmacology textbooks. It generally was agreed that no adequate pharmacology textbook for surgical technologists existed. As the discussion progressed and we complained about the situation, a question was posed: "Well, are you going to be part of the problem or part of the solution?" This third edition of the textbook is our continuing response to that question. It offers a distinct combination of subject matter. The text is organized into three units, each focusing on information specific to the surgical environment. Students will learn a framework of pharmacologic principles to apply the information in surgical situations; review basic math skills; learn commonly used medications by category, with frequent descriptions of actual surgical applications; and learn basic anesthesia concepts, not previously presented at this level, to function more effectively as a surgical team member.

Special learning tools used in this text include the following:

- Learning Objectives, stated at the beginning of each chapter
- Key Terms, which are then boldfaced in the chapters
- Insight boxes that offer additional information on the subject
- Illustrations, including surgical photographs, designed to familiarize the student with the surgical environment
- Tables and boxes that condense information to facilitate learning
- Chapter Key Concept summaries and Chapter Review questions that emphasize critical content
- Tech Tips and Make It Simple features to aid in understanding
- Advanced Practices sections emphasizing the role of the surgical first assistant
- Drug Category Index by Surgical Specialty

These features have been developed to assist the student in learning this new and often unfamiliar material. Key terms are listed at the beginning of each chapter for quick reference, and students are encouraged to consult a medical dictionary as needed for routine medical terminology used throughout the text. Learning objectives are used to guide the students through the material, emphasizing important concepts. Additional learning activities available on the Evolve web site are designed to help students think about concepts from a broader perspective and to apply content at a more personal level, particularly their local clinical facilities.

The authors would appreciate comments and suggestions from practitioners, instructors, and students using this text. Please contact us through Elsevier, c/o Jennifer Janson, 3251 Riverport Lane, Maryland Heights, MO 63043.

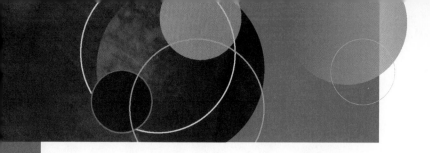

Acknowledgments

We would like to acknowledge and sincerely thank the following people for their valuable input and assistance in the development and completion of this third edition of our textbook. Thanks to the staff at Elsevier for continuing to share our vision and for helping us make this textbook's third edition a reality. We are especially grateful to Jennifer Janson, Kristen Mandava, and Kelly Brinkman for their expertise and guidance throughout the entire project. Thanks to our students for good-naturedly using various drafts of this text and for their helpful input. Our gratitude goes to Dorothy Corrigan, CST, for helping us realize the need for our text and challenging us to "be the solution."

Our special thanks goes to Renee Nemitz, CST, RN; Jeffrey Ware, CST/CFA; and Clifford W. Smith, MSN, RN, ONC, CRNFA, CRNP, for their contributions of the Advanced Practices sections.

Our sincere gratitude goes to the operating room crew at Brigham and Women's Hospital including Karyn Domenici, RPh and Claire Fitzgerald O'Shea, RN, MS, for their generous contributions to this project.

Unit Three of this third edition was revised in gratitude and loving memory of June Gross, CRNA (1939-2010) – friend, mentor, and patient advocate, whose insight was invaluable in the second edition of this text.

Acknowledgments

Contents

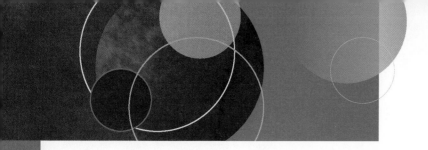

UNIT 1

INTRODUCTION TO PHARMACOLOGY

As a surgical technologist, you will mix and measure medications and deliver them to and from the sterile field. This means you will be dealing with *pharmacology*—the science of drugs. In Unit One, we look at general pharmacologic information, including how medications are measured, what kinds of medications are used, what laws pertain to them, how they are labeled, and how they are administered to the surgical patient. Chapter 1 gives a look at the medications themselves—their sources, names, classifications, routes by which they are administered, and their forms. This chapter provides a framework of pharmacologic terms, concepts, and principles—a framework that helps you understand current information about medications and prepares you to assimilate new information effectively. In Chapter 2, we focus on laws, regulations, and medication labels. You will see the importance of laws to regulate medications and the information found on medication labels, what types of laws exist, and which government agencies enforce the laws. You will also learn what acts govern your scope of practice in regard to medications. In Chapter 3, we address precision because it is critical to delivering exactly the right quantity and strength of any medication. Thus, we review mathematics that you need to do the job. We include a refresher on basic computation techniques and a review of the measurement systems used in medicine. Patient safety depends on accuracy, and the surgical technologist is the last line of defense against medication errors at the sterile field. Then in Chapter 4, we concentrate on methods you will use when handling medications, including aseptic technique, proper medication identification, and clear labeling of all medications on the sterile field.

CHAPTER 1

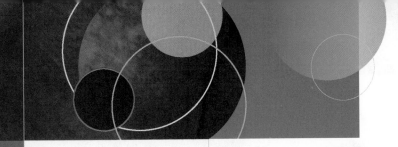

Basic Pharmacology

OBJECTIVES *After completing this chapter, you should be able to:*

1. Define terms and abbreviations related to pharmacology.
2. List sources of drugs and give an example of each.
3. List several drug classification subcategories.
4. Discuss medication orders used in surgery.
5. List the parts of a medication order.
6. Describe the drug distribution systems used in hospitals.
7. List types of drug forms.
8. Discuss the medication administration routes used in surgery.
9. Describe the four processes of pharmacokinetics.
10. Discuss aspects of pharmacodynamics.

KEY TERMS

absorption
adverse effect
agonist
antagonist
bioavailability
biotechnology
biotransformation
bolus
contraindication
distribution
duration
emulsion
enteral
excretion
hypersensitivity
idiosyncratic effect
indication
local effect
onset
parenteral
pharmacodynamics
pharmacokinetics
plasma protein binding
reconstituted
side effect
solubility
solution
suspension
synergist
systemic effect
topical

The science of pharmacology is a diverse study of the interaction between chemicals and biological systems. In the broadest sense, it includes toxicology, food science, agriculture, and medicine. When chemicals are used to treat diseases, we call them drugs or medications. Medical pharmacology is a rapidly expanding field of study because new drugs are being developed nearly every day. An understanding of basic principles in pharmacology can help the surgical technologist deal with such constant developments. Students should seek to build a framework of principles so they can incorporate new information more easily. When a new drug is introduced into surgical practice, the surgical technologist should be able to understand information about the drug by applying the principles of pharmacology. This chapter presents an introduction to the foundations of pharmacology that can be applied throughout a professional career in surgical technology.

DRUG SOURCES

Drugs in use today come from three main sources: natural sources, chemical synthesis, and biotechnology. Natural sources include plants, animals, and minerals. The study of drugs derived from natural sources is called *pharmacognosy*.

At one time, plants were nearly the only source of medicines available. Today, only a few prescription drugs relevant to surgical practice are still derived directly from plant sources (Fig. 1-1). Examples of current drugs made from plants include atropine from the roots of the belladonna plant (*Atropa belladonna*; deadly nightshade), digitalis from the leaves of the purple foxglove, and morphine from the seeds of the opium poppy (Table 1-1). The trend toward alternative medicines has initiated a closer look at plants as sources of important and helpful chemicals in the natural state (Insight 1-1). Chemicals produced by plants also hold great promise in the development of drugs to treat cancer. One such drug is paclitaxel (Taxol), which is derived from *Taxus baccata* and is used to treat breast cancer.

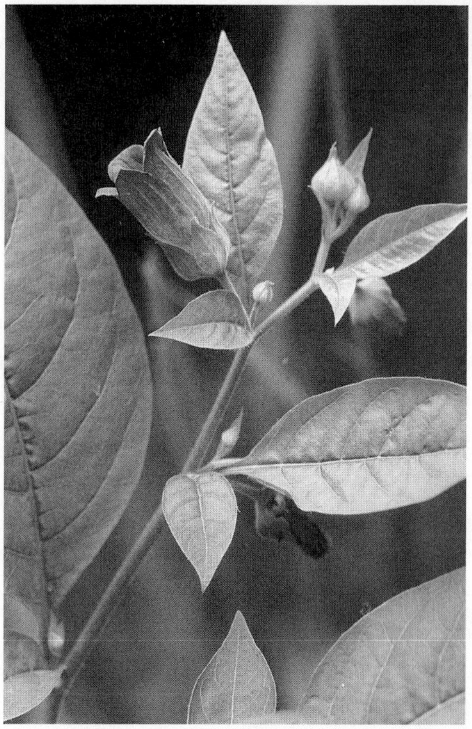

Figure 1-1 *Atropa belladonna. (Courtesy of Martin Wall Photography © 2010.)*

Animals provide a source for some drugs, particularly hormones. Cattle and hog endocrine glands were the best available source of hormones prior to the advent of biotechnology. We describe drugs derived from hogs as *porcine* and

Table 1-1 EXAMPLES OF PLANT-DERIVED DRUGS RELEVANT TO SURGICAL PRACTICE

Drug	Category	Plant
Atropine	Anticholinergic	*Atropa belladonna*
Cocaine	Local anesthetic	*Erythroxylum coca*
Digoxin	Cardiac agent	*Digitalis purpurea*
Ephedrine	Sympathomimetic	*Ephedra sinica*
Morphine	Analgesic	*Papaver somniferum*
Papaverine	Smooth muscle relaxant	*Papaver somniferum*
Pilocarpine	Parasympathomimetic	*Pilocarpus jaborandi*

IN SIGHT 1-1 In Search of New Drugs

Sometimes the quest for new drugs involves some very old sources. It has long been said that a glass of wine is good for you, and archeologists know the ancient Egyptians thought the same. While excavating the 5100-year-old tomb of Pharaoh Scorpion I, more than 700 jars were discovered in one of the chambers. Some of the jars contained wine residue with medicinal additives. These additives might have come from a relative of the present day wormwood (*Artenisia sieberi*), blue tansy, herbs, and tree resins. The jars were imported from several sites in the ancient world, in what we know today as Israel and Palestine. These jars demonstrate how humans from thousands of years ago had turned to their natural environments for effective plant remedies. It will take our modern technology to isolate these active components. Scientists are working with doctors to see if any of these compounds might be useful today—perhaps in the fight against cancer.

those from cattle as *bovine.* Thus, thyroglobulin (Proloid)—a purified extract of hog thyroid gland—is porcine in origin, whereas thrombin (Thrombogen)—a topical hemostatic—is bovine in origin. The early form of insulin is both bovine and porcine because it was obtained from the pancreas of cattle and hogs. Estrogen was another hormone obtained from an animal source. Conjugated estrogen (Premarin) was obtained from the urine of pregnant horses and so is referred to as *equine* in nature.

Minerals, such as calcium, magnesium, and silver salts in several forms, are used in some pharmacological agents. For example, Tums and Mylanta are antacids that contain calcium (Tums) and magnesium (Mylanta) hydroxides. Silver sulfadiazine (Silvadene cream) is an antimicrobial agent used in dressings for burn patients that contains silver salts. Even gold is used, as in aurothioglucose (Solganal), an antiarthritic agent.

The second major source of drugs is chemical synthesis in the laboratory. There are two ways for drugs to be *synthesized,* that is, put together. *Synthetic drugs* are drugs that are synthesized from laboratory chemicals. *Semisynthetic drugs* are drugs that start with a natural substance that is extracted, purified, and altered by chemical processes. The vast majority of modern drugs are either synthetic or semisynthetic. Meperidine (Demerol) is an example of a synthetic drug; it is made from chemicals, yet its pain-relieving effects are similar to those of opium. Many types of penicillin—such as amoxicillin—are semisynthetic drugs. The penicillin group of drugs was originally derived from a natural mold *(Penicillium),* the active substance of which is extracted and purified in the chemical laboratory. Another example of semisynthetic drugs is the aminoglycoside group of antibiotics, the active substance of which is obtained from the bacterial species *Streptomyces.*

An increasing source of drugs has been provided by the science of biotechnology. The term **biotechnology** is used to refer to the concepts of genetic engineering and recombinant DNA technology. The science of biotechnology has many applications in pharmacology and has provided significant improvements in the treatment of various conditions. Biotechnology is a process that allows scientists to produce proteins from bacteria—proteins that were previously available only from animals. Molecular biologists use bacteria as tiny factories to produce the proteins they need to make drugs. They do this by altering the DNA of bacteria such as *Escherichia coli (E. coli).* How? By physically inserting a gene into the DNA of a single *E. coli* cell—a gene that *codes for* (tells the cell to make) a certain protein (Fig. 1-2). When the

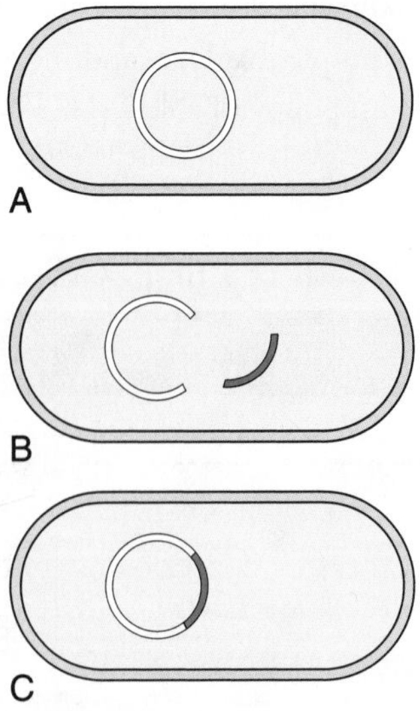

Figure 1-2 **Biotechnology. A,** *Escherichia coli* DNA. **B,** Desired gene is inserted into bacterial DNA. **C,** Bacterial DNA with recombinant gene.

bacterial cell has this gene incorporated into its DNA, it becomes a miniature copying machine, producing daughter cells that have daughter cells that have daughter cells—each with the new gene and each producing the desired protein. As this reproduction process occurs very rapidly, large volumes of the desired protein can be obtained quickly. The specific protein is extracted and purified in the laboratory and prepared for administration into a patient. Molecular biologists also use cultures of mammalian cell lines, such as genetically altered Chinese hamster ovary (CHO) cells to produce various therapeutic proteins. In general, CHO cells provide more stable gene expression and higher volumes of the desired proteins than bacterial cells and are becoming the primary choice of cell lines for pharmacological use.

Among the drugs produced by biotechnology are human insulin (Humulin), human growth hormone (Nutropin), human thyroid-stimulating hormone (Thyrogen), and the thrombolytic agent alteplase (Activase). Such genetically engineered proteins do not cause the adverse side effects—for example, immune or allergic reactions—often seen in the long-term use of drugs from animal sources. Drugs such as these are always administered by injection; they cannot be taken orally because they are proteins, which are digested when consumed.

DRUG CLASSIFICATIONS

Drug classifications are used to group similar drugs, or drugs that are used for similar purposes. We can classify drugs by what they do, what they affect, and what they are; thus, common classification categories include the following:

- *Therapeutic action:* what they do for a patient; for example, analgesics relieve pain.
- *Physiologic action:* what they do in the body; for example, histamine receptor antagonists block histamine production.
- *Affected body system:* what they affect; for example, cardiovascular agents affect the heart and circulatory system.
- *Chemical type:* what they are; for example, barbiturates are a class of chemical compounds derived from barbituric acid.

Drugs can be cross-referenced in multiple classification categories. For example, ranitidine (Zantac) is categorized therapeutically as an antacid, physiologically as a histamine receptor antagonist, and by body system as a gastric agent. Each classification category has several subcategories, as shown in Table 1-2. Drugs having multiple therapeutic effects are classified in more than one subcategory. For example, aspirin relieves pain, fever, and inflammation, so it is classified as an analgesic,

Table 1-2 DRUG CLASSIFICATION CATEGORIES AND SUBCATEGORIES

Therapeutic Action	Physiologic Action	Body System	Chemical Type
Analgesic	α-adrenergic blocker	Cardiovascular agent	Barbiturate
Anticoagulant	Cholinergic	Dermatologic agent	Benzodiazepine
Antiemetic	Diuretic	Ophthalmic preparation	Hormone
Antihistamine	Hemostatic	Urinary tract agent	Narcotic
Antihypertensive	Histamine receptor antagonist		Oxytocic
Anti-inflammatory	Muscle relaxant antagonist		Steroid
Antineoplastic	Narcotic antagonist		
Antipyretic	Tranquilizer		
Antispasmodic	Vasoconstrictor		
Sedative			
Thrombolytic			

an antipyretic, and an anti-inflammatory agent—three different therapeutic subcategories. Therapeutic-action subcategories of drugs frequently used from the sterile back table include antibiotics, anticoagulants, anti-inflammatory agents, and local anesthetics.

MAKE IT SIMPLE

The classification subcategories are far more helpful to the surgical technologist in practice because most subcategory titles will provide clues to the use or purpose of a medication. Use medical terminology word-building techniques to define the subcategories and help you determine a medication's purpose. For example: anesthetic; "an-" means without and "-esthesia" means sensation. So, an anesthetic agent causes a loss of sensation.

Subcategories of the classification physiologic action help in the understanding of how particular drugs work. For example, a vasoconstrictor will cause contraction of the walls of blood vessels and restrict blood flow. Anticonvulsants are used to treat epileptic seizures and so are more accurately identified as anti-epileptics. Some anticonvulsants such as phenytoin (Dilantin) have been found useful as adjuncts in pain management. Emetics are given to stimulate rapid emptying of the stomach, termed emesis, but are not frequently administered in current practice because simpler means are available to produce emesis.

Additionally, the subcategories of the classification *body system* may be helpful in clarifying appropriate surgical uses. For example, if a medication is subcategorized as an ophthalmic agent, it may be specially formulated for use in the eye only. An *otic* medication is specially formulated for use in the ear.

Drugs are also classified by how they may be obtained. The distinction between prescription and nonprescription or over-the-counter (OTC) drugs is a legal classification. In addition, some prescription medications are subcategorized as controlled substances. Legal classifications are discussed in detail in Chapter 2.

MEDICATION ORDERS

PRESCRIPTIONS

When treatment requires a specific drug, a licensed physician or designee such as a physician's assistant (PA) or nurse practitioner (NP) writes a prescription for the drug. State governments have the power to regulate which medical professionals write prescriptions, so there are variations in practice from state to state. Figure 1-3

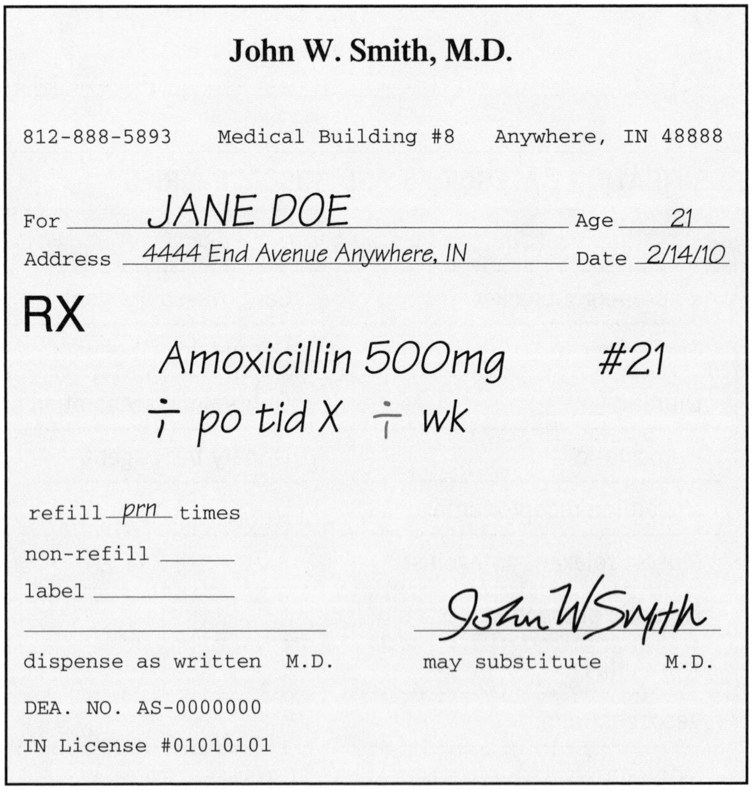

John W. Smith, M.D.

812-888-5893 Medical Building #8 Anywhere, IN 48888

For JANE DOE Age 21

Address 4444 End Avenue Anywhere, IN Date 2/14/10

RX

Amoxicillin 500mg #21

i̅ po tid X i̅ wk

refill prn times

non-refill

label

dispense as written M.D.

John W Smith

may substitute M.D.

DEA. NO. AS-0000000

IN License #01010101

Figure 1-3 A typical prescription form.

shows a typical written prescription form. As shown, prescriptions must include the date, name of the patient, name of the drug, dosage, route of administration, and frequency or time of administration. It must also bear the prescriber's signature. Notice that the printed form contains the name, address, telephone number, and DEA number of the prescriber. The Drug Enforcement Administration (DEA) requires that this number be listed on any prescription for a controlled substance (see Chapter 2). A written prescription usually designates the drug by trade name but may indicate that a generic substitution is permissible. When writing prescriptions, physicians (or their designees) use abbreviations and symbols (Table 1-3) for directions, dosages, frequency, and administration routes. Pharmacists interpret these symbols and give the drugs to the patient, along with instructions for proper use. Many pharmacies use computer database systems that provide specific, detailed printouts to the patient of such important drug information as side effects, precautions, normal usage, and storage. Prescriptions such as shown are not generally used during a patient's hospitalization, so have little or no use during surgery.

Table 1-3 ABBREVIATIONS FOR MEDICATION ADMINISTRATION DIRECTIONS

Abbreviation	Meaning
aa	Of each
ad	To, up to
ad lib	As desired
amt	Amount
c̄	With
KVO, TKO	Keep vein open, to keep open
npo, NPO	Nothing by mouth (os)
per	By means of, by
Rx	Take
s̄	Without
sig	Label
sos	Once if necessary
stat	Immediately

Written prescriptions occasionally present difficulties when interpreting handwriting. The introduction of electronic prescribing or *e-prescribing* may significantly reduce medication errors due to misinterpretation of poorly handwritten prescriptions. E-prescribing is the process of generating, transmitting, and filing of prescriptions through a computer-based system. These systems also provide ready access to important prescriber safety information such as patient medication history and allergies.

HOSPITAL MEDICATION ORDERS

In the hospital setting, any medications to be administered to the patient must be ordered by a licensed physician or designee and written on a physician's order sheet or entered into the electronic prescribing system. In surgery, the medication order may be one of several types.

Standing Orders

A standing order, or *protocol,* is used for common situations requiring a standard treatment. For example, institutions participating in the Surgical Care Improvement Project (SCIP) may have a standing order in place stating that all patients undergoing specified general surgery procedures are to receive 1 to 2 g of cefoxitin (Mefoxin) IV one hour prior to the incision. In the operating room, surgeon's preference cards contain standing orders for specific surgical procedures. For example, Dr. Vigil's preference card for abdominal aortic aneurysm (AAA) repair may include a standing order for 5000 units of heparin in 1000 mL of NaCl for topical irrigation. A standing order of this type informs the operating room team that the indicated medication should be ready on the sterile back table as a standard part of the setup for that procedure.

Verbal Orders

Verbal orders are commonplace in surgery, as a surgeon may request a particular drug to be administered either from the sterile field or by the anesthesia provider. For example, during an AAA repair Dr. Vigil may give a verbal order to the anesthesia provider to administer 5000 units of heparin intravenously three minutes prior to cross-clamping the aorta. Verbal orders in surgery are usually for a one-time single administration of a medication. The verbal order is documented in the patient's record.

STAT Orders

Often given verbally, STAT orders indicate that a drug is to be administered immediately and one time only. The most common use of STAT orders in surgery is during cardiac arrest resuscitation or other emergent situations.

PRN Orders

PRN stands for *pro re nata,* which means that the drug may be given as needed. For example, during septoplasty performed under local anesthesia, meperidine (Demerol) may be administered PRN to reduce patient discomfort.

In surgery, medications routinely needed during a procedure are listed on the surgeon's preference card. As shown in Figure 1-4, the preference card should list all pertinent information, such as drug strength and quantity. Surgical medication orders on preference cards usually contain the drug name, strength, and dosage.

REGIONAL MEDICAL CENTER
SURGEON PREFERENCE CARD AND REQUISITION

Patient name: Jane Doe
Procedure date: 01/31/10
Scheduled time: 0730
Surgeon: Meier, C.
Procedure: Cataract extraction with IOL, left eye.

Item code	Item description	Req.	Quantity Picked	Chgd
		STERILE SUPPLIES		
001957	Steridrape 1060 3M	1		
005006	Skin scrub tray	1		
000574	Glove sterile 71/2	1		
005890	Custom pack -cataract	1		
011005	Phaco tubing Kit	1		
		INSTRUMENTS		
009505	Cataract set - Meier	1		
011013	Phaco handpiece	1		
011014	I.A.instruments	1		
		MEDICATIONS		
002365	BSS 15 mL	2		
002367	BSS Plus 500 mL	1		
218965	Dexamethasone 4 mg	1		
218966	Celestone 3 mg	1		
012164	Ancef 50 mg	1		
010433	Micochol	1		
359003	Lidocaine 2% 50 mL w/epi 1:200,000	1		
359004	Bupivacaine 0.5%	1		
010492	Epinephrine 1:1000 1 mL	1		
437283	Wydase 150 units	1		
455849	Healon 0.85 mL	1		
238934	Tobradex ointment	1		
567392	Vancomycin 10 mg	1		

SURGEON SPECIAL REQUESTS

- Add 0.3 mL epinephrine, 2 mg dexamethasone, and 10 mg of vancomycin to 500 mL bottle of BSS plus.
- Add remaining dexamethasone (2 mg) to celestone for injection at end of case.
- Do not add Wydase to anesthetic agent until just prior to use.
- Combine 2% lidocaine w/epi (5 mL), bupivacaine 0.5% (5 mL), and Wydase 150 units for injection.

Figure 1-4 A computerized surgeon's preference card lists medications required for the procedure.

IN SIGHT 1-2 Practical Math—Calculating Drug Dosages at the Sterile Back Table

Dosage = strength × volume

Some drugs are available in various strengths, such as lidocaine. How much of the drug is given depends on the strength *and* the volume. The same dosage of lidocaine can be given in different ways. For example, 30 mL of 1% lidocaine delivers the same dosage as 15 mL of 2% lidocaine or 60 mL of 0.5% lidocaine.

Unlike medication orders given in nursing care units, the surgeon administers all medications at the sterile field, so route of administration and frequency are not usually stated on surgeon's preference cards.

Many abbreviations are used to represent drug forms, dosages, routes, and timing of administration. Dosages are stated in a particular unit of measure, usually in the metric system, and abbreviated, such as 300 mg, 10 mL, or 1000 units. The dosage of a medication is the medication strength (usually expressed as a percent) multiplied by the volume administered (Insight 1-2).

For example, lidocaine (Xylocaine) may be injected for local anesthesia and therefore is listed on the preference card as "lidocaine plain 1%—30 mL." This indicates that a 30-mL vial of a 1% solution of lidocaine without epinephrine should be delivered to the sterile back table and prepared for use. It may not be necessary to use the entire 30 mL during the procedure, so the surgical technologist in the scrub role reports the final amount (volume) used to the circulator who records the dose.

For regular hospital medication orders, the route of administration is usually abbreviated; for example, if a drug is to be given intravenously, it is designated as IV. The frequency or time of administration is also clearly stated and is often abbreviated; for example, if the drug is to be taken twice a day, it is designated bid. Table 1-4 lists common abbreviations used to represent frequency of drug administration. Again, most surgeons' preference cards do not list the route or frequency because the surgeon is administering all medications given at the surgical site.

⚠ CAUTION

Some abbreviations have been associated with an increased risk of misinterpretation and possible medication errors. The Joint Commission, which accredits hospitals and other health care institutions, requires accredited facilities to publish a "do not use" list for potentially dangerous abbreviations, acronyms, and symbols (see Chapter 2, Table 2–2). Before using what you may think are standard abbreviations, consult this list at your facility.

Table 1-4 ABBREVIATIONS FOR FREQUENCY OF MEDICATION ADMINISTRATION

Abbreviation	Meaning
bid	Twice a day
h, hr	Hour
prn, PRN	As necessary *(pro re nata)*
q	Every
qh	Every hour
q2h	Every 2 hours
qid	Four times a day
tid	Three times a day
stat	Immediately

DRUG DISTRIBUTION SYSTEMS

Dispensing prescription drugs is the responsibility of a licensed pharmacist. That is, pharmacists must *release* drugs, either directly to patients or to the physician or surgeon who orders them. In hospitals, drugs are often released for secure storage in various patient care areas so they can be distributed as necessary.

{NOTE} *In all medical facilities, controlled substances (such as morphine) must be stored in a secure location once they have been released from the pharmacy. Individual institutional policies are put in place to account for and document the use of controlled substances.*

Distribution systems for drugs used in surgery vary among institutions. In large hospitals with many operating rooms, a satellite pharmacy (Fig. 1-5) within the surgical suite may dispense drugs as needed for each procedure. Other, often smaller, facilities may maintain a medication room or cabinet where they store frequently

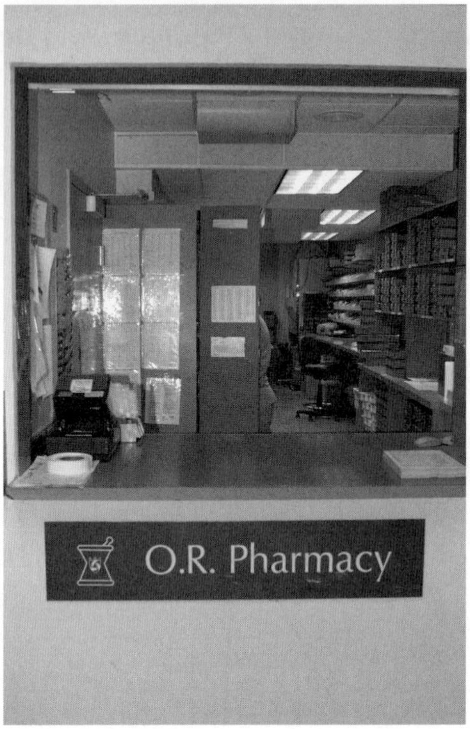

Figure 1-5 A satellite pharmacy in surgery.

used drugs, such as antibiotics and local anesthetics. In addition, some hospitals use a system of mobile drug carts, which must be exchanged for restocking after the drugs are used. For example, emergency-response drug carts, known as *crash carts,* are used for cardiac arrest and other emergency situations. Such carts may be restocked on an exchange basis to assure the immediate availability of all necessary drugs. Computer-automated dispensing systems are also used for medication distribution in surgery. These systems have been developed to minimize medication administration errors. A bar code-scanning system allows an approved user access to particular medications ordered for a particular patient.

DRUG FORMS OR PREPARATIONS

Drugs are available in several different forms or preparations. Drugs may be in solid, semisolid, liquid, or gas form. The form of drug administered affects both the onset of drug actions and the intensity of the body's response to the drug. Liquids, for instance, tend to act more quickly than solids, and gases or vapors tend to act even faster. Drug form also dictates route of administration. For example, the antibiotic neosporin comes in ointment (semisolid) form, which must be applied topically only. Some drugs are available in more than one form. For example, lidocaine (Xylocaine) is available in jelly for topical application and in solutions of various strengths for injection. The names of drug forms are often abbreviated in drug orders. Table 1-5 lists several common abbreviations for drug forms.

Table 1-5 ABBREVIATIONS FOR DRUG FORMS OR PREPARATIONS

Abbreviation	Meaning
cap	Capsule
gtts	Drops
soln	Solution
susp	Suspension
tab	Tablet
ung	Ointment

SOLIDS

Many drugs come prepared in solid form. These drugs may be in capsule (cap) or tablet (tab) form and are administered orally. Capsules are gelatin cases containing a drug in powder or granule form; tablets are a compressed form of the drug, usually combined with inert ingredients. Capsules and tablets are rarely used in surgery, because oral administration is required. In most cases surgical patients must be kept NPO (from the Latin *nil per os,* nothing by mouth), or they may be under a general anesthesia and unable to swallow.

Some drugs come in powder form and are contained in glass vials. Such powders must be mixed with a liquid **(reconstituted)** to form a solution that can be administered by injection. For example, several antibiotics administered in surgery are powders that must be reconstituted with sterile water or a sodium chloride solution (saline) to make an injectable solution. Other drugs, such as dantrolene (Dantrium)—an infrequently used yet important skeletal muscle relaxant—also come in powder form and must be reconstituted before use (see Chapter 16).

SEMISOLIDS

Semisolid preparations include creams, foams, gels, and ointments. Creams consist of active ingredients in a water base while ointments contain active ingredients in an oil, lanolin, or petroleum base. Gels (such as K-Y Jelly) are thicker than creams, but are still water based. Examples of semisolid drugs used in surgery include lidocaine (Xylocaine) jelly for topical anesthesia, Silvadene cream for burns, estrogen cream for vaginal packing, and neosporin ointment for wound dressing.

LIQUIDS

Several types of liquid drug preparations are available. Many liquid medications are available in solution. A **solution** is a mixture of drug particles (called the solute) fully dissolved in a liquid medium (called the solvent such as water or saline). Several common solutions are used from the sterile back table, including normal saline (0.9% NaCl) irrigation, antibiotic irrigation solutions, and heparin irrigation solution. Liquid nasal sprays such as oxymetazoline (Afrin) may also be used from the sterile back table.

Drugs may also be in **suspension.** A suspension is a form in which solid undissolved particles float (are suspended) in a liquid. Suspensions should be shaken prior to administration to evenly distribute particles throughout the liquid. Suspensions used from the sterile back table include Cortisporin otic, used in ear surgery, and Celestone, an anti-inflammatory used in ophthalmology.

> **TECH TIP**
>
> Just before handing a medication in suspension to the surgeon, simply roll the syringe or vial between your fingers or palms to mix the suspended particles evenly.

Another type of liquid medication form is an **emulsion,** in which the medication is contained in a mixture of water and oil bound together with an emulsifier. Emulsions can be either water in oil or oil in water, depending on the medication's solubility. The most common emulsion used in surgery is propofol (Diprivan), an intravenous sedative-hypnotic agent used for anesthesia (see Chapter 15).

Drugs in liquid form may also be administered orally, as *elixirs* (sweetened solutions of alcohol) or *syrups* (sweetened aqueous solutions). But elixirs and syrups are rarely, if ever, used in surgery because of the NPO status for surgical patients.

GASES

The only common medications available in gas form are inhalation anesthetic agents. These agents include nitrous oxide and volatile liquids such as desflurane (Suprane) (see Chapter 15). The volatile liquid agents are vaporized through an apparatus on the anesthesia machine into gas form for administration.

DRUG ADMINISTRATION ROUTES

Medications are formulated for administration by a specific route. In addition to the drug form, the route by which a drug is given can affect onset time and body response. Drugs may be administered by many different routes, only a few of which are used commonly in surgery. Medication orders state route of administration, usually in abbreviated form (Table 1-6). The three major categories of medication administration routes are **enteral, topical,** and **parenteral**. The enteral route indicates that the medication is taken into the gastrointestinal tract, primarily by mouth (orally). Topical medications are applied to the skin surface or a mucous membrane–lined cavity. The term *parenteral* indicates any route other than the digestive tract, the most common of which are subcutaneous, intramuscular, and intravenous.

> **MAKE IT SIMPLE**
>
> Use medical terminology word-building techniques to help you understand the terms *enteral* and *parenteral*. The root word or combining form "enter/o-" means intestines, and the adjective ending "-al" means pertaining to. The combining form "/o" is not used when the suffix begins with a vowel, so the word enteral means pertaining to the intestines or intestinal tract. The prefix "para-" indicates beside or beyond (the "a" is dropped when the root word begins with a vowel) so the term *parenteral* means outside, or *not in*, the intestinal tract.

The oral route (PO, from the Latin *per os*, "by mouth") is the simplest and most common way to administer many drugs. Tablets or capsules are swallowed and readily absorbed through the lining (mucosa) of the gastrointestinal tract. Certain drugs may irritate the gastrointestinal mucosa and should therefore be given with food. Other drugs may be inactivated by

Table 1-6 ABBREVIATIONS FOR DRUG ADMINISTRATION ROUTES

Abbreviation	Meaning
IM	Intramuscular
IV	Intravenous
PO, po	Per os, orally

increased amounts of digestive enzymes and so are best taken between meals. When drugs are administered orally, onset of action is usually slower and duration of effect is usually longer than with other routes. Some drugs, however, are completely inactivated by the digestive process and therefore must not be given orally. Insulin, a hormone, and heparin, an anticoagulant, are not effective when administered orally.

The oral route is rarely used in surgery because the patient must be kept NPO before surgery and because many patients are under general anesthesia during surgery and so are unable to swallow. An exception is oral administration of a small amount of sodium citrate (Bicitra), which used to be given preoperatively to neutralize gastric acid (see Chapter 13).

Some medications are available in topical preparations, which are intended for application to the skin or a mucous membrane–lined cavity. Some topical agents work at the site of application; this is called a **local effect.** Some topical medications exert a **systemic effect,** that is, throughout the entire body. Examples of topical medications with local effect include steroid creams for rashes and antibiotic ointment for cuts. Applied to the affected area, these agents work directly on the immediate site. Topical medications that exert a systemic effect include hormone replacement therapy (estrogen and progestin), birth control (estrogen and progesterone), and motion sickness (scopolamine) transdermal patches. Even though these types of agents are applied to an area of the skin, once absorbed the agents will have an effect on the entire body. Blood supply to the topical administration area impacts the speed of absorption. Topical medications are absorbed slowly through the skin, but are absorbed rapidly when applied to blood supply–rich mucous membranes.

{NOTE} *Some medications, though taken orally, are actually topical in that the tablet (pill) is held in the mouth, either in the cheek (buccal) or under the tongue (sublingual), and allowed to dissolve. The medication is absorbed through the mucous membrane of the mouth and does not pass directly into the gastrointestinal tract.*

Several topical medications are used in surgery. Antibiotic ointments, such as neosporin, may be used on the surgical incision as part of the postoperative wound dressing. Estrogen cream may be applied to vaginal packing used as a pressure dressing after a vaginal hysterectomy.

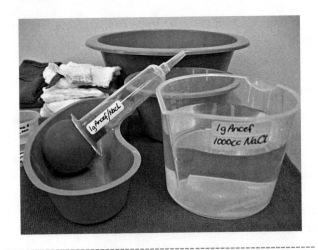

Figure 1-6 Antibiotic irrigation used during surgery is an example of a topical application of a medication.

Topical antibiotic irrigation is common in surgery, in which case an antibiotic solution is poured or squirted into the surgical site (Fig. 1-6). In many vascular procedures, a solution of heparin (an anticoagulant; see Chapter 9) is used as a topical irrigation to prevent the formation of blood clots in operative vessels during surgery.

{NOTE} *Vascular procedures may also involve using intravenous heparin for systemic effect. But when used as a topical irrigation, heparin exerts a more significant local effect, because the operative vessel is usually clamped off, preventing systemic absorption of the agent.*

Instillation of a medication into a mucous membrane–lined cavity, such as the eye, nose, or urethra, may also be considered a topical route or application. A number of medications are instilled into body cavities intraoperatively, situations unique to surgery. For example, tetracaine (Pontocaine) drops may be instilled into the eye for local anesthesia for cataract extraction, phenylephrine (Neo-Synephrine) may be instilled into the nasal cavity for vasoconstriction during sinusoscopy, or lidocaine (Xylocaine) jelly may be instilled into the urethra as topical anesthesia for cystoscopy. During diagnostic gynecologic laparoscopy, a methylene blue solution may be instilled via a cervical cannula into the uterus. This procedure is known as a tubal dye study or chromotubation and is used to assess tubal patency in patients with infertility. The methylene blue solution fills the uterus and exits through the uterine tubes into the pelvic cavity when the tubes are patent (open). The laparoscope is used to observe the blue solution exiting the tubal fimbria. If the tubes are blocked by scarring, the solution cannot enter the pelvic cavity. Another example of medication instillation occurs during operative cholangiography. Although not as frequently performed currently due to the availability of endoscopic retrograde cholangiopancreatography (ERCP), intraoperative cholangiography involves the instillation of a radiographic contrast media into the common bile duct to detect gallstones under x-ray. If present, common bile duct stones will be evident on radiograph as shadows in the radiopaque contrast media. For additional information on diagnostic agents, see Chapter 6.

Inhalation is a means of medication administration that can be considered topical. Some asthmatic drugs are administered through a respiratory inhaler or through a nebulizer—a device that converts liquid drugs into an inhalable mist. The drug is absorbed in the bronchi of the lungs, providing local relief of bronchoconstriction. In surgery, anesthetic gases and vapors are administered via inhalation, but these drugs exert systemic rather than local effects.

Most medications used in surgery are administered parenterally. The most common parenteral routes are subcutaneous, intramuscular, and intravenous. Subcutaneous injections are given beneath the skin into the subcutaneous tissue layer. Common sites for subcutaneous injections are the upper lateral aspect of the arm, the anterior thigh, and the abdomen. Depending on blood supply, absorption from subcutaneous tissue is fairly rapid. Only a few drugs are administered subcutaneously in surgery; for example, heparin may be injected subcutaneously preoperatively in some cases to help prevent pulmonary embolism.

A few drugs used in surgery are administered intramuscularly (IM). Intramuscular injections are usually given into a large muscle mass, such as the deltoid, gluteal, or vastus lateralis. Intramuscular absorption is usually rapid due to the large absorbing surface and good blood supply. An example of a drug given IM in surgery is ketorolac (Toradol), a nonsteroidal anti-inflammatory drug (NSAID) used for postoperative pain relief.

Probably the most common example of the parenteral route used at the surgical site is the administration (injection) of a local anesthetic agent for intraoperative pain control. Local anesthesia during a surgical procedure may be accomplished with an agent such as lidocaine (Xylocaine), which is injected into multiple tissue layers as needed. Quite frequently, a longer-acting local anesthetic (such as bupivacaine) is used to inject the surgical site for postoperative pain control. For a more detailed discussion of local anesthetics, see Chapter 14.

Most medications administered parenterally during surgery are given intravenously (IV), that is, within a vein, as shown in Figure 1-7. A small catheter is inserted into a vein and connected to tubing called an infusion set. The infusion set is attached to a bag of intravenous fluid for administration. Drugs may then be injected as needed into sites along the tubing. Drugs may be given all at once, as a **bolus,** or by slow infusion. Absorption is immediate for medications administered intravenously because the agent goes directly into the bloodstream.

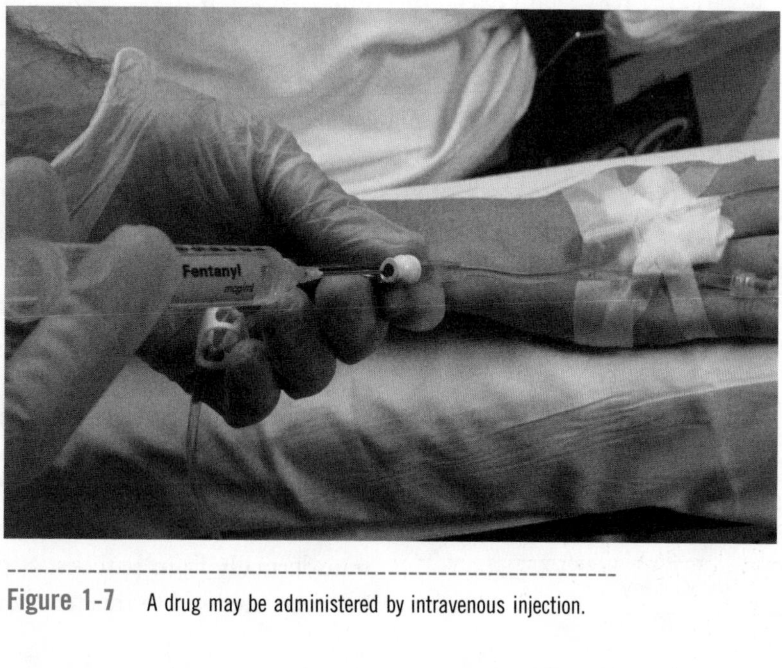

Figure 1-7 A drug may be administered by intravenous injection.

Other parenteral routes are used less frequently. *Intradermal* injections are given between layers of skin, as seen in tuberculin skin testing and allergy testing. A local anesthetic may be injected intradermally prior to placing an intravenous catheter, thereby reducing discomfort at the insertion site. *Intra-articular* injections (into the joint space) of anti-inflammatory agents or local anesthetics may be given after arthroscopy. *Intrathecal* injections of anesthetics or contrast media are administered into the spinal subarachnoid space to diffuse into cerebral spinal fluid (CSF). During cardiac arrest resuscitation, a drug such as epinephrine may be injected directly into the heart; this is called an *intracardiac* injection.

PHARMACOKINETICS

The study of **pharmacokinetics** focuses on how the body processes drugs, and the science of **pharmacodynamics** examines how the action of the drug affects the body. The science of pharmacokinetics studies a medication from administration through four basic physiologic processes—absorption, distribution, biotransformation, and excretion (Table 1-7). The patient's general health has a significant effect on how the body processes drugs. For example, if the patient's blood supply, liver function, or kidney function is compromised, the ability to process medications is also compromised.

ABSORPTION

To be effective, a drug must first be absorbed into the body. **Absorption** is the process by which a drug is taken into the body and moves from the site of administration into the blood. Drugs are absorbed from the site of administration into the bloodstream and enter systemic circulation. Speed of absorption, or absorption rate, varies by administration route and by blood supply to the area. **Solubility** of the drug (its ability to be dissolved) also affects the absorption rate. If a drug is in solid form, it must dissolve before it can be absorbed. Drugs in suspensions absorb faster than solid drugs, and solutions absorb faster than suspensions. For example, a solution instilled in the conjunctiva will absorb more quickly than an ointment applied to the conjunctiva.

Oral absorption varies depending on the drug's chemical structure as well as the pH (acidity) and motility of the gastrointestinal tract. If the digestive tract is highly motile, as in patients with diarrhea, ingested drugs may not be adequately absorbed. Conversely, if the patient is constipated drugs may be fully absorbed, sometimes to toxic levels. Intramuscular absorption is rapid if water-based drug solutions are injected and is slower if the solution is an oil-based emulsion. The amount and vascularization of muscle mass also affects the rate of absorption of medications given IM. Intravenous absorption is immediate because drugs are injected directly into the bloodstream. The absorption rate of drugs given subcutaneously depends on blood supply to the area of injection.

{NOTE} *Rapid drug absorption can be undesirable in surgery when local anesthetics are used. The anesthetic agent must stay in the desired area to exert its desired effect. Thus, a* vasoconstrictor, *usually epinephrine, may be added to the anesthetic agent to narrow the small blood vessels in the local area and delay absorption of the anesthetic agent into systemic circulation. Local vasoconstriction will prolong the anesthetic agent's effect (see Chapter 14).*

Absorption of drugs given by inhalation, especially inhalation anesthetics, is rapid, because of the huge numbers of capillaries in the alveoli of the lungs. Some drugs administered by inhalation (such as steroids for asthma) are specifically formulated for local effect, and so do not absorb rapidly. Mucosal tissues provide excellent absorption for some drugs because of the number of capillaries just under the mucosal surface. Common mucosal administration sites include the respiratory tract, oral cavity, and the conjunctiva.

Although most drugs are not absorbed easily through skin, some are specifically formulated to overcome the skin barrier. Such drugs are administered transdermally from patches. Scopolamine patches, for instance, are used to treat motion sickness; they release

Table 1-7 THE FOUR PROCESSES OF PHARMACOKINETICS

Process	Body System
Absorption	Body system varies by administration route (e.g., integumentary, gastrointestinal, respiratory)
Distribution	Circulatory system
Biotransformation	Liver
Excretion	Kidney

the drug slowly so it may be absorbed through skin over a period of hours.

Thus, absorption of a medication depends on the formulation of the drug, the route of administration, and the extent of blood supply to the site of administration.

DISTRIBUTION

Once a drug has been absorbed into the bloodstream, it is transported throughout the body by the circulatory system. Drug molecules eventually diffuse out of the bloodstream to the site of action in the process called **distribution**. The term **bioavailability** indicates the degree to which the drug molecule reaches the site of action to exert its effects. Several factors affect a drug's bioavailability including the acid-base balance (Insight 1-3). Because drugs are carried to all parts of the body, their effects can be seen in locations other than the intended area. The amount of drug reaching the site of action depends on the general condition of the patient's circulatory system, on the effective blood flow to the intended area (tissue perfusion), and on the extent of plasma protein binding. Areas with high blood flow include the heart, liver, and kidneys and tissues with low blood flow include bone, fat and skin. For example, since bone has very limited blood flow, intravenous antibiotics often have little effect in treating bone infections. In addition, two barriers exist that limit the distribution of certain drug molecules to particular sites. The placental barrier allows some molecules to pass to the fetus, while restricting others. The blood-brain barrier also limits passage of certain molecules into brain tissue.

Plasma Protein Binding

Not all drug molecules in the bloodstream are available to bind at the site of action. Some drug molecules bind to proteins (albumins and globulins) contained in plasma—the liquid portion of blood—via a process known as **plasma protein binding.** Both the amount of plasma protein in the blood and the binding characteristics of the drug determine the extent to which a drug is bound. Some drugs are highly bound (up to 99%), some are only minimally bound, whereas others are not bound at all. Highly bound drug molecules have a longer duration of action, because they stay in the body longer, and a lower distribution to the site of action. The only drug molecules available to exert effects on the body are unbound molecules. Unbound drug molecules are considered *bioactive.*

Plasma protein binding is usually nonspecific; that is, plasma proteins can bind with many different drug molecules. It is also competitive in that drug molecules also compete with other drug molecules for protein-binding sites, changing the amount of available drug significantly. Potential hazards arise if patients are taking different drugs that compete for the same binding sites. For instance, if a patient taking warfarin sodium (Coumadin), a highly bound anticoagulant, takes aspirin, the aspirin will bind with the same plasma protein sites, making more warfarin available than is needed (Fig. 1-8). If more than the expected amount of warfarin is available, overmedication and excessive anticoagulation may occur. Other highly-bound drugs used in surgery include propofol (Diprivan), fentanyl, and diazepam.

Plasma protein binding is reversible. When the concentration of unbound drug in blood is lowered, either by metabolism or excretion, bound molecules are released from binding sites. The extent of plasma protein binding can prolong a drug's effects and contribute to drug-drug interactions.

BIOTRANSFORMATION

The circulatory system also distributes drugs to the liver, the major structure of the biliary system. In the liver, the chemical composition of a drug is changed by a process

INSIGHT 1-3 Bioavailability and Acid-Base Balance

A number of factors affect the bioavailability of a drug, including the size of the drug molecule (smaller molecules pass more easily through plasma membranes), lipid solubility (lipophilic molecules pass easier than hydrophilic molecules), and ionization of the drug molecule. Non-ionized molecules pass through plasma membranes easier than ionized molecules. Acid-base balance also plays a role in drug bioavailability. An example of this concept in surgery occurs when a local anesthetic (a weak base) is injected into an infected wound (an acidic environment). The local anesthetic agent becomes ionized (a basic pH in an acidic condition) and cannot enter the lipid membrane of nerves to reach the site of action. If the agent doesn't enter the membrane, it cannot reach its site of action and therefore cannot produce its intended effect.

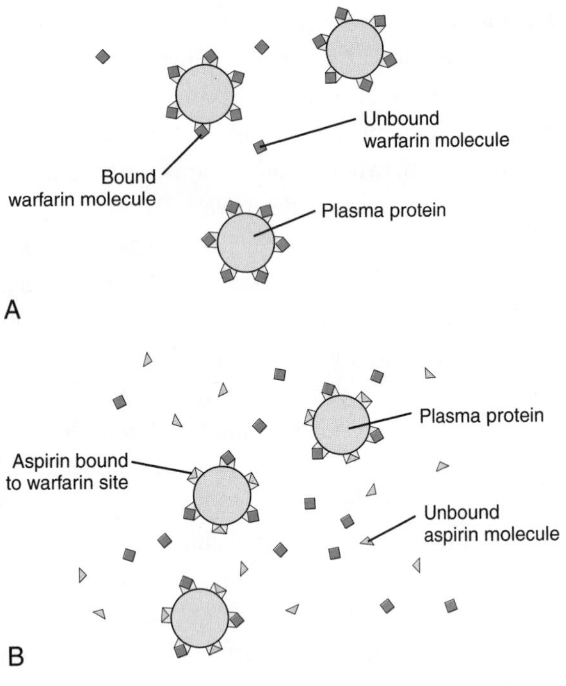

Figure 1-8 **Plasma protein binding of aspirin and warfarin. A,** Warfarin binds to specific receptor sites on plasma proteins. **B,** Aspirin binds to the same receptor sites, making more warfarin available.

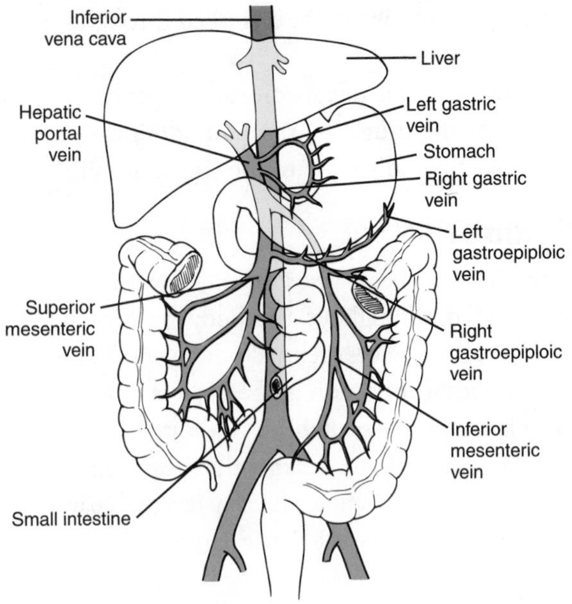

Figure 1-9 Drugs administered orally are distributed to the liver for metabolism by the hepatic portal circulation.

called metabolism or **biotransformation.** The goal of biotransformation is to change lipid-soluble drug molecules into water-soluble molecules that can be more easily excreted. The liver is the primary site for biotransformation, but for some drug molecules this process may take place in other locations such as plasma, lungs, gastrointestinal (GI) tract, or kidneys. Biliary biotransformation takes place when liver cells (hepatocytes) containing enzymes break down some drug molecules into other molecules called metabolites. The effectiveness of liver enzymes depends on several factors, including patient age, concurrent drug therapy, organ disease (e.g., cirrhosis), and nutritional status. Only unbound (bioactive) drug molecules can be biotransformed. Whereas some drugs are completely broken down and some are not broken down at all, most drugs are at least partially biotransformed.

Some drugs are really *prodrugs;* this means they are administered in an inactive form, which is biotransformed into an active drug to produce the needed effect. Examples of prodrugs include the thrombolytic anistreplase (Eminase) and the anti-glaucoma agent dipivefrin (Propine). Dipivefrin is also an example of a drug that is not broken down by the liver but at the site of administration (the eye). Dipivefrin is a prodrug that is biotransformed into epinephrine in the eye by enzyme hydrolysis. Hydrolysis is the addition of water to break chemical bonds of a larger molecule to form two smaller molecules (in this case into epinephrine and pivalic acid).

All drugs taken orally enter the liver through the hepatic portal circulation (Fig. 1-9) prior to entering systemic circulation. The hepatic portal circulatory system is the venous drainage of the upper gastrointestinal tract, carrying molecules absorbed by the gut into veins leading to the liver. Many drugs undergo a first-pass effect, which means they may be altered or nearly inactivated when passing through the liver, potentially reducing the drug's effectiveness. Once liver enzymes begin to transform drug molecules, however, the enzymes are less able to break down additional amounts of the drug; thus, repeated dosing may be used to overcome the first-pass effect. Drugs administered parenterally or sublingually are not subject to the first-pass effect.

EXCRETION

Medications taken into the body are eliminated in the process called **excretion.** Some drug molecules are eliminated in the bile, feces, or skin, but most unchanged drugs and metabolites are excreted by the kidneys and eliminated in urine (Fig. 1-10). Notable exceptions to urinary excretion are the volatile anesthetic agents, which are excreted by the lungs. The circulatory system carries blood to the kidneys, where it is filtered and returned to general circulation. Two renal processes remove drug

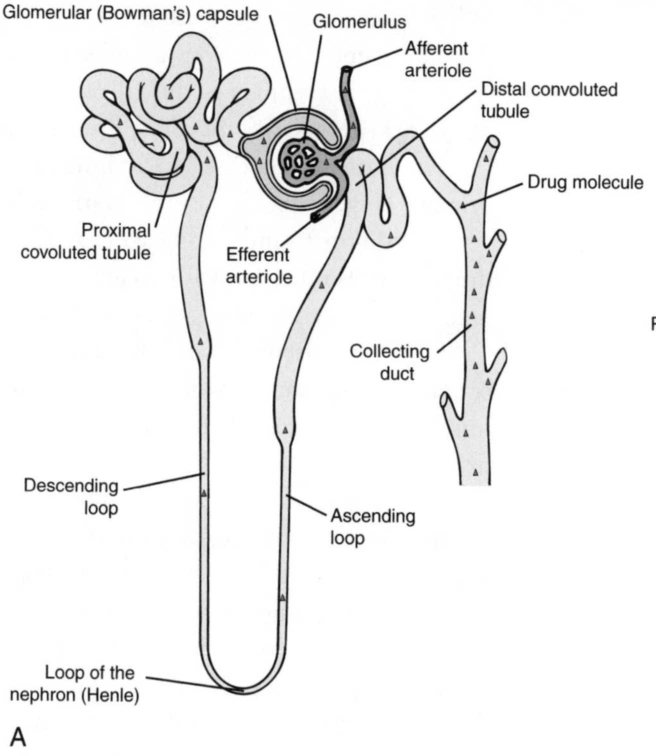

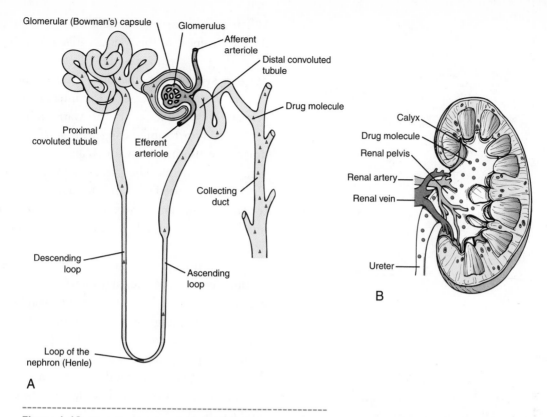

Figure 1-10 Most drugs are excreted by the kidneys. Drugs are removed in the nephrons **(A)**, and eliminated by the kidneys **(B)**.

molecules and metabolites from the body: glomerular filtration and tubular secretion. Only drug molecules *not* bound to plasma proteins (that is *bioactive* molecules) will be filtered out of blood plasma reaching the glomerulus. How much unbound drug is filtered out depends on the glomerular filtration rate (GFR), which depends on blood pressure and blood flow to the kidneys. Tubular secretion uses cellular energy to force drugs and their metabolites from the bloodstream for elimination. Some drugs, depending on their characteristics and the pH of urine, may be reabsorbed and returned to circulation by tubular reabsorption. Factors influencing renal elimination of drug molecules include presence of kidney disease, such as renal failure, the pH of urine, and the concentration of drug molecules in the plasma.

PHARMACODYNAMICS

As stated previously, pharmacodynamics is the study of how drugs exert their effects on the body, at both the molecular and physiological levels. The human body responds to different drugs in varying degrees and at various rates. Drugs may also have more than one effect on the body and this is taken into consideration when prescribing medications.

MAKE IT SIMPLE

Pharmacokinetics is the study of what the body does to drugs (how the body processes drugs).

Pharmacodynamics is the study of what drugs do to the body (how drugs affect the body).

Drugs must be able to reach the site of action and interact with cells to produce therapeutic effects. In most cases, drugs bind to specialized proteins, or receptors, on cell membranes. Some drugs are specific in action and some are nonspecific. Interaction with the target site produces the intended effect, whereas interaction with other cells may produce what are called side effects.

Drug molecules with specific mechanisms interact with specific receptors sites on cell membranes. This specificity has been described by the lock-and-key analogy; the lock is the receptor site on the cell membrane (usually a protein complex), and the drug molecule is the key that fits in that specific lock. Very few drugs are exactly specific to a certain receptor; instead, most drug molecules will react with several types of receptors.

Agonists are drugs that bind to or have an affinity (attraction) for a receptor and cause a particular response (Fig. 1-11). This can be compared to the analogy of a key

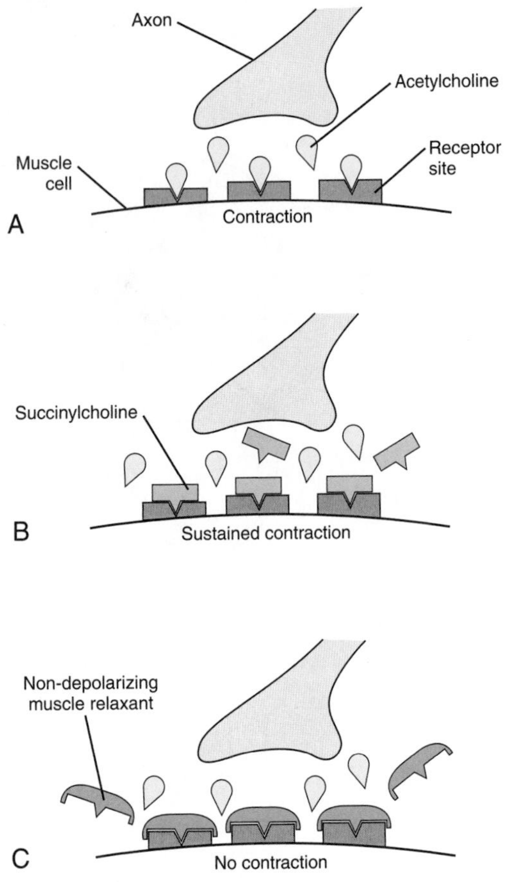

Figure 1-11 **Receptor site agonist and antagonist action. A,** Acetylcholine is a natural agonist. **B,** Succinylcholine is a chemical agonist. **C,** Nondepolarizing muscle relaxants act as antagonists.

opening a lock. Natural agonists include neurotransmitters, such as acetylcholine, and hormones. Some drugs such as succinylcholine act as chemical agonists. Drugs that bind to a receptor and prevent a response are called **antagonists** (see Fig. 1-11). Antagonists are also called receptor blockers. Following the lock and key analogy, an antagonist can be thought of as a key that fits the lock, but can't open it (cause a response). Antagonists may be competitive, that is, bind to sites and prevent the agonist from reaching the site, or noncompetitive in that the antagonist alters the target site, preventing the agonist from causing the intended effect.

Drug antagonism is responsible for many drug interactions, some of which are not desired. Many patients are on multiple drug therapy, so potential exists for several drug-drug interactions. Multiple drugs may cancel each other out or reduce each other's effects. Vitamin K is given as an antidote for warfarin if the patient has been over-anticoagulated because vitamin K cancels out the effect of warfarin. An example of a drug that reduces the effect of another drug is the antibiotic amoxicillin. When it is given to a patient on oral contraceptives, the effectiveness of the contraceptive is reduced.

A drug that enhances the effect of another drug is called a **synergist.** Some drug-drug interactions may cause a dramatic increase in the intended effect of the primary drug, as seen in aspirin-warfarin interactions.

In addition to interacting with another drug, some drugs may also interact with vitamins, minerals, and/or herbal supplements. The effect of tetracycline, for example, is compromised when it is taken with dairy products containing calcium. However, it is important to keep in mind that most drugs do not interact with foods or other drugs.

Not all drug actions are receptor-type interactions. Antibiotics, for example, may interfere quite specifically with certain aspects of bacterial cell metabolism, such as penicillin inhibiting the formation of bacterial cell wall (see Chapter 5). Some drugs interact specifically with certain enzymes rather than receptor sites on a cell. A drug molecule may bind with a particular enzyme and either inhibit or stimulate the enzyme's activity to produce the desired effect.

An example of a nonspecific (i.e., not a drug-receptor complex) interaction is a drug molecule's ability to change the chemical environment surrounding the target cell. For example, mannitol—an osmotic diuretic—increases the osmotic pressure of urine; this means it reduces the reabsorption of water and produces large amounts of dilute urine. Antacids such as sodium bicarbonate chemically neutralize acid in the stomach. The anticoagulant heparin neutralizes the electric charge on a plasma protein that is needed to initiate blood clotting.

Several terms are used to clarify aspects of pharmacodynamics and the surgical technologist should become familiar with the common terms as applied to the surgical patient. The reason or purpose for giving a medication is called the **indication,** while reasons against giving a particular drug are called **contraindications.** For example, a particular antibiotic may be indicated for a bacterial infection, but is contraindicated when the patient has a known hypersensitivity to that antibiotic.

Some important terms should be understood regarding the timing of expected drug effects. The time between administration of a drug and the first appearance of effects is called the **onset.** A drug's onset can be affected by the administration route, the absorption rate, and the efficiency of distribution to the site of action. The time between administration and maximum effect is called the time to peak effect. Steady state, or equilibrium, is achieved when the amount of drug entering the body is equal to the amount of drug being eliminated. The time between onset and disappearance of drug effects is called the **duration.** A drug's duration of action, or drug half-life, refers to the length of time the drug concentration is in the therapeutic range. Some drugs have a very short duration of action such as Diprivan (6-8 minutes), while other drugs have a long duration of action such as warfarin (a single dose is active for 2-5 days).

A number of terms are used to describe the body's response or reaction to medications. A **side effect** is a predictable but unintended effect of a drug. Side effects are rarely serious, but usually unavoidable. An example of a side effect is the drowsiness that often occurs when antihistamines are used.

Adverse effects are undesired, potentially harmful side effects of drugs. Adverse effects include nausea and vomiting, drug toxicity, hypersensitivity, and idiosyncratic (unusual) reactions. Drug toxicity may be the result of accidental overdosing or failure of the body to process the drug properly, as seen in patients with kidney or liver dysfunction. In cases of drug toxicity, the primary effect of the drug may be exaggerated, such as excessive anticoagulation when taking coumarins. Some drugs may be particularly toxic (usually in high doses) to a specific organ, such as the liver, kidney, or even the ear. For example, some antibiotics are known to be ototoxic in high doses; that is, they have the potential to damage the hearing mechanism. Acetaminophen can cause hepatotoxicity and ibuprofen can cause nephrotoxicity.

Drug **hypersensitivity** is an adverse effect resulting from previous exposure to the drug or a similar drug. A patient may become sensitized to a drug after one or more doses, then exhibit an allergic response on subsequent administration of the drug. An allergic response may be immediate, with symptoms ranging from mild to severe. Mild allergy symptoms include the appearance of raised patches on the skin (wheals) with itching, commonly known as hives. A severe allergic reaction, called anaphylaxis, can result in swollen bronchial passages and possible circulatory collapse (see Chapter 16). Delayed allergic reactions can occur days or weeks after a drug is taken and can include fever and joint swelling.

Another type of adverse effect is called **idiosyncratic.** Idiosyncratic drug effects are rare and unpredictable adverse reactions to drugs. Most idiosyncratic drug reactions are thought to occur in people with some genetic abnormality, causing either an excessive or an inadequate response to a drug. For example, malignant hyperthermia (see Chapter 16) is a life-threatening response to certain drugs, attributable to a genetic defect. The emerging science of pharmacogenetics (see Chapter 2) may someday help identify and prevent some idiosyncratic drug effects.

In the fascinating science of pharmacodynamics, some specific mechanisms of drug actions are known, but much remains to be discovered regarding many physiologic interactions involved in drug therapy.

ADVANCED PRACTICES FOR THE SURGICAL FIRST ASSISTANT

CHAPTER 1—Basic Pharmacology

Key Terms

drug dependence
H&P
potentiation
tachyphylaxis
therapeutic levels
tolerance

MEDICATION ORDERS

As a physician extender, one of surgical first assistant's duties may be to write out the physician's prescriptions and medication orders. Then, the physician will clarify, verify, and sign them. It is imperative for the surgical first assistant to have a working knowledge of commonly accepted and approved medical abbreviations, and the basic components of a medication order. (See abbreviations in this chapter, and refer to Chapter 2 for the current listing of "do not use" abbreviations.) The surgical first assistant should never act outside of the Scope of Practice in medication prescriptions or administration.

A physician's medication orders and prescriptions, in addition to his or her signature, consist of the same components: *name* of the patient, *medication* name, medication *dosage*, the *route* of administration, the *frequency* or *time* of administration, and the *date* the order was written. For some orders, usually those found in the clinical setting, the *time* the order was written must also be included as well as any special notations. Notice the first five components are essentially the five rights of medication administration. (See the "five rights" and additional information in Chapter 4.) These are closely checked every time a medication is prepared and administered in order to assure patient safety. It is very important to include all components of the prescription or medication order; if any are omitted, the order is considered invalid and is not a legal order.

Safeguarding prescription pads is an important priority. Not only is this a safe practice, but also a legal consideration. Prescription pads may be a carbon-copy type, which will have a copy for the patient's record, or carbonless. In this case, a copy of the prescription can be made for the chart. If a multiple-line prescription pad is used, the surgical first assistant or physician can obliterate the unused lines to prevent any alteration of the original prescription. Prescription pads should never be used as notepads, but only for writing prescriptions. Other orders, such as for laboratory tests, should be on a laboratory request form.

ASSISTANT *ADVICE*

*It is good practice to review the patient's **H&P** (history and physical) preoperatively. Care must be taken to verify the patient's history to include any OTC or herbal medications. Many patients do not consider these medications as part of their medical history, yet they can cause serious complications and interactions with other drugs.*

CAUTION

All prescription pads must be secured in a safe location, no matter if they are in the clinical or office setting. The physician should never sign prescription blanks in advance.

The surgical first assistant may be involved in routine preoperative, immediate postoperative, and dismissal orders and/or prescriptions. For example, preoperative orders may include shaving the operative site and verifying the patient has had prophylactic antibiotics; immediate postoperative orders address monitoring vital signs, intravenous fluids, antibiotics, pain medications, and wound management such as bleeding, drains, and tubes. Dismissal orders may include pain medications, antibiotics, follow-up appointments, and wound care at home.

ASSISTANT *ADVICE*

Traditionally there have been four clinically accepted vital signs: temperature, pulse, respirations, and blood pressure. Pain has been added to this group as a fifth vital sign to more accurately and efficiently assess the patient's needs.

CAUTION

The international system of units (SI) abbreviations is used in this text. Note that milligrams is abbreviated as mg, and milliliters as mL. These appear to be similar, but are NOT interchangeable. Milligram (mg) is a unit of weight, whereas milliliter (mL) is a unit of volume. Confusing the two can have serious consequences in dosage calculations.

Medication Effects on the Patient

There are several factors that affect drug activity in the body. These include drug administration, disintegration, pharmacokinetics, pharmacodynamics, and individual differences among patients. Drug administration involves the route, the achievement of **therapeutic levels** (see next paragraphs) in the bloodstream, and medication errors. Disintegration is how readily the drug is broken down, or dissolved. Pharmacokinetics, as described in this chapter, refers to the way drugs are moved through the body and pharmacodynamics is how a drug works or its mechanism of action. This involves the drug-receptor cell interaction. Finally, there are physiologic and psychologic differences to consider. These include age, gender, genetics, diet and nutrition, disease, and other medications the patient may be taking.

When two or more medications are administered to a patient, the drugs will have no effect upon each other, or they will increase each other's effect, or decrease each other's effect. Some medications are also affected by food, because food in the stomach can decrease absorption of the drugs. As discussed in this chapter, drugs may be agonists, synergists, or antagonists. Other terms that apply to these principles are **potentiation**, competitive antagonist, noncompetitive antagonist, and partial agonist. Potentiation occurs when two drugs are taken together and their effect is greater than the effect of either drug given alone. Competitive antagonist is an agent with an affinity for the same receptor site as the agonist and this competition inhibits the action of the agonist. Noncompetitive antagonist is an agent that combines with different parts of the receptor mechanism and inactivates the receptor so that the agonist can't be effective, regardless of its concentration in the patient's system. A partial agonist is an agent that has an affinity but may antagonize the action of other drugs that have greater ability to produce a specific result, regardless of dosage.

It is important to remember that everyone reacts differently to the same medication, and some patients may develop inadvertent responses. Medication **tolerance** is a phenomenon in which the body has decreased responsiveness to a medication through repeated exposure to the agent. Many medications can produce tolerance but it is most commonly seen in opiates, and various other CNS depressants. Tolerance can develop not only through the use of the medication, but also to a medication with similar pharmacological properties (particularly those that act on the same receptor sites). Tolerance levels will vary from person to person and in order to maintain therapeutic levels, the physician will order blood tests and may have to increase the dosage. A therapeutic level is defined as the amount of a drug in the bloodstream needed to achieve and maintain a desired effect. Reversal of a medication tolerance can be achieved by discontinuing the agent.

Another type of tolerance is termed **tachyphylaxis.** This is a unique situation in which tolerance may occur after only one or two doses. Tachyphylaxis can develop very quickly and the patient's initial response to the medication cannot be reproduced, even with a larger dose of the agent.

Drug Dependency

Through a suggestion from the World Health Organization (WHO) the terms addiction and habituation have been replaced with the term ***drug dependence.*** The general term of drug dependence avoids the social stigma associated with drug abuse. Drug dependency is defined as a physiological and psychological compulsion to take a drug periodically or continuously, despite its negative or dangerous effects. However, a physical dependence is not always an addiction. For example, some drugs (medications) are prescribed for high blood pressure or for their anti-inflammatory actions. They can cause the body to physically depend upon their effects, but this is not considered an addiction. Other drugs cause addiction without medication value, such as heroin. Tolerance to a drug is usually part of addiction.

ASSISTANT *ADVICE*

It is important to use the blood levels and numbers as guidelines, and to LISTEN to the patient for a full understanding of the medications' effects.

Advanced Practices Bibliography

Fulcher E, Fulcher R, Soto C: *Pharmacology principles and applications*, ed 2, 2009, Saunders/Elsevier.

Jansen SC, Peppers MP: *Pharmacology and drug administration for imaging technologists*, ed 2, St. Louis, 2006, Mosby/Elsevier.

Mosby's medical dictionary, ed 8, St. Louis, 2009, Mosby/Elsevier.

Rothrock JC, Seifert PC: *Assisting in surgery: patient-centered care*, U.S., 2010, Competency and Credentialing Institute, Denver, CO.

Advanced Practices Internet Resources

Boston University School of Medicine, Pharmacology and Experimental Therapeutics, Glossary of Terms and Symbols Used in Pharmacology: *www.bumc.bu.edu/Dept/Content.aspx?DepartmentID=65&PageID=7797*

Google Health, Drug Dependence: *https://health.google.com/health/ref/Drug+dependence*

Greenwich Medical Media Ltd., Basic Pharmacology: *www.nurse-prescriber.co.uk/education/modules/pharmacology/pharmacy3.htm*

Information about Drugs: Adapted from Engs, R.C. Alcohol and Other Drugs: Self Responsibility, Tichenor Publishing Company, Bloomington, IN, 1987. © Copyright Ruth C. Engs, Bloomington, IN, 1996: *www.indiana.edu/~engs/rbook/drug.html*

U.S. Drug Enforcement Administration: *www.dea.gov*

Advanced Practices: Learning the Language (Key Terms)

Using your textbook or a standard medical dictionary, look up and write the definitions of each term.

- drug dependence
- H&P
- potentiation
- tachyphylaxis
- therapeutic levels
- tolerance

Advanced Practices: Review Questions

1. When writing a medication order, it is the Surgical Assistant's duty to:
 A. sign and initial the order for the physician
 B. have the physician verify, clarify, and sign it
 C. verify the four components are present on the order
 D. have the physician sign it before checking the order

2. Prescription pads are
 A. signed in advance by the physician
 B. kept in an area where they can be easily accessed
 C. used to order blood work
 D. kept in a secure place

3. Which of the following has been added to the four basic vital signs?
 A. Pain
 B. Heart rate
 C. Respirations
 D. Pupil reaction

4. If a prescription is written on a carbonless pad, it is good practice to
 A. have the physician sign it ahead of time
 B. make a copy of the prescription for the chart
 C. obliterate the signature line to prevent forgery
 D. write two prescriptions and keep one for future use

5. Therapeutic levels are verified by
 A. checking the patient's reaction to the medications
 B. patient's symptoms abating
 C. taking the patient's vital signs
 D. testing the patient's blood

KEY CONCEPTS

- Knowledge of basic principles of pharmacology can provide the surgical technologist with a solid foundation on which to build an understanding of the many drugs used in surgery.
- Drug sources include natural sources such as plants, animals, and minerals, as well as drugs developed in the chemistry and molecular biology laboratory.
- Drug classification subcategories are helpful in identifying the purpose or use of a drug.
- Medication orders may be in various forms in surgery, and must be interpreted precisely. The surgical technologist should also be able to use different drug distribution systems, depending on the system in use at the clinical facility.
- Drugs come in many forms or preparations, and surgical technologists must be able to recognize the type needed for the intended purpose.
- Pharmacokinetics is the study of the four basic steps the body uses to process drugs: absorption, distribution, metabolism, and excretion.
- The study of how drugs exert their effects is called pharmacodynamics. Most drugs interact with receptors on target cell membranes to produce the desired effect.
- Many important terms are used to describe aspects of pharmacodynamics.

Bibliography

Fulcher E, Fulcher R, Soto C: *Pharmacology principles and applications*, ed 2, 2009, Saunders/Elsevier.

Kester M, Karpa K, Quraishi S, et al: *Elsevier's integrated pharmacology*, St. Louis, 2007, Mosby/Elsevier.

Moscou K, Snipe K: *Pharmacology for pharmacy technicians*, St. Louis, 2009, Mosby/Elsevier.

Nagelhout J, Plaus K: *Nurse anesthesia*, ed 4, St. Louis, 2009, Saunders/Elsevier.

Stoelting R, Miller R: *Basics of anesthesia*, ed 5, 2007, Churchill Livingstone/Elsevier.

Internet Resources

Institute for Safe Medical Practices, List of Error-Prone Abbreviations, Symbols, and Dose Designations: www.ismp.org/Tools/errorproneabbreviations.pdf.

The Joint Commission, Official "Do Not Use" List: www.jointcommission.org/NR/rdonlyres/2329F8F5-6EC5-4E21-B932-54B2B7D53F00/0/dnu_list.pdf.

RxList, The Internet Drug Index: www.rxlist.com/script/main/hp.asp.

Taylor L: *Plant based drugs and medicines*, Raintree Nutrition, Inc. www.rain-tree.com/plantdrugs.htm.

U.S. Food and Drug Administration: www.fda.gov/.

LEARNING THE LANGUAGE (KEY TERMS)

Using your textbook or a standard medical dictionary, look up and write the definitions of each term.

absorption
adverse effect
agonist
antagonist
bioavailability
biotechnology
biotransformation
bolus
contraindication
distribution
duration
emulsion
enteral
excretion
hypersensitivity
idiosyncratic effect
indication
local effect
onset
parenteral
pharmacodynamics
pharmacokinetics
plasma protein binding
reconstituted
side effects
solubility
solution
suspension
synergist
systemic effect
topical

REVIEW QUESTIONS

1. What are the sources of drugs used today? State examples.
2. Why are drug classification subcategories more helpful to the surgical technologist than the four major categories used to classify drugs?
3. What types of medication orders are used in surgery?
4. What type of drug distribution system is used in your local clinical facility? If you aren't in your clinical rotation yet, what type of system do you think might be in use there?
5. Which types of drug forms do you have in your home medicine cabinet?
6. What is the most common medication administration route used in surgery?
7. How does the body process drugs?
8. How is a side effect different from an adverse effect?

CRITICAL THINKING

Scenario 1

Mrs. Lopez is a 52-year-old woman with type 1 diabetes. She has been taking insulin for 10 years. Recently, she has developed some reactivity to the insulin she has always taken. Her physician has prescribed Humulin instead of regular insulin. Humulin is a drug that has been developed using biotechnology.

1. What might she have been reacting to in the regular insulin?
2. Why might switching to Humulin solve her problem?
3. How is Humulin produced using biotechnology?

Scenario 2

Mr. Dhang is a 75-year-old man taking Coumadin for recurrent deep vein thrombosis (DVT). He recently began experiencing frequent, almost daily headaches but has not consulted his physician. He has started taking aspirin to treat his headaches.

1. Why is taking aspirin while on Coumadin a problem?
2. How does the presence of aspirin alter the effect of Coumadin?
3. What adverse effects might you expect to see?

CHAPTER 2

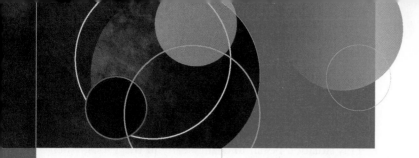

Medication Development, Regulation and Resources

OBJECTIVES *Upon completion of this chapter you should be able to:*

1. Discuss international, federal, and state roles in regulating drugs.
2. Define medication development and testing.
3. Discuss pharmacogenetics and pharmacogenomics.
4. Distinguish between brand, generic, and chemical medication names.
5. List information found on medication labels.
6. Obtain medication information from pharmacology resources.

KEY TERMS

AHFS drug information
contraindication
controlled substances
DEA
Facts and Comparisons
FDA
indication
The Joint Commission
narcotics
OTC
PDR
pharmacogenetics/pharmacogenomics
prescription drugs
USP-NF
World Health Organization

As a surgical technologist, you should be aware of federal, state, and local roles in regulating drugs and their administration. In this chapter, then, we'll present a broad overview of federal drug legislation, federal agencies, as well as a general discussion of international, state, and local regulations. Because new medications are approved for use regularly, we'll also briefly consider the process that leads to this approval—testing, study, and using genetic technology. Finally, we'll look at available medication references, which will help you obtain information useful to your practice as a surgical technologist.

MEDICATION REGULATION

Throughout history, some individuals have misrepresented, misused, and abused medicinals such as herbs, chemicals, and drugs. As societies progressed, their governments recognized the need to regulate or control the use of these substances. Before the 20th century, medications of all kinds were sold freely in the United States, both to physicians and consumers. Thus, neither physician nor consumer had any real proof of the medication's safety or effectiveness. Medicines were sold by "medicine men" in traveling shows, in stores, and even by mail order. There was no legal requirement for a physician's prescription. This situation began to change early in the 1900s, when the federal government stepped in to protect consumers and to regulate the pharmaceutical industry. The states, too, established practice acts to regulate the dispensing and administration of medications (Insight 2-1).

INSIGHT 2-1 Alternative Medications

Alternative healing therapies are now being accepted into the concepts of Western medicine. They may be defined as treatments for which scientific evidence of safety and usefulness are lacking. The current medical system is based on the conventional approach of theory, knowledge, and research. This is termed "biomedicine," or theoretical medicine: the clinical medicine based on principles of natural sciences such as biology, chemistry, and etc. However, in the 1990's, consumers began to look outside of the traditional approach toward alternative medicines. In 1992, the U.S. Congress established the Office of Alternative Medicine (OAM) within the National Institutes of Health. In 1998, this office became the National Center for Complementary and Alternative Medicine (NCCAM). Its mission is to define the usefulness and safety of complementary and alternative medicines (CAM) and their roles in improving health care. NCCAM defines CAM as a group of diverse medical and healthcare interventions, practices, products, or disciplines that are not generally considered part of conventional medicine. Now more funding and research projects for information are possible. The NCCAM has categorized alternative healing and complementary medicines into five main areas: alternative medical systems, mind-body interventions, biologically based therapies, manipulative and body-based methods, and energy therapies.

An alternative medical system is a set of practices based on a philosophy different than Western biomedicine and includes: Asian systems, folk health care, herbal medicines, massage, energy therapy, acupressure, acupuncture, and qigog. A traditional system from India is known as Ayurveda which aspires to restore the individual's harmony of body, mind, and spirit. Native American, Middle Eastern, Tibetan, Central and South American, and African cultures also have developed traditional alternative medical systems. Other examples include naturopathic and homeopathic medicine. Naturopathic practices are based on the belief that the human body has an innate healing ability. These practices use diet, exercise, lifestyle changes and natural therapies to enhance the body's ability to ward off and combat disease. Homeopathic medicine is based on the concept the "like cures like." Patients are treated with heavily diluted preparations which claim to cause effects similar to the symptoms presented. Homeopaths also use aspects of the patient's physical and psychological state in recommending remedies.

Mind-body explores the concept that the mind has an ability to affect the body (mental healing). These interventions include meditation, some types of hypnosis, music and art therapy, dance, and prayer. Biologically based therapies include dietary supplements such as herbs and orthomolecular therapies. Herbs are considered as dietary supplements and so are regulated by the Department of Agriculture and the FDA. However, in this category, herbs are not subject to the strict regulations that apply to medications. Orthomolecular therapies use different chemical concentrations to treat disease. These include magnesium, melatonin, and megadoses of vitamins. Manipulative and body-based methods include chiropractic methods, osteopathy, and massage. And finally, energy therapies include biofield and electromagnetic field therapies. Biofield therapies are those that focus on fields which come from the body and include acupuncture, Reiki, qigong, and therapeutic touch. Electromagnetic fields come from sources other than the body and include magnetic fields, alternating current fields, or direct current fields. While these fields have yet to be proven, the therapies are used with patients who have arthritis, cancer, or pain.

INTERNATIONAL LAWS

International regulation of medications is under the authority of the **World Health Organization** (WHO), a specialized agency of the United Nations. It acts as the coordinating authority on international public health, providing technical assistance in the drug field, and promoting research on drug abuse. Its tasks include combating disease and promoting the general health of all people. The WHO publishes a report annually, *The World Health Report*, which combines expert assessment with a focus on a specific subject. This is to provide countries and all donor agencies with information to help them make policies and funding decisions. The WHO does not enforce laws concerning drugs, so drug control is different from country to country. Some countries have more stringent laws, some less strict, than the United States. As a result, drugs are often available in some countries before they have been approved for use in others. The WHO also publishes *Guidelines for Safe Surgery* which includes such topics as: antibiotic prophylaxis, types of adverse drug reactions and their treatment/prevention, cause of errors in delivery of perioperative medications, management of blood loss, and safe delivery of anesthesia.

FEDERAL LAWS

Federal regulation of medications was initially intended to protect consumers from harmful, impure, untested, and unsafe medications. Thus, when the Pure Food and Drug Act was passed in 1906, it set standards for quality and required the proper labeling of medications. In 1938, the federal government began to address drug effectiveness. It passed the Food, Drug, and Cosmetic Act, which required animal testing of medications. Now prior to selling a new medication, pharmaceutical companies had to apply for approval to market the medication, and that approval was contingent on proof that the medication was effective on animals. The Durham-Humphrey Amendments to the Food, Drug, and Cosmetic Act were passed in 1952. These amendments required a physician's order to dispense certain medications, called **prescription drugs**, and established an over-the-counter (**OTC**) category of medications that did not require a prescription. However, even OTC drugs are studied to make sure they are safe for public use without a physician's guidance. Their labels must include sufficient warnings and instructions. Then, in 1970, the Controlled Substance Act was passed. It designated certain medications as **controlled substances.** See Box 2-1 for a summary of these and other federal drug laws and their timelines.

The Controlled Substances Act of 1970 established classifications, known as schedules, of medications that had potential for abuse. These medications are specifically labeled so as to be easily identified. A large C signifies the drug as a controlled substance, and a Roman numeral designating its class (from I to V) appears with the C (Fig. 2-1). Five schedules (Table 2-1) were determined, based on the level of abuse and dependence potential and on appropriate medical uses for the medication. Drugs such as LSD are listed on the C-I schedule; they have high abuse potential and no accepted

Box 2-1 FEDERAL DRUG LAWS

Pure Food and Drug Act (1906)

- Required all drugs marketed in the United States to meet minimal standards of uniform strength, purity, and quality
- Required that preparations containing morphine be labeled
- Established two references of officially approved drugs: the *United States Pharmacopeia* (*USP*) and the *National Formulary* (*NF*)*

Federal Food, Drug, and Cosmetic Act (1938; Amended in 1952 and 1965)

- Established the U.S. Food and Drug Administration (FDA)
- Established specific regulations regarding warning labels on preparations, (e.g., cautions about a drug's capacity to cause drowsiness or become habit-forming)
- Stated that both prescription and nonprescription drugs must be effective and safe
- Stated that all labels must be accurate and include the generic name
- Required FDA approval of all new drugs
- Designated which drugs could be sold over-the-counter (OTC), (i.e., without a prescription)

Controlled Substances Act (1970)

- Established the U.S. Drug Enforcement Administration (DEA)

Continued

- Set tighter controls on drugs capable of being abused (controlled substances), (e.g., depressants, stimulants, and narcotics)
- Required stricter security controls for anyone (physicians, pharmacists, hospitals) who dispenses, receives, sells, or destroys controlled substances
- Set limits on the use of prescriptions: established guidelines for the number of times a drug can be prescribed in a period of time, and set rules on which preparations may be prescribed over the telephone to the pharmacy
- Required that each prescriber register with the DEA, obtaining a DEA number to be used on prescriptions
- Identified drugs that can be abused and that are addicting, classifying them into schedules according to the degree of danger

* These two publications have since been combined and are referred to as the *USP-NF*.

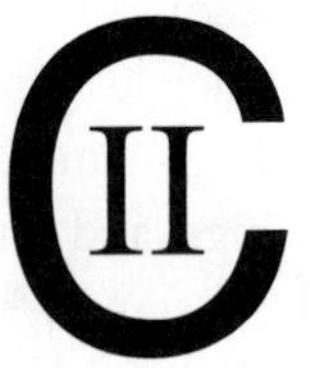

Figure 2-1 Symbol for a controlled substance with a schedule of II.

medical use. Controlled substances from the C-II schedule have high abuse potential, but also have accepted medical uses, as in the surgical setting. C-II controlled substances that are frequently used in surgery include alfentanil, cocaine, and morphine. Medications listed as C-III have moderate abuse potential, while medications on schedules C-IV and C-V have low abuse potential.

In 1983, the **Drug Enforcement Administration (DEA)** of the Department of Justice was established to enforce the Controlled Substances Act. It sets standards for handling controlled substances and has the legal authority to enforce those standards. Institutional policies and procedures for storing and handling controlled substances must comply with DEA standards, and documentation requirements must be strictly followed. When hospitals administer **narcotics**, for example, they must keep careful records of the amount of medication used as well as the date, the patient, the person administering the medication, and the person obtaining it. Physicians or other health professionals who administer, dispense, or prescribe controlled substances are required to have a current state license and register with the DEA. The DEA assigns each a registration number that is used to track controlled substances dispersed to patients.

Table 2-1 SCHEDULES OF CONTROLLED SUBSTANCES*

Schedule	Examples	Description
C-I	Heroin, LSD, PCP, marijuana	Drugs with high abuse potential and severe physical and psychologic dependence. No medicinal use, research only.
C-II	Alfentanil, opium, cocaine, codeine, morphine	High potential for drug abuse. Accepted medical use, but can lead to physical and psychological dependency. Specific restrictions.
C-III	Anabolic steroids, products with low amounts of codeine	Potential for drug abuse less than in previous categories. Medically accepted for use. High psychologic dependence, low physical dependence.
C-IV	Diazepam, lorazepam, Phenobarbital	Potential for dependency. Medically accepted for use. Limited psychologic and physical dependence.
C-V	Many antitussive and antidiarrheal agents	Very limited potential for dependence. Medically accepted for use. Many are OTC medications.

**Drugs may be moved from schedule to schedule on the list. A current schedule of all drugs controlled by the DEA can be obtained from that office at www.deadiversion.usdoj.gov/schedules/index.html.*

Federal Agencies

There are two federal agencies that contribute policies for health care workers' (and public) safety and these policies can influence drug regulation in the health care field. The Occupational Safety and Health Administration (OSHA) is an agency within the U.S. Department of Labor. OSHA's mission is to assure the safety and health of American workers by setting and enforcing standards. An example of how OSHA interacts with surgical technologists is the Occupational Exposure to Bloodborne Pathogens Standard which went into effect in 2001. OSHA estimates that between 590,000 and 800,000 needle sticks/sharps injuries occur annually which put people (including surgical technologists) at risk for contracting hepatitis B, hepatitis C, and HIV. This standard states each employer must have a plan that ensures immediate and confidential post-exposure treatment and follow-up procedures in accordance with current CDC guidelines. The CDC, or the Centers for Disease Control and Prevention, is an agency under the U.S. Department of Health and Human Services. It is recognized as the leading federal agency for protecting the health and safety of people, and for providing credible information to enhance health decisions. It serves as the national focus for developing and applying disease prevention and control. In 1995, the CDC issued a report of a study recommending prophylactic medication treatment as soon as possible after a needle stick or sharps injury (less than 2 hours from the time of exposure). This treatment is known as post-exposure prophylaxis or PEP and is of importance to surgical technologists. Since the original report was published, it has been updated several times because of the approval of new antiretroviral drugs and the availability of new information on the treatment of HIV. Post-exposure prophylaxis (PEP) is the use of antiretroviral drugs as soon as possible after a significant occupational exposure to blood or other high risk body fluids that are likely to be infected with HIV. While these antiretroviral drugs are not found in the surgical setting, they should be familiar to those health care workers who are at risk. One treatment regimen recommends taking zidovudine (ZDV, previously called AZT), 600 mg every day ck in divided doses and lamivudine (3TC), 150 mg two times per day for a total of four weeks. These medications are available as Combivir, which can be taken as one tablet twice a day ck. There are other medications and regimes also recommended. These include the antiretrovirals tenofovir DR (Viread), emtriatabine (Emtriva), stavudine (d4T, Zerit), and didanosine (Videx).

{NOTE} *You must be familiar with and strictly follow needle stick/sharps injuries protocol as set forth by your surgical technology program and also all policies relating to these incidents at your clinical sites.*

STATE PRACTICE ACTS

State governments must comply with federal regulations. When federal and state laws concerning medications conflict, the stricter of the laws prevail. State laws known as *practice acts* govern the ordering, dispensing, and administration of medications. Such laws vary from state to state. For example, state laws regulate who—physicians, physician assistants, nurse practitioners—may prescribe drugs. They also regulate pharmacy practices, specifying how medications are to be dispensed and by whom (usually a licensed pharmacist). Drug substitution laws, for example, specify if a pharmacist may automatically substitute a generic equivalent for a prescribed medication if not indicated otherwise.

Physicians can "lend" or delegate some of their functions to others. For example, the surgical technologist functions as a "physician extender"—an extra pair of hands, so to speak. As such, he or she performs medication-handling duties under the delegatory power of the physician. Each state controls the limits of this delegatory power through the Medical Licensing Board.

{NOTE} *As a surgical technologist, you should be knowledgeable about the medication handling and administration laws in your own state. State practice acts are public information; this means you can read these acts yourself in order to be correctly informed. This is important because the delegatory power and its interpretations differ from state to state. For instance, many people believe that only nurses may administer medications to patients. However, in many states, credentialed allied health professionals such as perfusionists, respiratory therapists, and medical assistants routinely administer medications legally. The surgical technologist must have direct knowledge of, and function within, the legal standards of medication administration determined by the state in which he or she practices.*

LOCAL POLICIES

When state laws do not specifically address the practice of surgical technology, published institutional policies should be used to determine the scope of practice.

The role of the surgical technologist in drug handling is usually specified in institutional policies, which have local authority. The surgical technologist must be thoroughly familiar with medication administration policies and closely adhere to their stated limits. If current policies are outdated, or do not reflect the scope of practice appropriate to the education and expertise of the surgical technologist, the institution should revise or update them as appropriate. The surgical technologist's job description may also contain relevant information regarding medication handling and administration.

CAUTION

Under no circumstances should a surgical technologist exceed the limits of the facility's published job description. These job descriptions are subject to revision, as needed, to reflect current practice standards.

THE JOINT COMMISSION

The Joint Commission (formerly known as The Joint Commission on Accreditation of Healthcare Organizations, or JCAHO) evaluates and accredits approximately 16,000 health care organizations and programs in the United States. These organizations include general and rehabilitation hospitals, critical access hospitals, ambulatory care providers such as outpatient surgery centers and office-based surgery facilities. Thus the Joint Commission is the predominant standards-setting organization, and facilities that obtain its accreditation demonstrate their commitment to meeting certain performance standards.

Among the Joint Commission's standards are National Patient Safety Goals (NPSG). These goals are established annually and address issues such as infection control, Universal Protocol for Preventing Wrong Site, Wrong Procedure, Wrong Person Surgery™, and medical errors. During 2009, an extensive review of the NPSG and the process for development of the goals was undertaken. Due to this review, there are no new NPSG developed for 2010. This review addresses the challenges that some goals represent and the need for additional information about effective approaches. Beginning January 1, 2004, these goals were expanded to include a list of "dangerous" abbreviations, acronyms, and symbols that should not be used in the clinical setting. This list was confirmed in May 2005 and is an effort to improve the effectiveness of communication among caregivers and to address the many inherent problems associated with misread abbreviations that contribute to medication errors. This list applies to all handwritten, patient-specific documentation, computer, and pre-printed forms. Accredited facilities are required to develop a "Do Not Use" list and must include terms as specified by the Joint Commission (see Table 2-2). Many facilities not only include these required terms, but have expanded their lists. It is important to check your facility's "Do Not Use List."

DRUG DEVELOPMENT

Prior to legal regulation, drugs could be manufactured, sold, and administered without scientific proof of safety, quality, or effectiveness. Today, all drugs must undergo stringent testing and provide proof of safety and effectiveness before release. This process can take as long as 15 years and cost more than $800 million dollars per drug. The federal Food and Drug Administration **(FDA)** is an agency within the Department of Health and Human Services that consists of centers and offices. The Center for Drug Evaluation and Research (CDER) regulates the pharmaceutical industry, ensuring that basic standards are followed. These regulations include prescription drugs, OTC drugs, biological therapeutics, and generic drugs. The CDER evaluates all new drugs before they are sold and also monitors the more than 10,000 existing drugs on the market. It observes television, radio, and printed drug ads for accuracy, as well as providing health professionals with information for consumers. To do this, the FDA inspects the facilities where drugs are made, reviews new drug applications, investigates and removes unsafe drugs from the market, and requires proper labeling of drugs.

U.S. FOOD AND DRUG ADMINISTRATION PREGNANCY CATEGORIES

The FDA has developed a classification system related to medication effects on the unborn child, or fetus. This classification is useful for surgical medications in some medical situations: for example, a pregnant woman who develops acute appendicitis and requires surgery. In medication literature and reference books, most medications have a pregnancy category listed. Categories A and B are considered to be within safe limits for medication use during pregnancy, with special attention given to the first trimester of the pregnancy (the first three months) (Table 2-3).

Table 2-2 THE JOINT COMMISSION'S OFFICIAL "DO NOT USE" LIST[1]

Do Not Use	Potential Problem	Use Instead
U (unit)	Mistaken for "0" (zero), the number "4" (four) or "cc"	Write "unit"
IU (International Unit)	Mistaken for IV (intravenous) or the number 10 (ten)	Write "International Unit"
Q.D., QD, q.d., qd (daily)	Mistaken for each other	Write "daily"
Q.O.D., QOD, q.o.d, qod (every other day)	Period after the Q mistaken for "I" and the "O" mistaken for "I"	Write "every other day"
Trailing zero (X.0 mg)*	Decimal point is missed	Write "X mg"
Lack of leading zero (.X mg)		Write "0.X mg"
MS	Can mean morphine sulfate or magnesium sulfate	Write "morphine sulfate" Write "magnesium sulfate"
MSO4 and MgSO4	Confused for one another	

ADDITIONAL ABBREVIATIONS, ACRONYMS, AND SYMBOLS

(For possible future inclusion in the official "Do Not Use" List)

Do Not Use	Potential Problem	Use Instead
> (greater than) < (less than)	Misinterpreted as the number "7" (seven) or the letter "L" Confused for one another	Write "greater than" Write "less than"
Abbreviations for drug names	Misinterpreted due to similar abbreviations for multiple drugs	Write drug names in full
Apothecary units	Unfamiliar to many practitioners Confused with metric units	Use metric units
@	Mistaken for the number "2" (two)	Write "at"
Cc	Mistaken for U (units) when poorly written	Write "mL" or "ml" or "milliliters" ("mL" is preferred)
μg	Mistaken for mg (milligrams) resulting in one thousand-fold overdose	Write "mcg" or "micrograms"

[1] Applies to all orders and all medication-related documentation that is handwritten (including free-text computer entry) or on pre-printed forms.

**Exception: A "trailing zero" may be used only where required to demonstrate the level of precision of the value being reported, such as for laboratory results, imaging studies that report size of lesions, or catheter/tube sizes. It may not be used in medication orders or other medication-related documentation.*

Pharmaceutical companies are continually developing new medications, and each must undergo required testing prior to FDA approval. This testing is an extensive process. All new medications are first tested on animals to determine if they are safe to administer to humans. At least two species of mammals, of both genders, must be used for this initial stage of drug testing. During this process, researchers look for toxic effects and determine safe dosage levels. Once the medication has proven safe in animals, the drug company applies to the FDA for permission to begin human testing which consists of four primary phases (plus a phase for investigational new drug studies) (Insight 2-2).

Table 2-3 U.S. FOOD AND DRUG ADMINISTRATION PREGNANCY CATEGORIES

Category	Description
A	No risk to fetus per studies.
B	No risk in animal studies, and well controlled studies in pregnant women not available. It is assumed there is little or no risk.
C	Animal studies: a risk to the fetus. Controlled studies on pregnant women not available. Risk versus benefit of the drug must be determined,
D	A risk to the human fetus has been proved. Risk versus benefit must be determined.
X	A risk to the human fetus has been proved. Risk outweighs the benefit, and drug should be avoided during pregnancy.

Note: *These categories are being reviewed for possible revision; please check the FDA website for the most current information.*
Source: www.fda.gov.

IN SIGHT 2-2 Phases of Human Medication Testing

Phase 0: This phase is a recent designation in accordance with the FDA's Guidance on Exploratory Investigational New Drug studies. It is also known as human microdosing and is designed to "speed up" development of promising drugs. This is a way to establish if the drug or agent has the expected outcome from preclinical studies. Phase 0 will be used for exploratory, first-in-human trials. It features the administration of a single small dose of the study drug to a limited number of subjects (usually 10-15) in order to gather preliminary data on the drug's pharmacokinetics and pharmacodynamics (see Chapter 1). Phase 0 testing is not designed to report on the safety or efficacy of a drug, because the dose given is too low to cause any therapeutic effect. Drug development companies use these studies to decide which drugs have the best effects in humans to take forward for further development and testing. Some experts question the usefulness of this phase.

Phase I: Clinical Pharmacology In the clinical pharmacology phase, the new medication is given to a small group (20-80) healthy volunteers, or those who have the problem that the drug manufacturer is hoping to treat. This group is usually males between the ages of 18 and 45. This phase is used to determine the dose level for symptoms of medication toxicity in humans and can take 1 to 2 years.

Phase II: Clinical Investigation In the clinical investigation phase, the medication is given to a larger group (usually several hundred) of patients presenting with the disease or condition the medication was developed to treat. The clinical investigation phase is used to establish medication effectiveness and to determine optimum dosage and dose range. It can take 1 to 3 years.

Phase III: Clinical Trials In the clinical trial phase researchers continue to note medication effectiveness, safety, and side effects in large studies. In this phase, which begins only if no serious side effects occur in Phase II, the new medication is given to hundreds or thousands of patients, usually in large medical research facilities. The medication's effectiveness is verified and its actions are characterized by various types of scientific studies. Several kinds of studies may be conducted. For instance, in *double-blind studies,* half of the testing group receives the medication and the other half receives an inactive substance called a placebo. Neither the subject patients nor the prescribing physicians know which group received the placebo until the study has been completed. The results of these and other studies must be thoroughly documented. This phase can take several years to complete.

Phase IV: Post-marketing Study The post-marketing study phase occurs after the medication is released for use in treatment of the specified condition. In this phase the drug company continues to monitor the medication, gathering results from prescribing physicians. This continuing evaluation of the medication includes results from those patients excluded from the previous phases, such as pregnant patients and the elderly. This data must be gathered, analyzed, and reported to the FDA in order to document the medication's safety and effectiveness comprehensively. The time frame for this phase varies with the medication/study being done.

Twenty-first century technology is allowing scientists and pharmaceutical companies to test medications in a different way. **Pharmacogenetics** is the study of genetic factors in predicting a medication's action and how it could vary from its intended response. The term is the mixing of pharmaceuticals and genetics. Pharmacogenetics is vital technology because people have different genetic make-ups and do not respond identically to medication dosage or intended therapy. Genetic factors can alter the metabolism of a medication and either enhance or diminish its action. Thus, a patient can have a positive response, a negative response, or no response at all to a medication. **Pharmacogenomics** refers to the general study of all genes and genetic technology that determine medication behavior. However, the distinction between these two terms is so slight that they are used interchangeably. As technology allows scientists to catalog more genetic variations found within the human genome, pharmaceutical companies can create medications based on this knowledge. This could facilitate new medication discovery, develop "drug markers" to target specific diseases, revive previously failed medication candidates and match them with a specific population, and facilitate the medication approval process which would lower the costs and risks of clinical trials. The drawbacks to pharmacogenetics are the complexity and cost of genetic research and educating health care providers in the use of this technology.

MARKETING

During development, the drug company assigns a generic name to the new medication. Later, it selects a company trade name, which it uses for marketing purposes once the medication gains FDA approval. The **United States Pharmacopeia and National Formulary (USP-NF)** assigns an official name to the new medication; this is usually the generic name. Once a drug has been approved for release, the pharmaceutical company responsible for the medication's development has exclusive rights to market that medication under its trade name for twenty years. This process allows the drug company to recover development costs. However, this patent is issued before clinical trials begin, and so the drug time of the patent maybe from seven to twelve years. After these exclusive rights have expired, other companies may begin to market a generic equivalent with a different trade name.

MEDICATION LABELING

As previously mentioned the Federal Pure Food and Drug Act of 1906 established proper labeling of medications. It is important to correctly obtain (read) the information found on medication labels. It is recognized that surgical technologists do not directly administer medications to the patient. However, you will be obtaining medications for the sterile field and playing an important part in correct medication identification and avoiding medication errors. Medication labels display pertinent information that the surgical technologist must read and interpret accurately.

Brand and Generic Names of the Medication

The manufacturer's name for a medication is called the brand, trade, or proprietary name. It is selected by the pharmaceutical manufacturer and used to market the medication. It is usually the most prominent word on the label. It may be in large or bold type, is always capitalized, and is very visible to promote the product. The name is followed by the ® sign which means the name and the formula are registered. Directly under the brand name is the generic (nonproprietary) or official name, in lower case letters. The generic name is not owned by any one company, so it is not capitalized. On some labels the generic name may be placed inside parentheses. It is given to the medication by the USP and by law, the generic name must be identified on all medication labels. On the Keflin® label (Fig. 2-2), the brand name appears in large letters set off in a black background. The generic name is cephalothin sodium and is printed underneath the brand name.

{NOTE} *Each medication has several names—usually its brand name, its generic name, and also its chemical name. The chemical name has meaning for chemists. It is a precise, systematic description of the chemical composition and molecular structure of the medication.*

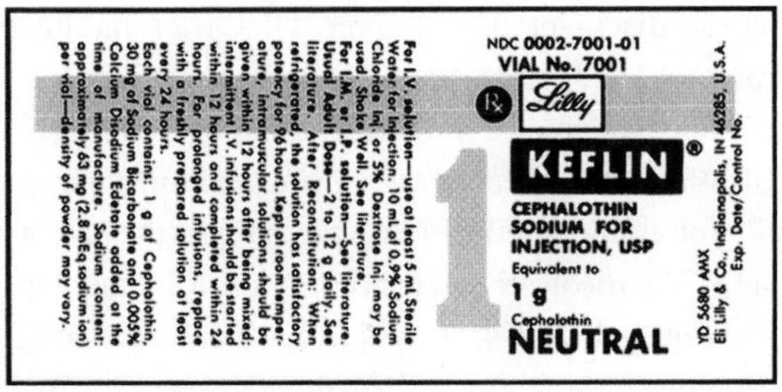

Figure 2-2 Keflin® label. *(From Ogden SJ:* Calculation of drug dosages, *ed 7, St. Louis, 2003, Mosby.)*

Chemical names can be found in references such as the Physicians' Desk Reference, *but are not normally found on medication labels.*

CAUTION

On some medication labels, only the generic name appears. Be sure to cross-check medication names if you are unsure of their generic equivalents. Many generic spellings are very similar, yet the medications are vastly different and an error could be fatal to the patient. Also, it is important to recognize that some variations may exist between generic medications produced by different manufacturers.

Manufacturer's name: This is also displayed on the label to advertise the company. See the word "Lilly" on the Keflin® label.

Dosage strength: This number on the label refers to dosage weight or the amount of the medication in a specific unit of measurement. On the Keflin® label the dosage strength of medication in the bottle is given as 1 gram (1 g).

Form: This identifies the composition of the medication. As discussed in Chapter 1, solid forms are tablets and capsules. Some are in powdered, or granular, form and can be combined with food or beverages. This is usually found in the medical rather than the surgical setting as for post-operative pain medications that the patient can take at home. Other medications must be reconstituted, or liquefied by being dissolved in a solution such as sterile water or sterile normal saline. These medications are then measured in an exact liquid volume such as milliliters (mL) or cubic centimeters (cc). They may be crystalloid (a clear solution) or a suspension (solid particles in a liquid that separate in the container). On the neomycin and polymyxin B sulfates otic label (Fig. 2-3), the word *suspension* tells us the solution must be shaken to dilute the particles before it is administered to the patient (as discussed in Chapter 1). Other medication forms include creams, patches, and suppositories.

Supply dosage: This refers to dosage strength and medication form. Read it as "X measured units per quantity." For liquid medications, the supply dosage is the same as the medication's concentration. On the heparin sodium label (Fig. 2-4), there are 1000 units per milliliter of solution. Note also that heparin sodium is the generic name of the medication and so has no ® registration mark.

Total volume: This is the full quantity contained in the bottle or vial, or its total fluid volume. For solids it is the total number of individual items in the package. On the heparin label, there is a total volume of 30 mL as this medication is in liquid form.

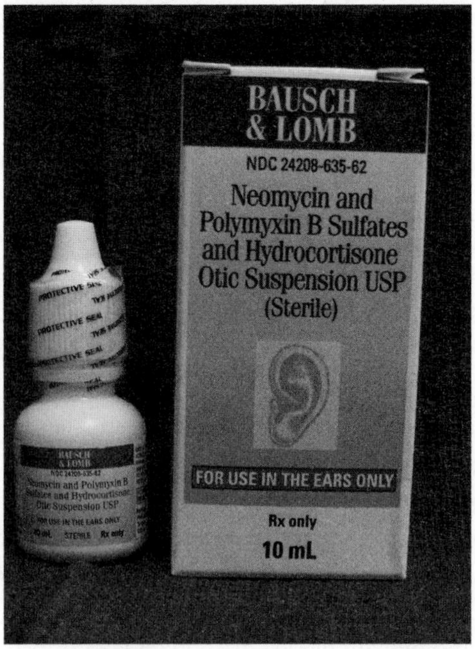

Figure 2-3 Neomycin and polymyxin B sulfates and hydrocortisone otic suspension USP label.

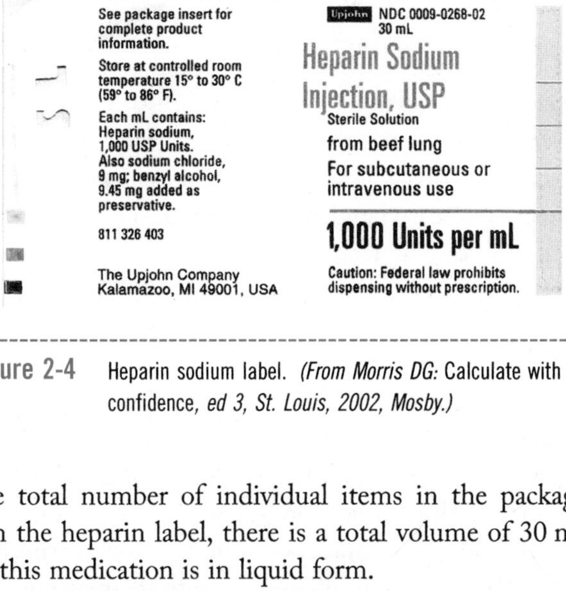

Figure 2-4 Heparin sodium label. *(From Morris DG:* Calculate with confidence, *ed 3, St. Louis, 2002, Mosby.)*

Administration route: This refers to the method of medication delivery to the patient or body site. Refer to Chapter 4 for further information on medication administration. On the neomycin and polymyxin B sulfates label, it states for use in the ears only. The Keflin label states for injection and the heparin lists subcutaneous or intravenous use.

Label alerts: Manufacturers may print warnings on the packages such as "refrigerate" or "protect from light." Suspension medications would carry the warning to "shake well before use." This would be found on the neomycin and polymyxin B sulfates label. Another

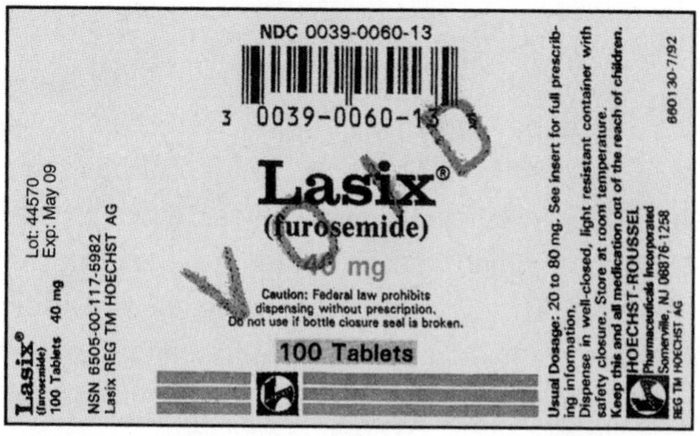

Figure 2-5 Lasix label. *(From Ogden SJ:* Calculation of drug dosages, *ed 7, St. Louis, 2003, Mosby.)*

example of an alert is red on the label of a local anesthetic agent such as lidocaine. This would signify the presence of epinephrine (adrenaline) in the medication.

MAKE IT SIMPLE

Red on the label of a local anesthetic agent means it contains epinephrine.

Expiration date: Medications should be used, discarded, or returned to the pharmacy by this date. This is very important information and it is usually presented as a month/year (as 5/09 on the Lasix® label [Fig. 2-5], which would indicate the medication can be used until May 1, 2009). If this medication were obtained from pharmacy for a procedure, it should not be used as it is *outdated.* It should be returned to the pharmacy and another obtained with a date that is not passed.

CAUTION

If a medication is expired, it may have reduced potency or effectiveness. It can become chemically altered and provide a lethal effect to the patient.

Lot or control numbers: Federal law requires all medication packages to be identified with a lot or control number. If a medication is recalled this number identifies the specific group of packages to be removed from shelves. The Lasix label gives the lot number as 44570 (see Fig. 2-5).

Bar code symbols: These are used in sales and they document medication dosing for record keeping. They may have future use to automate medication documentation to the patient's bedside, much like the scanners are used in stores today. You can see a bar code on the Keflin label.

National Drug Code (NDC): Federal law requires every prescription medication have an identifying number. It must appear on every manufacturer's label and is printed as NDC-••••-••••-••. Note the code on the top of the Keflin® label as NDC 0002-7001-01.

United States Pharmacopeia (USP) and National Formulary (NF): These codes are found on manufacturer-printed labels. These are two different official national lists of approved medications. Each manufacturer follows special guidelines that determine when to include these initials on the label. Initials are placed after the generic drug name. Note the initials "USP" on the heparin sodium and Keflin® labels (Insight 2-3).

MEDICATION REFERENCES

When a medication has been approved for use, the pharmaceutical company must publish comprehensive information regarding it. This information must appear in package inserts and in compiled reference works. In addition, many medication information resources are available to medical, nursing, and allied health professionals. There are dozens of textbooks on pharmacology and various specialty areas within that science.

IN SIGHT 2-3 Medications Under the Labels

The medications used as examples in the medication labeling section are the ones you will see used in the surgical setting or for the surgical patient. The first medication, Keflin, is an antibiotic. It may be used preoperatively, intraoperatively, or postoperatively to help fight infections. Refer to Chapter 5 for more on antibiotics. The next medication, neomycin and polymyxin B sulfates otic drops, is also an antibiotic with other medications mixed in, that is, hydrocortisone. Hydrocortisone is a steroid used to decrease the body's inflammatory response. Refer to Chapter 5 and also Chapter 8. The next, heparin sodium, is an anticoagulant that is used on vascular procedures. Refer to Chapter 9 for more on medications that affect the vascular system. The last medication mentioned is Lasix, a diuretic. It is used in neurosurgery to decrease intracranial pressure. Refer to Chapter 7 for more on diuretics and their actions.

IN SIGHT 2-4 **Ancient Medical References**

There are ancient medical references that can be traced back as early as c. 3000 BCE for pharmacology by the Egyptians, Mesopotamians, peoples of India and China. Two papyri of ancient Egypt are the Ebers Papyrus (c. 1550 BCE) and the Edwin Smith Papyrus (16th century BCE). The Ebers Papyrus describes more than 700 medical compounds and lists more than 811 prescriptions. It is thought to be a copy of a much earlier text that dates to 3000 BCE. The Edwin Smith Papyrus is a manuscript on trauma surgery that also addresses the prevention and cure of infection with honey and moldy bread. It tells how to stop bleeding with raw meat. In Mesopotamia (the Persian Gulf area c. 2500 BCE) more than 800 clay tablets have been discovered, written in cuneiform, which describe more than 500 remedies. The *Pen Tsao-Ching* from China (c. 2750 BCE) has more than 1000 medicinal compounds and 11,000 prescriptions which are attributed to the Emperor Shen Nung. The *Dravyaguna*, an ancient Aryuvedic manuscript from India, includes information on how to obtain and prepare hundreds of medicinal herbs. One of the most well-known medical manuscripts comes from first century Greece. Dioscorides was a physician and pharmacist who described some 600 medicinal plants, including aloe, belladonna, ergot, and opium in his writings titled *De Materia Medica* (Regarding Medical Matters). Some of the compounds described in these ancient medical references are still in use today.

Moreover, several pharmacology resources are expressly designed for use in clinical practice. Each surgery department should have such references readily available to the staff (Insight 2-4).

PHYSICIAN'S DESK REFERENCE

One of the most frequently used pharmacology resources is the *Physicians' Desk Reference*, or **PDR**. It provides easy access to information on several thousand medications used in medical and surgical practice. The PDR is published annually and contains seven color-coded sections:

- Section 1 (white)–An alphabetical list of drug manufacturers, the address, emergency phone number, and some available products
- Section 2 (pink)–A comprehensive, alphabetical index of brand and generic drug names
- Section 3 (blue)–A list of drugs by prescribing category, such as antibiotics, analgesics, and so on
- Section 4 (gray)–A photographic identification section supplied by each manufacturer of actual size tablets, capsules, and other drug forms
- Section 5 (white)–A product information section that includes the same information as found in the package inserts for the major products of the manufacturers
- Section 6 (white)–An alphabetical listing on diagnostic test medications and products
- Section 7 (white)–A miscellaneous section that includes keys to the controlled substances categories and to FDA use-in-pregnancy ratings, a list of poison control centers, an FDA directory, drug information centers, look-alike/sound-alike drugs, and adverse event report forms.

The product information section (section 5), which is the largest part of the book, contains the manufacturer's information on approximately 3000 medications. Medications are listed alphabetically by manufacturer. Each entry includes data on **indications** (why it is used), effects, dosage, administration routes, methods, and frequency. It also includes warnings regarding side effects and **contraindications**. The PDR also publishes separate references for non-prescription medications and ophthalmic medications. Its website at *www.pdrhealth.com/* offers readers information on a variety of topics, such as prescription medications, OTC medications, herbals and supplements, Health Information Centers, and clinical trials. There is a link on the home page for health care professionals, which offers free PDR.net access.

{NOTE} *The information presented in the PDR is the same as that found in the manufacturer's package insert. Students may easily obtain package inserts for medications used in surgery. You can get them as medications are opened or from the pharmacy at your clinical site.*

UNITED STATES PHARMACOPEIA AND NATIONAL FORMULARY

The *USP-NF* is the official medication list recognized by the United States government. It is actually two publications—the Pharmacopeia and the Formulary—combined into three volumes. It is available in print, on CD, and on line at www.usp.org/USPNF/. The *USP-NF* lists standards for medication quality, safety, and effectiveness; it also contains information on the physical and chemical characteristics of listed medications. Used primarily by drug companies and pharmacists, the *USP-NF* is issued annually by the United States Pharmacopeial Convention (a national committee of pharmacists, pharmacologists, physicians, chemists, biologists, and other scientific professionals). The *United States Pharmacopeia/Dispensing Information* (*USP-DI*) is a related clinical reference divided into several volumes including one for health care professionals. This includes pharmacology, precautions to consider, side and adverse effects, and general dosing information. Another volume gives medication information directed to the patient (client). It is written in understandable language and includes administration of medications, medication effects, indications, adverse reactions, guidelines for dosages, and what to do for missed doses. It should be noted there is also an *International Pharmacopeia* which is revised every five years with supplements published in between. It was first published in 1951 by the WHO and appears in English, Spanish, and French with CD-ROM and online availability.

AMERICAN HOSPITAL FORMULARY SERVICE (AHFS) DRUG INFORMATION

This reference is published annually and updated quarterly by the American Society of Health-System Pharmacists, Bethesda, Md. The **AHFS** provides accurate information on almost all prescription medications marketed in the United States. Medications are listed according to therapeutic medication classification. The information includes chemistry and stability, pharmacological actions, pharmacokinetics, uses, cautions and precautions, contraindications, drug interactions, acute toxicity, dosage and administration, and preparation of the medications. This text is considered unbiased because it does not contain information supplied only by the pharmaceutical company that manufactures the medications. Online data can be accessed via the website at www.ashp.org/ahfs/.

THE MEDICAL LETTER

The *Medical Letter* on medications and therapeutics is published biweekly by the Medical Letter, Inc. in New York. This is a nonprofit publication for physicians and other allied health professionals. It issues two newsletters, *The Medical Letter on Drugs and Therapeutics* and *Treatment Guidelines from the Medical Letter*. They cover medications for the treatment of diseases such as HIV, and cover new medications recently approved by the FDA. The information includes pharmacokinetics, clinical studies, dosage, adverse effects, and interactions. The website is www.medicalletter.org.

FACTS AND COMPARISONS

Facts and Comparisons is a loose-leaf edition that contains thousands of prescription and OTC medications, as well as thousands of comparison charts and tables. It can also be found on CD-ROM and online at www.FactsandComparisons.com. It is a reference for drug actions, indications, warnings and precautions, dosage and route of administration, adverse reactions, overdosage, interactions, contraindications, and patient (client) information. Medications are grouped by therapeutic category and it also includes information on investigational medications. Facts and Comparisons is available as an annual subscription that includes monthly updates via a newsletter.

HOSPITAL PHARMACIST

Another valuable source of information on drugs is the clinical pharmacist. Consulting and educating has become an important part of pharmacy practice. The pharmacist is consulted when any question arises regarding medications, especially those that are newly approved.

DATABASES

A vast amount of information regarding medications, their proper use, possible drug side effects and interactions, and other important clinical considerations is available via computer. Databases, such as *Micromedix* and Facts and Comparisons *CliniSphere*, are helpful tools that medical professionals use to access current pharmacological information. Drug manufacturers also include drug information on their websites. Helpful Internet addresses include the following:

The American College of Clinical Pharmacy at www.accp.com/
The American Heart Association at www.amhrt.org/
The American Medical Association at www.ama-assn.org/

The Centers for Disease Control and Prevention at www.cdc.gov/
Clinical Pharmacology at www.clinicalpharmacology.com
Drug Store News at www.drugstorenews.com
Facts and Comparisons at www.factsandcomparisons.com
Internet Drug Index at www.rxlist.com/
Micromedix at www.micromedix.com
The National Cancer Institute at www.cancer.gov
The National Institute of Health (NIH) at www.nih.gov/
The National Library of Medicine at www.nlm.nih.gov/
The Occupational Safety and Health Administration at www.osha.gov/
Pharm Web at www.pharmweb.net/
The Pharmaceutical Information Network at www.virtualref.com
Pharmacy Times at www.pharmacytimes.com
RX Med at www.rxmed.com
U.S. Pharmacist at www.uspharmacist.com
U.S. Pharmacopeia at www.usp.org
The World Health Organization at www.who.org

CAUTION

Keep in mind that medication information can be posted on the Internet by anyone, so the information may not always be accurate. It is a good idea to check reliable sources such as governmental websites, and always verify information from two different sources. Other drug resource material is easily accessible by computer, including the *USPDI, PDR,* current journal articles, and manufacturer's bulletins.

KEY CONCEPTS

- Federal regulations of medications protect consumers.
- The Federal Pure Food and Drug Act sets standards for quality and proper medication labeling.
- The Food, Drug and Cosmetic Act requires animal testing of medications.
- The Controlled Substances Act Established schedules for medications.
- The U.S. Drug Enforcement Administration (DEA) enforces the Controlled Substances Act.
- The U.S. Food and Drug Administration (FDA) developed a classification system related to medications' effects upon the unborn child.
- State practice acts govern the ordering, dispersal, and administration of medications.
- The role of the surgical technologist in medication handling may be specified by institutional policy.
- The Joint Commission (formerly JCAHO) evaluates and accredits health care facilities and sets policies such as National Patient Safety Goals.
- Genetic factors are being used to predict a medication's action on patients, thus being useful in medication development.
- Medications must undergo testing that involves several phases (including animal testing) before being given FDA approval.
- There are numerous medication references and databases that include the ones found on the Internet that can be accessed for information.

Bibliography

Fulcher E, Fulcher R, Soto C: *Pharmacology principles and applications*, ed 2, 2009, Saunders/Elsevier.
Junge T: From concept to creation: a look at the drug discovery, development and approval process, *Surg Technol* 41(1): 13–20, 2009.
Moscou K, Snipe K: *Pharmacology for pharmacy technicians*, St. Louis, 2009, Mosby/Elsevier.

Internet Resources

American Association of Acupuncture and Oriental Medicine: http://www.aaaomonline.org/.
American Association of Naturopathic Physicians: http://www.naturopathic.org/content.asp?contentid=59.
Centers for Disease Control and Prevention: www.cdc.gov.
Facts and Comparisons: www.factsandcomparisons.com.
Human Genome Project Information: www.ornl.gov/sci/techresources/human_genome/medicine/pharma.shtml.
National Acupuncture Foundation: http://www.nationalacupuncturefoundation.org/pages/about.html.
National Center for Complementary and Alternative Medicine (NCCAM): http://nccam.nih.gov/about/.
Qigong Research and Practice Center: http://www.qigonghealing.com/qigong/whatis.html.
SpringerImages, Medicine and Public Health: http://www.springerimages.com/Images/MedicineAndPublicHealth/5-10.1186_1472-6882-8-14-2.
TeensHealth, "Complementary and Alternative Medicine": http://kidshealth.org/teen/your_body/medical_care/alternative_medicine.html#.
The Joint Commission: www.jointcommission.org.

The Joint Commission, Official "Do Not Use" List: www.jointcommission.org/patientsafety/donotuselist.
Thomson Reuters, Micromedex: www.micromedex.com.
U.S. Department of Labor, Occupational Safety and Health Administration: www.osha.gov.
U.S. Drug Enforcement Administration: www.dea.gov.
Washington Acupuncture Center: http://www.acupuncture-florida.com/lee.html.
WebMD, Complementary Medicine - Alternative Medical Systems: http://www.webmd.com/balance/tc/complementary-medicine-alternative-medical-systems.
World Health Organization: www.who.int/.
World Health Organization, Patient Safety, Safe Surgery Saves Lives: www.who.int/patientsafety/safesurgery/en/.

LEARNING THE LANGUAGE (KEY TERMS)

Using your textbook and/or a medical dictionary, look up and write the definitions of each term.

AHFS drug information
contraindication
controlled substances
DEA
Facts and Comparisons
FDA
indication
The Joint Commission
narcotics
OTC
PDR
pharmacogenetics/pharmacogenomics
prescription drugs
USP-NF
World Health Organization

REVIEW QUESTIONS

1. How does the federal government regulate medications?
2. What is the significance of the Pure Food and Drug Act of 1906?
3. What is the role of the FDA in drug regulation?
4. Why is the separation of drugs into five schedules important?
5. What is the role of The Joint Commission in medication regulation? OSHA? CDC?
6. Use at least two medication references to research the indications and the side effects of the following medications.
   a) Heparin sodium
   b) Lasix
   c) Keflin
7. Why is it important for the surgical technologist to have an understanding of medications, even though he or she does not directly administer them to the patient?

CRITICAL THINKING

1. How does the DEA affect clinical practice?
2. Name three medications the surgeon uses during a procedure that are prepared on the back table.
3. How are medications for procedures obtained at your clinical site?

Case Study Scenario

The surgery is scheduled as an excision of a cyst from the right lower back. The surgeon requests Xylocaine 1% with epinephrine, Demerol, and Versed for the local procedure.

1. What are the generic names for these medications?
2. Xylocaine is available in what strengths?
3. Which of these medications is/are narcotics? What is/are the controlled substances schedules?
4. Which of the medications would have red on the label? What does this signify?

CHAPTER 3 Pharmacology Math

OBJECTIVES *Upon completion of this chapter, you should be able to:*

1. Convert civilian time to military time.
2. Define terminology, abbreviations, and symbols used in basic mathematics and measurement systems.
3. Use fractions in conversions and calculations.
4. Read and write decimals accurately.
5. Use decimals in conversions and calculations.
6. Convert between fractions and decimals.
7. Define percentages.
8. Convert between percentages and decimals, and between percentages and fractions.
9. Define ratios and proportions.
10. Use ratios and proportions to solve problems.
11. Convert temperatures between the Fahrenheit and Celsius scales.
12. Define the metric system of measurement and explain how it is used as the international standard
13. Identify other systems of measurement and their medical applications.
14. Identify symbols of measurement, and measurement equivalents.

KEY TERMS

Celsius scale	Fahrenheit scale	percentage
civilian time	fraction	proportion
decimal point	metric system	ratio
exponent	military time	relative value

In this chapter we look at basic mathematics, including military time, fractions, decimals, percentages, and ratios and proportions. We review how to solve simple problems, perform fundamental calculations, and make important conversions. Many surgical technology students are familiar with these principles; this chapter is designed as a refresher for students who need to practice their mathematical skills. Each rule is explained, and then examples are given to illustrate its principle. In addition there are exercises, including specific surgical technology story problems, for students to practice the mathematical operations. This chapter also introduces students to measurement systems and how they are used in the medical setting. Students use basic mathematical skills to perform conversions in the systems of measurement. Knowledge of metric measurements and basic mathematical skills are necessary in pharmacology as they are used during surgical procedures, particularly when using implants, grafts, and assisting the surgeon as medications are administered from the sterile field.

MAKE IT SIMPLE

Go to the end of this chapter and take the Math Evaluation Pretest. This pretest has a variety of math skills that are explained in the chapter. If you discover areas where you believe you are weak, review those sections of this chapter to strengthen your skills.

MILITARY TIME

Hospitals and other medical institutions, along with law enforcement and the military, use a precise method of expressing time called international or **military time.** Military time uses a 24-hour scale without AM or PM designations (Figure 3-1). It is similar to **civilian time** in the morning hours from midnight until noon. After noon, it increases in one-hour increments from 12 while civilian time starts over again with 1.

To convert military time to civilian time after noon, subtract 12. For example, 1900 hours becomes 7:00 PM. ($19 - 12 = 7$). To convert civilian time to military time after noon, add 12. For example, 1:00 PM becomes 1300 hours ($1 + 12 = 13$).

Military time is pronounced differently than civilian time. For example, 5:00 AM in civilian time, or 5 o'clock in the morning, is 0500 in military time and is pronounced as oh-five-hundred or zero-five-hundred. In surgery, a procedure scheduled for 4 o'clock in the afternoon would be "sixteen hundred hours" (1600) in military time. If the incision for this 4 o'clock case is made at 4:46 PM, it would be written as 1646 and pronounced as sixteen forty six hours in military time. Table 3-1 provides conversions between civilian and military times.

What if an event occurs at 9 minutes after midnight? In civilian time it would be written as 12:09 AM. In military time, it would be written as 0009 and pronounced as "zero-zero-zero-nine hours." If the event occurs at 9 minutes after noon, in civilian time it would be written as 12:09 PM. In military time, it would be written as 1209 and pronounced as "twelve-oh-nine hours."

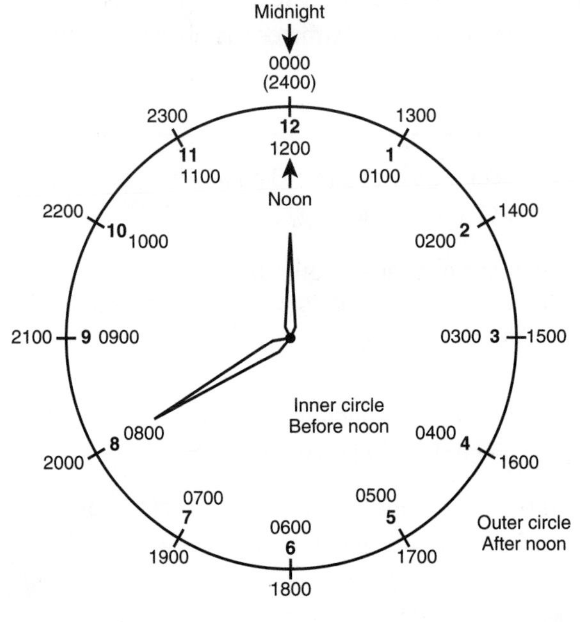

Figure 3-1 **Military/civilian clock.** This 24-hour clock shows the time as 1140 (or 11:40 AM) and 2340 (or 11:40 PM).

Table 3-1 MILITARY AND CIVILIAN TIMES

Civilian Time	Military Time	Civilian Time	Military Time
Midnight*	0000	Noon	1200
1:00 AM	0100	1:00 PM	1300
2:00 AM	0200	2:00 PM	1400
3:00 AM	0300	3:00 PM	1500
4:00 AM	0400	4:00 PM	1600
5:00 AM	0500	5:00 PM	1700
6:00 AM	0600	6:00 PM	1800
7:00 AM	0700	7:00 PM	1900
8:00 AM	0800	8:00 PM	2000
9:00 AM	0900	9:00 PM	2100
10:00 AM	1000	10:00 PM	2200
11:00 AM	1100	11:00 PM	2300

**Midnight can be written two ways in military time: 2400 and read as "twenty four hundred," or 0000 and read as "zero hundred."*

MAKE IT SIMPLE

Notice that military time uses four digits to indicate the hours and minutes: the first two digits represent hours and the last two represent minutes.

{NOTE} *Midnight can be written two ways in military time: 2400 and read as "twenty four hundred," or 0000 and read as "zero hundred."*

FRACTIONS

A **fraction** is a number that represents one or more equal parts of a whole. The word comes from the Latin *fractio,* which means "to break into pieces." A fraction is a quotient—a number that can be written in an a/b or $\frac{a}{b}$ form, where b is never equal to 0. We say that a and b are the terms of the fraction where a is the *numerator* and b is the *denominator.*

EXAMPLE

One-half = 1/2 = $\frac{1}{2}$ =

$\frac{1}{2}$ $a = 1$ is the numerator; $b = 2$ is the denominator

Five-sixths = 5/6 = $\frac{5}{6}$ =

$\frac{5}{6}$ $a = 5$ is the numerator; $b = 6$ is the denominator

Five-eighths = 5/8 = $\frac{5}{8}$ =

$\frac{5}{8}$ $a = 5$ is the numerator; $b = 8$ is the denominator

We use fractions to express division of a whole into equal parts:

- The denominator tells how many equal parts into which the whole is divided.
- The numerator tells how many equal parts we are interested in.

EXAMPLE

Imagine a pie divided into 6 equal parts, and 5 of those equal parts are eaten (Fig. 3-2).

$\frac{5}{6}$ 5: number of eaten parts; 6: number of equal parts into which the whole pie is divided

So

- $\frac{5}{6}$ of the pie is eaten
- $\frac{1}{6}$ of the pie remains

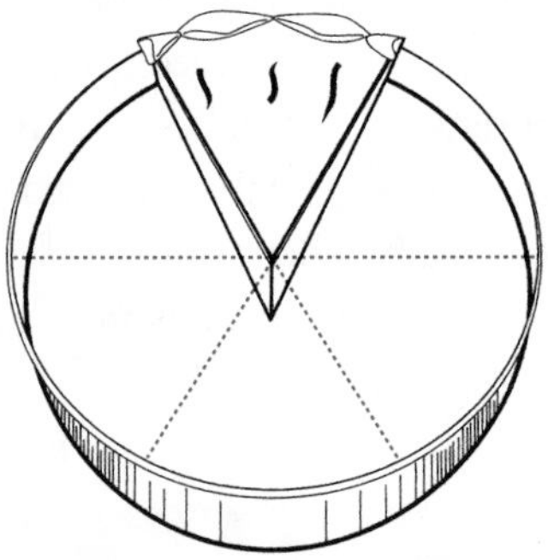

Figure 3-2

The larger the denominator, the smaller the pieces (fractions) in the whole.

{NOTE}

$\frac{1}{2}$ is greater than $\frac{1}{3}$
$\frac{1}{3}$ is greater than $\frac{1}{4}$
$\frac{1}{4}$ is greater than $\frac{1}{5}$
$\frac{1}{5}$ is greater than $\frac{1}{6}$
and so on.

MAKE IT SIMPLE

If the denominators of two fractions are the same, the one with the higher numerator determines the higher fraction. If the numerators are the same, the one with the lower denominator determines the higher fraction.

EXAMPLE

Imagine a circle divided into 8 equal parts, and 5 of those equal parts are shaded (Fig. 3-3).

$\frac{5}{8}$ 5: number of shaded equal parts; 8: number of equal parts into which the whole circle is divided

So

- $\frac{5}{8}$ of the circle is shaded
- $\frac{3}{8}$ of the circle is not shaded

If the numerator and the denominator are equal to each other, the fraction is equal to 1

EXAMPLES

$\frac{1}{1} = \quad \frac{2}{2} = \quad \frac{5}{5} = \quad \frac{100}{100} = \quad \frac{3569}{3569} = 1$

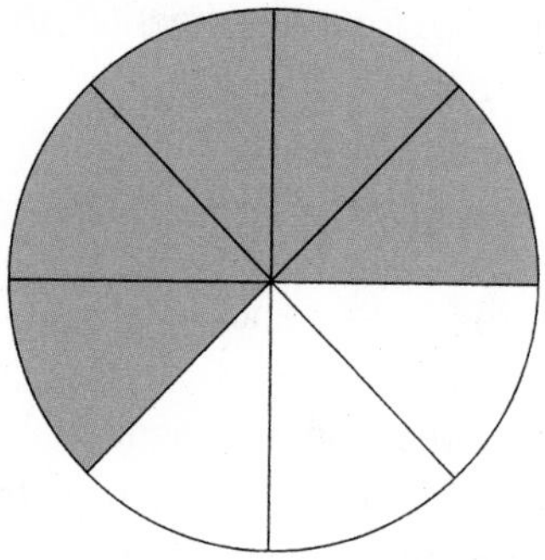

Figure 3-3

If the numerator is less than the denominator, the value of the fraction is less than 1. Then the fraction is a proper fraction.

EXAMPLES

$\frac{2}{3}$ $\frac{3}{4}$ $\frac{3}{5}$ $\frac{99}{100}$

If the numerator is greater than the denominator, the value of the fraction is more than 1. Then the fraction is an improper fraction.

EXAMPLES

$\frac{3}{2}$ $\frac{4}{3}$ $\frac{12}{6}$ $\frac{15}{10}$

A mixed number is a combination of a whole number with a fraction.

EXAMPLES

$1\frac{1}{2}$ $2\frac{1}{3}$ $5\frac{3}{7}$ $8\frac{49}{50}$

{NOTE} *Any time the numerator of a fraction is zero, the value of the fraction is zero.*

You can change a mixed number to an improper fraction in three steps.

Given the mixed number $2\frac{1}{2}$,

Step 1: Multiply the denominator of the fraction by the whole number:

$$\text{Whole number} \times \text{denominator} = 2 \times 2 = 4$$

Step 2: Add the numerator to the result obtained in Step 1:

$$\text{Numerator} + (\text{step 1 result}) = 1 + 4 = 5$$

Step 3: Use the result obtained in Step 2 as the numerator of the new fraction; use the original denominator as the new denominator:

$$\frac{\text{Step 2 result}}{\text{Original denominator}} = \frac{5}{2} = \frac{5}{2}$$

Thus, the mixed number of $2\frac{1}{2}$ is the same as the improper fraction $\frac{5}{2}$. You can change an improper fraction to a mixed number in 4 steps. Given an improper fraction $\frac{8}{5}$,

Step 1: Divide the numerator by the denominator:

$$\frac{\text{Numerator}}{\text{Denominator}} = \frac{8}{5} = 1\text{ R3} \quad \text{(i.e., 1 with 3 left over)}$$

Step 2: Use the whole number obtained in Step 1 as the whole number of the mixed fraction:

$$\text{Whole number} = \text{Step 1 whole number} = 1$$

Step 3: Use the remainder (R) obtained in Step 1 as the numerator of the new fraction; use the original denominator as the new denominator:

$$\text{Fraction} = \frac{\text{Step 1 remainder}}{\text{Original denominator}} = \frac{3}{5} = \frac{3}{5}$$

Step 4: Put the whole number and the fraction together to get the mixed number:

$$1 \text{ and } \frac{3}{5} = 1\frac{3}{5}$$

Thus, the improper fraction $\frac{8}{5}$ is the same as the mixed number $1\frac{3}{5}$.

If you multiply or divide the numerator and the denominator of a fraction by the same nonzero number, you get an equivalent fraction.

EXAMPLE

$$\frac{3}{4} = \frac{3 \times 2}{4 \times 2} = \frac{6}{8}$$

$$\frac{6}{8} = \frac{6 \div 2}{8 \div 2} = \frac{3}{4}$$

Thus, $\frac{3}{4}$ and $\frac{6}{8}$ are equivalent fractions.

A fraction is in its *lowest terms* when no nonzero number except 1 can be evenly divided into both the numerator and the denominator. Reducing fractions to their lowest terms is ALWAYS the last step in mathematical problem solving.

EXAMPLE

In the fraction $\frac{10}{12}$, both the numerator and the denominator can be evenly divided by 2. When this is accomplished, the resulting fraction, $\frac{5}{6}$ is an equivalent fraction to the original and also its lowest terms.

ADDITION AND SUBTRACTION OF FRACTIONS

To add (or subtract) fractions whose denominators are the same, just add (or subtract) the numerators and keep the denominators the same.

EXAMPLE

$$\frac{2}{5}+\frac{1}{5}=\frac{2+1}{5}=\frac{3}{5} \qquad \frac{2}{5}-\frac{1}{5}=\frac{2-1}{5}=\frac{1}{5}$$

To add (or subtract) fractions whose denominators are not the same, first convert the fractions to equivalent fractions with the lowest common denominators, then add (or subtract) the numerators. This can be done in 3 steps. Given the problem $\frac{1}{2}+\frac{1}{3}=?$,

Step 1: Find the lowest common denominator of $\frac{1}{2}$ and $\frac{1}{3}$. The lowest number divisible by both 2 and 3 is 6, so six is the lowest common denominator.

Step 2: Change the fractions to equivalent fractions using 6 as the new denominator:

$$\frac{1}{2}=\frac{1\times 3}{2\times 3}=\frac{3}{6}$$

and

$$\frac{1}{3}=\frac{1\times 2}{3\times 2}=\frac{2}{6}$$

Step 3: Now perform your operation, add the two new fractions as they have the same denominators (remember to always reduce to lowest terms):

$$\frac{3}{6}+\frac{2}{6}=\frac{5}{6}$$

In this example, $\frac{5}{6}$ is in lowest terms

EXAMPLES

$\frac{1}{2}-\frac{1}{3}=\frac{3}{6}-\frac{2}{6}=\frac{1}{6}$

$\frac{3}{4}+\frac{1}{8}=\frac{6}{8}+\frac{1}{8}=\frac{7}{8}$

To add (or subtract) mixed numbers, convert the mixed numbers to improper fractions, find the lowest common denominator, and add (or subtract) as usual. Then convert the answer, if it is an improper fraction, to a mixed number. This can be done in 4 steps.

Given the problem $4\frac{2}{3}+1\frac{1}{6}=?$,

Step 1: Convert the mixed numbers to improper fractions.

$$4\tfrac{2}{3}=\tfrac{14}{3} \quad \text{and} \quad 1\tfrac{1}{6}=\tfrac{7}{6}$$

Step 2: Find the lowest common denominator of $\frac{14}{3}$ and $\frac{7}{6}$. The lowest number divisible by both 3 and 6 is 6, so 6 is the lowest common denominator.

Step 3: Change the fractions to equivalent fractions using 6 as the new denominator.

$\frac{14}{3}=\frac{14\times 2}{3\times 2}=\frac{28}{6}$ and 7/6 already has 6 as its denominator

Step 4: Now perform your operation and add the two new fractions as they have the same denominators (and convert back to a mixed number as that is the lowest term for this fraction):

$$\frac{28}{6}+\frac{7}{6}=\frac{28+7}{6}=\frac{35}{6}=5\frac{5}{6}$$

EXAMPLES

$9\frac{3}{4}-2\frac{1}{3}=\frac{27}{4}-\frac{7}{3}=\frac{81}{12}-\frac{28}{12}=\frac{53}{12}=4\frac{5}{12}$

$2\frac{1}{5}+2\frac{1}{10}=\frac{11}{5}+\frac{21}{10}=\frac{22}{10}+\frac{21}{10}=\frac{43}{10}=4\frac{3}{10}$

MULTIPLICATION AND DIVISION OF FRACTIONS

To multiply two fractions, multiply the numerators by the numerators and the denominators by the denominators. The results are the new fraction/answer. Remember to always reduce to lowest terms.

EXAMPLES

$$\frac{2}{3}\times\frac{1}{4}=\frac{2\times 1}{3\times 4}=\frac{2}{12}=\frac{1}{6}$$

$$\frac{1}{7}\times\frac{1}{8}=\frac{1\times 1}{7\times 8}=\frac{1}{56}$$

To divide two fractions, invert the divisor, then multiply.

EXAMPLES

$$\frac{1}{5}\div\frac{3}{8}=\frac{1}{5}\times\frac{8}{3}=\frac{8}{15}$$

$$\frac{5}{12} \div \frac{1}{3} = \frac{5}{12} \times \frac{3}{1} = \frac{15}{12} = 1\frac{3}{12} = 1\frac{1}{4}$$

{NOTE} *To remember the rule for division of fractions:*
The number you are dividing by
Turn upside down and multiply.

To multiply or divide mixed numbers, first convert them to improper fractions, then multiply or divide.

EXAMPLES

$$1\tfrac{1}{4} \times 2\tfrac{1}{8} = \frac{5}{4} \times \frac{17}{8} = \frac{85}{32} = 2\tfrac{21}{32}$$

$$\frac{2}{12} \div 3\tfrac{1}{3} = \frac{5}{2} \div \frac{10}{3} = \frac{5}{2} \times \frac{3}{10} = \frac{15}{20} = \frac{3}{4}$$

DECIMALS

Decimal numbers are written by placing digits (0, 1, 2, 3, 4, 5, 6, 7, 8, 9) into place value columns that are separated by a **decimal point**, as shown in Table 3-2. The place value columns are read in sequence from left to right as multiples of decreasing powers of 10:

- Numbers to the left of the decimal point represent values greater than 1.
- Numbers to the right of the decimal point represent values less than 1.
- The number sequence is added.

The number 652.345 is represented as:

hundreds		tens		ones	decimal point ↓	tenths		hundredths		thousandths
(6 × 100)	+	(5 × 10)	+	(2 × 1)	•	(3 × 1/10)	+	(4 × 1/100)	+	(5 × 1/1000)
600	+	50	+	2	•	3/10	+	4/100	+	5/1000

Table 3-2 DECIMAL PLACE VALUES

Ten thousands			10^4
Thousands			10^3
Hundreds			10^2
Tens			10^1
Ones			10^0
Decimal point			
Tenths			10^{-1}
Hundredths			10^{-2}
Thousandths			10^{-3}
Ten thousandths			10^{-4}
Hundred thousandths			10^{-5}
Millionths			10^{-6}
or			
Ten thousands	10,000.	=	10^4
Thousands	1,000.	=	10^3
Hundreds	100.	=	10^2
Tens	10.	=	10^1
Ones	1.	=	10^0
Decimal point	.	=	
Tenths	0.1	=	10^{-1}
Hundredths	0.01	=	10^{-2}
Thousandths	0.001	=	10^{-3}
Ten thousandths	0.000 1	=	10^{-4}
Hundred thousandths	0.000 01	=	10^{-5}
Millionths	0.000 001	=	10^{-6}

{NOTE} *Notice that each place value is a power of 10. This can also be written using* ***exponents****. These are shortcuts to showing multiplication of a number times itself. For example, 10 × 10 can be written as* 10^2. *Any number with an exponent of 0 is equal to one. So,* $10^0 = 1$. *The above multiples of ten can be written as:*

$$(6 \times 10^2) + (5 \times 10^1) + (2 \times 10^0) + (3 \times 10^{-1}) + (4 \times 10^{-2}) + (5 \times 10^{-3})$$

Remember:

$$10^2 = 10 \times 10 \text{ or } 100$$
$$10^1 = 10$$
$$10^0 = 1$$
$$10^{-1} = 1/10$$
$$10^{-2} = 1/100$$

The decimal 652.345 can be read as "six hundred fifty-two point three four five." It can also be read as "six hundred fifty-two and three hundred forty-five thousandths." Notice that:

- The word "and" is used for the decimal point.
- The decimal fraction is named for the rightmost place in the place column sequence.
- The suffix *-th* is used to signify fractions.

EXAMPLES

5.45 is read as five "and" forty-five hundredths
7.0 is read as seven or seven "and" 0 tenths

The **relative value** of a decimal number is determined by looking at the spaces to the left of the decimal point. The more spaces, the higher the value. When comparing two decimal numbers with the same spaces to the left of the decimal point, the first place where they differ determines the relative value of each number. To compare decimal numbers, write the numbers with each decimal point aligned. For example, compare 45.67 and 46.78.

EXAMPLES

Write 4**5**.67
4**6**.78

Begin with the numbers to the left of the decimal and compare. In these numbers, 6 is larger than 5. As the larger number determines the higher value, 4**6**.78 is larger than 4**5**.67.

Compare 45.67 and 45.78. Now both numbers to the left of the decimal point are the same. So we must look at the numbers to the right of the decimal point.

Write: 45.67
45.78

Begin with the numbers to the right of the decimal point and compare. In these numbers, 7 is larger than 6. As the larger number again determines the higher value, 45.**78** is larger than 45.**67**.

ADDITION AND SUBTRACTION OF DECIMALS

To add or subtract decimal numbers, line up the decimal points and carry out the calculations.

EXAMPLES

24.531 + 2.798 =

↓ align the decimal points

```
  24.531
   2.798
  ------
  27.329
```

5.04 − 1.213 =

```
   5.040 ← add a zero as a place holder
 − 1.213
   -----
   3.827
```

{NOTE} *Adding zeros to the right of a number on the right side of the decimal point does not change its value. Adding zeros to the left of a number on the left side of the decimal point does not change its value.*

MULTIPLICATION AND DIVISION OF DECIMALS

To multiply two decimals, carry out the multiplication, then add the number of decimal places from the right of the decimal point in the original two numbers. This total is the number of decimal places from the right of the decimal point in the product (answer).

EXAMPLES:

```
  0.07      2 decimal places
 × 2.1     +1 decimal place
 -----
   007
  014
 -----
 0.147      3 decimal places
```

```
  0.00051       5 decimal places
   × 0.04      +2 decimal places
 ---------     ----------------
 0.0000204      7 decimal places
   └┘────────── add zeros
```

To divide decimals by whole numbers, carry out the long division. Align the decimal point of the quotient directly above that of the dividend.

EXAMPLES:

```
   3.09
5)15.45
  15
    45
    45
     0
```

```
  3.3
3)9.9
  9
   9
   9
   0
```

If the divisor is a decimal, convert it to a whole number before dividing. To do this, move the decimal point of the divisor and that of the dividend the same number of places to the right.

EXAMPLES:

```
                  2.5
2.5)6.25  =  25.)62.5
                  50
                 125
                 125
                   0
```

One place value

Divisor → Whole number

(1) 2.5 × 10 = 25

(2) 6.25 × 10 = 62.5

Dividend

```
                 20.
.25)5  =  25.)500.
               50
               00
```

Two place values

Divisor → Whole number

(1) .25 × 100 = 25

(2) 5 × 100 = 500

Dividend

When more than one operation (addition, subtraction, multiplication, division, exponents) must be carried out, use the order of operations:

Parentheses
Exponents
Multiplication
Division
Addition
Subtraction

MAKE IT SIMPLE

To remember the order of operations, use the phrase, "Please excuse my dear Aunt Sally," or the initials PEMDAS.

To convert fractions to decimals, divide the numerator by the denominator.

EXAMPLES:

```
        0.25                 0.666...
1/4 = 4)1.00     2/3 = 3)2.0000    = 0.66 (line over 66)
        8                 1 8
        20                 20
        20                 18
         0                 20
```

$\frac{1}{4} = 1.00 \div 4 = 0.25$; $\frac{2}{3} = 2.0000 \div 3 = 0.666... = 0.\overline{66}$

{NOTE} *When the answer is a nonterminating repeating number, you may signify this with a line over the repeating numerals.*

To convert decimals to fractions, the decimal numeral expressed becomes the numerator and the decimal place (tenth, hundredths) becomes the denominator.

EXAMPLES:

.95 — 95 is the decimal expressed and becomes the numerator. 1/100 or hundredths is the decimal place expressed and becomes the denominator

thus, $.95 = \frac{95}{100}$

.05 — 05 is the decimal expressed and becomes the numerator. 1/100 or hundredths is the decimal place expressed and becomes the denominator

thus, $.05 = \frac{5}{100} = \frac{1}{20}$ (always reduce to lowest terms)

{NOTE} *To round to the nearest tenth, carry the division out to the next decimal value after tenths, which is hundredths. If this number is 5 or greater, round the number in tenths up. If this number is less than 5, the number in tenths place remains the same.*

To compare the values of two or more decimals to determine which is larger (or smaller), place the decimals in a column and align the decimal points. Fill in with zeros to the *right* of the decimal point so all decimals have the same number of digits. The larger decimal will have the largest digit in the greatest column (the decimal place farthest left).

EXAMPLES:

Compare 0.000350 and 0.000082.
0.000350
0.000082

Align them with equal numbers of digits. As the 3 is in the ten-thousandths place and the 8 is in the hundredth-thousandths place, the 3 is larger. Thus, 0.000350 is the larger decimal.

Compare 0.012 and 0.0045.
0.0120
0.0045

Align them with equal numbers of digits. As the 1 is in the hundredths place and the 4 is in the thousandths place, the 1 is larger. Thus, 0.012 is the larger decimal.

PERCENTAGES

Percentages are special types of fractions that mean "per every hundred." Thus the denominator of a percent is always understood to be 100 and is shown by the symbol % rather than being written.

A percent can be written as a fraction by putting the number expressed as the numerator and the denominator as 100. It can be written as a decimal by putting down the number expressed and moving the decimal point two places to the left, thus signifying hundredths.

MAKE IT SIMPLE

It is easier to calculate percentages if they are first converted to fractions or decimals.

EXAMPLES:

$25\% = \frac{25}{100}$ or $\frac{1}{4}$

$25\% = .25$

$56\% = \frac{56}{100} = \frac{14}{25}$

$56\% = .56$

In other words, when you drop the % sign, either replace it with a denominator of 100 or a decimal place of hundredths. When you add the % sign, either drop the denominator of 100 or move the decimal point two places to the right.

EXAMPLE:

$.33 = 33\%$
$.33 = 33/100$
$.17 = 17\%$
$.17 = 17/100$

To find the percent of a number, change the percent to a decimal or fraction, replace the "of" with the times (×) sign, and multiply.

EXAMPLES:

10% of $100 =$
$.10 \times 100 = 10$

or .10 can be expressed as 10/100, which is reduced to $1/10 \times 100 = 10$

50% of $10 =$
$.50 \times 10 = 5$

or .50 can be expressed as 50/100, which is reduced to $1/2 \times 10 = 5$

Try these:

9 is what percent of 27?

$\frac{9}{27} = \frac{1}{3} = .333$ or 33.3%

5 is what percent of 25?

$\frac{5}{25} = \frac{1}{5} = .20 = 20\%$

Table 3-3 lists common fractions, decimals, and percentages.

RATIO AND PROPORTION

A **ratio** is a comparison of two numbers, a and b, expressed as:

$$a : b \text{ or } a/b \text{ or } \frac{a}{b}$$

EXAMPLES:

A two-to-one ratio is expressed as:

$$2 : 1 \text{ or } 2/1 \text{ or } \frac{2}{1}$$

A one-to-one thousand ratio is expressed as:

$$1 : 1000 \text{ or } 1/1000 \text{ or } \frac{1}{1000}$$

A **proportion** is a statement of equality between ratios: *a/b = c/d or a:b = c:d* See Insight 3-1 for more

Table 3-3 COMMON FRACTIONS, DECIMALS, AND PERCENTAGES

Fraction	Decimal	Percentage
$\frac{1}{2}$	0.5	50%
$\frac{1}{4}$	0.25	25%
$\frac{3}{4}$	0.75	75%
$\frac{1}{3}$	0.333*	$33\frac{1}{3}$%
$\frac{2}{3}$	0.666*	$66\frac{2}{3}$%
$\frac{1}{5}$	0.2	20%
$\frac{2}{5}$	0.4	40%
$\frac{3}{5}$	0.6	60%
$\frac{4}{5}$	0.8	80%
$\frac{1}{10}$	0.1	10%
$\frac{1}{1}$	1.0	100%

**0.333 and 0.666 are nonterminating decimals. This means the number patterns 0.333... and 0.666... go on forever.*

on ratios. In any proportion, the product of the means must equal the product of the extremes:

$$a \times d = b \times c$$

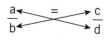

$\frac{a}{b} = \frac{c}{d}$ where a and d are the extremes and b and c are the means

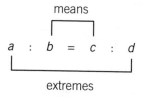

or

$a : b = c : d$ (means: b and c; extremes: a and d)

EXAMPLES:

$2 : 1 = 8 : 4$ (means: 1 and 8; extremes: 2 and 4)

means $1 \times 8 = 8$
extremes $2 \times 4 = 8$

$\frac{2}{1} = \frac{8}{4}$

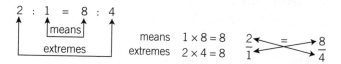

Proportions can be used to solve for an unknown term when the other three terms are known. This can be done in 4 steps:

Step 1: Let x be the unknown.

Step 2: Set up the proportion with the terms that are given (known).

Step 3: Multiply the means and the extremes.

Step 4: Solve for x.

EXAMPLES:

Given 2:3 = x : 9, what is x?

$\frac{2}{3} = \frac{x}{9}$	Let x be the unknown, set up the proportion
$3x = 2 \times 9$	Multiply the means and the extremes
$3x = 18$	
$x = 18/3$	Divide both sides of the proportion by the same number (3) in order to have x alone on one side
$x = 6$	Answer

Given 4:16 = 1 : x

$\frac{4}{16} = \frac{1}{x}$	Let x be the unknown, set up the proportion
$1 \times 16 = 4x$	Multiply the means and the extremes
$16 = 4x$	Divide both sides of the proportion by the same number (4) in order to have x alone on one side
$4 = x$	Answer

You can use ratios and proportions to calculate the quantities of medications. To do this, you must know that strength is a ratio—it is always expressed as units of substance per unit or units of volume—for example, the strength of meperidine (Demerol) may be 100 mg (milligrams) of meperidine per 1 mL (milliliter) of solution.

IN SIGHT 3-1 Ratios Used in Surgery

You will see a ratio expressed on a split thickness skin graft procedure with the skin graft mesher. The mesher uses plates or special rollers to cut "slits" into the donor skin graft. This meshing allows the graft to be enlarged when it is stretched. The graft can then cover a greater area of the recipient site and epithelial tissue will grow in between the slits. Meshers are available in a variety of expansion ratios such as 1:2, 1:3, and even 1:9.

And sometimes we express strength per hundred units of another substance. For example a 5% saline solution is 5 grams of sodium chloride (NaCl) per 100 grams of water.

{NOTE} *1 cubic centimeter (cc) of water weighs 1 gram, so a 5% solution of saline is also 5 grams per cubic centimeter (g/cc).*

EXAMPLE:

The doctor prescribed 50 milligrams of Demerol. The Demerol solution that the anesthesia provider has is a strength of 100 milligrams per milliliter (mg/mL). How many milliliters of that solution are needed?

This relationship can be expressed in the proportion 100 : 1 = 50 : x, or

$\frac{100 \text{ milligrams}}{1 \text{ milliliter}} = \frac{50 \text{ milligrams}}{x \text{ milliliters}}$	x is the unknown amount of solution needed, set up the proportion
$100 \times x = 50 \times 1$	Multiply the means and the extremes
$100x = 50$	Solve for x by dividing both sides of the proportion by 100 so x stands alone on one side
$x = 50/100$ or $\frac{1}{2}$ milliliter	Answer

You can also use proportions to solve other calculation problems. For example, the doctor will be giving the patient medications that are prescribed according to weight in kilograms (kg). You know the patient weighs 150 pounds (lbs), but how many kilograms is this?

First you must know three parts of the proportion, so you research and find that 1 kilogram is equal to 2.2 pounds.

This relationship can be expressed in the proportion 1: 2.2 = x : 150

$\frac{1 \text{ kg}}{2.2 \text{ lbs}} = \frac{x \text{ kg}}{150 \text{ lbs}}$	x is the unknown, and set up the proportion
$1 \times 150 = x \times 2.2$	Multiply the means and the extremes
$150 = 2.2x$	Divide both sides of the proportion by 2.2 to leave x alone on one side
$x = 68.18$ kg	Answer

Sometimes we can think of ratios in terms of parts of a whole. In this case, it is easy to think about percentages.

EXAMPLE:

You want to make up a 3 : 3 : 4 solution of saline, Lincocin, and Garamycin. (a) what percentage of the solution does each ingredient represent? (b) If you wanted to make up 200 milliliters of this solution, how many milliliters of saline would you use? Of Lincocin? Of Garamycin?

(a) A 3 : 3 : 4 solution means that there are three parts to three parts to four parts. That is, you need a total of 3 + 3 + 4 = 10 parts of whole solution

By convention, the parts are listed in the same order as the ingredients, so you have:

3 parts of saline in 10 parts of solution = 3/10 = 30/100 = 30%

3 parts of Lincocin in 10 parts of solution = 3/10 = 30/100 = 30%

4 parts of Garamycin in 10 parts of solution = 4/10 = 40/100 = 40%

Total parts of solution 100%

(b) You want 200 milliliters of solution, so you multiply each ingredients percentage by 200:

Saline (30%) .30 × 200 milliliters = 60 milliliters

Lincocin (30%) .30 × 200 milliliters = 60 milliliters

Garamycin (40%) .40 × 200 milliliters = 80 milliliters

Total 200 milliliters

You want to make up a 1 : 1 : 3 solution of saline, antibiotic a, and antibiotic b respectively. What percentage of the solution does each ingredient represent?

1 : 1 : 3 solution means one part to two parts to three parts. That is:

1 + 1 + 3 = 5 total parts in the solution

The parts are listed in the same order as the ingredients, so you have:

1 part of saline in 5 parts of solution = 1/5 = 20/100 = 20%

1 part of antibiotic a in 5 parts of solution = 1/5 = 20/100 = 20%

3 parts of antibiotic b in 5 parts of solution = 3/5 = 60/100 = 60%

Total parts of solution 100%

Another way to use proportions for calculations is to use the standard dilution equation. This is expressed as

$$\frac{C_1}{C_2} = \frac{V_2}{V_1} \text{ or } C_1 \times V_1 = C_2 \times V_2$$

where C stands for concentration in percent and V stands for volume. Thus,

C_1 = concentration 1

C_2 = concentration 2

V_1 = volume 1

V_2 = volume 2

EXAMPLE:

The procedure calls for 60 cubic centimeters (cc) of 1/2% contrast media. How much saline and how much contrast media do you need to make the required about of solution when you have 1%.

In this problem, you are being asked for a dilution, so you start by sorting out what you know from what you do not know:

$C_1 = \frac{1}{2}$ or .5% asked for contrast media
$C_2 = 1\%$ have on hand contrast media
$V_1 = 60$ asked for volume
$V_2 = x$ unknown volume of saline (solve this unknown first)

Now you can write the standard dilution equation as:

$$C_1 \times V_1 = C_2 \times V_2$$
$$\frac{1}{2} \times 60 = 1 \times x$$
$$30 = x$$
$$x = 30 \text{ cc of saline are needed}$$

But we are not finished with the problem. It also asks how much of the 1% contrast media we need also. If you add 30 cc of saline and the total amount you want is 60 cc, that means that 60 cc − 30 cc = 30 cc of the 1% contrast media is added.

TEMPERATURE CONVERSIONS

In medicine we use two scales to measure temperature (Fig. 3-4): the **Fahrenheit scale** and the **Celsius** (centigrade) **scale.** In the Fahrenheit scale, the boiling point of water is 212° F and its freezing point is 32° F. In the Celsius scale, the boiling point of water at 100° C and its freezing point is 0° C. Nine degrees on the Fahrenheit scale corresponds to 5 degrees on the Celsius scale. Using these ratios, the following formulas (Table 3-4) were developed to convert temperatures from one scale to the other.

$$C = 5/9(F - 32)$$
$$F = (9/5C) + 32$$

where *C* is the Celsius temperature and *F* is the Fahrenheit temperature.

Temperature is important in many aspects of the surgical setting, and readings may be given in Fahrenheit or Celsius degrees. The surgical patient's body temperature is of vital importance and is constantly monitored. Normal body temperature is 98.6° F or 37° C. Preoperatively, an elevated temperature could signify an infection or other health problem. This could result in the postponement of the surgical procedure. Intraoperatively, the body temperature is monitored by anesthesia personnel. An abnormal body temperature—whether below normal (*hypothermia*) or elevated (*hyperthermia*)—alters the basal metabolic rate, interfering with blood pressure, heart rate, circulation, and so on. Hyperthermia can also indicate life-threatening situations such as malignant hyperthermia (see Chapter 16). Postoperatively, temperature is monitored for the same reasons, and an elevated temperature at this time may indicate a wound

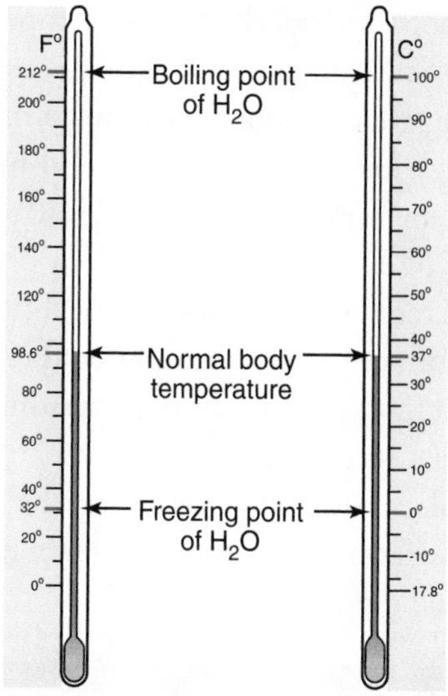

Figure 3-4 Fahrenheit and Celsius scales

Table 3-4 TEMPERATURE CONVERSIONS

To Convert From	Use the Formula	The Operation Means
Fahrenheit to Celsius	$C = \frac{5}{9}(F - 32)$	**1.** Subtract 32 from the Fahrenheit temperature. **2.** Multiply this number by 5/9.
Celsius to Fahrenheit	$F = \frac{9}{5}C + 32$	**1.** Multiply the Celsius temperature by 9/5. **2.** Add 32 to the result.

infection. Another surgical aspect of temperature is the sterilization of instruments and equipment. Here, temperature along with pressure and time is monitored for proper sterilization. Temperature is also important for the surgical environment. Each surgical room is kept at 68° F to 75° F (20° C to 24° C) to discourage the growth of bacteria that can cause surgical site infections. It is also important to keep the room at this temperature range for the comfort of surgical personnel who are working under surgical lights attired in full scrub apparel. A cool environment decreases the chance that perspiration will drip from a surgical team member onto the sterile field.

MAKE IT SIMPLE

Temperature of	F	C
Boiling water	212°	100°
Normal body temperature	98.6°	37°
Freezing point of water	32°	0°

MEASUREMENT SYSTEMS

While the surgical technologist does not administer medications directly to the patient, the technologist is responsible for obtaining medicines and mixing them for use in the sterile field. You may, for example, have to mix antibiotics in an irrigation solution. This may require you to calculate measurements, and perform some conversions. Therefore, you'll need to know conversion equivalents and be able to perform the calculations involved in such conversions.

The metric system of measurement is the most commonly used in medicine. However, there are other systems with which the surgical technologist should be familiar. They include the apothecary and household systems and measurements of some medications that are based upon their strengths.

THE METRIC SYSTEM

The **metric system** (also called the International System) is the *international standard* of weights and measures used by scientists and engineers everywhere. Developed by the French in the eighteenth century, today it is the preferred system for prescribing and administering medications. It is also utilized extensively in the health care field. The *United States Pharmacopeia,* for example, uses it exclusively and all specimens sent to pathology are weighed and measured in metric terms. The metric system allows a way to calculate small drug dosages, and most manufacturers use this system for calibration in the development of new drugs. Most medications used in surgery are dispensed utilizing the metric system of measurement.

In the metric system, length, volume, and weight (mass) are measured against certain defined units called *base units:*

Length—the *meter* (m)
Volume—the *liter* (L)
Weight—the *gram* (g)

Each of these base units is divided into smaller and larger units based on multiples of 10, and these multiples are indicated by prefixes (Table 3-5).

Any prefix can be used with any base unit to indicate a measurement. For example, 1 **m**m = .001 m, 1 **m**L = .001 L, and 1 **m**g = .001 g; similarly, 1 **k**m = 1000 m, 1 **k**L = 1000 L, and 1 **k**g = 1000 g. But you'll be most concerned with just a few of them—particularly, micro, milli, and centi.

Because the metric system is based on the decimal system, conversions are very easy. You just have to recognize the correct multiple of 10. Then you can use the appropriate unit conversion (Table 3-6).

Metric Comparisons

The meter is about 39.37 inches, just over a yard (36 inches). It's a linear measure used for lengths, including heights and widths. For example, patient height is measured in meters, while tumors, flaps, and defects are measured as lengths and widths—usually in

Table 3-5 METRIC PREFIXES

Prefix (Abbreviation)	Multiply Base Unit by
micro (μ)	.000001 (or 1/1,000,000)
milli (m)	.001 (or 1/1000)
centi (c)	.01 (or 1/100)
deci (d)	.1 (or 1/10)
Unit	Meter, liter, gram
deka (da)	10
hecto (h)	100
kilo (k)	1000

Table 3-6 UNIT CONVERSIONS

	Unit Conversion		
Length			
1 meter = 1000 millimeters	1 m/1000 mm = 1	or	1000 mm/1 m = 1
1 meter = 100 centimeters	1 m/100 cm = 1	or	100 cm/1 m = 1
1 meter = 1,000,000 micrometers (microns)	1 m/1,000,000 µm = 1	or	1,000,000 µg/1 m = 1
1 millimeter = 1000 micrometers (microns)	1 mm/1000 µm = 1	or	1000 µg/1 mm = 1
Volume			
1 liter = 1000 milliliters	1 L/1000 mL = 1	or	1000 mL/1 L = 1
1 kiloliter = 1000 liters	1 kL/1000 L = 1	or	1000 L/1 kL = 1
Weight (mass)			
1 gram = 1000 milligrams	1 g/1000 mg = 1	or	1000 mg/1 g = 1
1 gram = 1,000,000 micrograms	1 g/1,000,000 µg = 1	or	1,000,000 µg/1 g = 1
1 milligram = 1000 micrograms	1 mg/1000 µg = 1	or	1000 µg/1 mg = 1
1 kilogram = 1000 grams	1 kg/1000 g = 1	or	1000 g/ 1 kg = 1

centimeters or millimeters (hundredths or thousandths of meters). Note that when a length measure is multiplied by another length measure, the result is an area, which is a *square measure.* For instance, a defect that is 10 cm by 5 cm has an area of $5 \times 10 = 50\ cm^2$.

The meter is related to volume by *cubic measure.* When 1 centimeter is multiplied by itself three times—1 cm × 1 cm × 1 cm—it becomes the volume 1 cubic centimeter (1 cm^3), which is about the same size as a sugar cube. When length, width, and height (or depth) are multiplied together, the result is measured in cubic terms. Thus, a block of tissue that is 5 cm long, 3 cm wide, and 1 cm deep is $5 \times 3 \times 1 = 15\ cm^3$.

The liter is a fluid (or liquid) measure approximately equal to a quart (1 L = 1.06 qt). Most medicines in surgery are in liquid form, including intravenous and irrigation solutions (often measured in liters) as well as many antibiotic solutions (usually measured in milliliters or thousandths of liters). In medicine, however, we call a cm^3 a "cc" (short for cubic centimeter, of course). This liquid measure of volume is related to the solid measure by one simple definition: 1 cc = 1 cm^3 = 1 mL. You'll see and hear these terms used interchangeably. However, the abbreviation "mL" is used more often than "cc" because "cc" can be confused with other abbreviations such as "u" or "00."

The gram is a small unit of mass (or weight), which is much less than an ounce (30 g is about 1 oz). For a mental picture, consider a paper clip; it weighs about a gram. In this case it's easier to think in terms of kilograms. One kilogram is 2.2 pounds (picture a 2-lb can of coffee). It's worth knowing that 1 cc (1 mL) of water weighs 1 gram, which means that aqueous solutions measured in weight percent (g/100 g) can also be reckoned in grams per milliliter of solution. You'll encounter gram or milligram measures when working with drugs in powder form, such as antibiotics that must be reconstituted (dissolved) in water.

{NOTE} *You will use kilogram measures when calculating dosages determined by body weight. It is important to be able to convert a patient's weight from pounds (lbs) to kilograms (kg). There are 2.2 pounds in 1 kilogram, so to convert pounds to kilograms, divide the weight by 2.2.*

TECH TIP

One way to remember your pounds to kilograms conversion is to note you will weigh a lot less in the metric system. For example a patient who weighs 143 pounds only weighs 65 kilograms. So if your conversion comes out with the kilogram weight more than the pound weight, you know it is incorrect and you might have your conversion reversed.

The metric system is, by far, the most important measuring system in the world—and the most important to you. It lets you measure—and calculate with—small and large quantities of any kind without having to multiply by such ill-behaved conversion factors as 12 inches per foot, 2 pints in a quart (and 4 quarts in a gallon), and 16 ounces per pound. All you have to do is multiply and divide by 10, which is mostly a matter of moving the decimal point the correct number of places in the proper direction. Eventually, you'll find yourself thinking in it. But if you aren't already used to it, you'll find it helpful to compare metric measures with common measures. If, for example, you already know how long an inch is, you can easily picture that length as about 2.5 cm. Box 3-1 lists some of the more common equivalents, giving approximate conversions.

MAKE IT SIMPLE

One cubic centimeter (cc) is the amount of space occupied by one milliliter (mL) of liquid. Thus, 1 cc = 1 mL (Fig. 3-5).

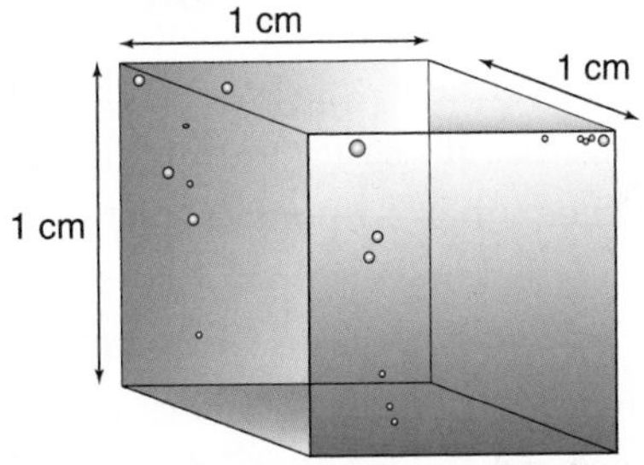

Figure 3-5 A cubic centimeter filled with water (1 cc = 1 mL here).

The apothecary and the household systems were used more in the past. It is not necessary to learn conversions from these measurement systems because medications are prepared and administered primarily from the metric system. These systems can be used for comparisons as they are more familiar until you are proficient with the metric system (Insight 3-2).

Figure 3-6 shows measuring equipment used in surgery.

OTHER STANDARDIZED MEASUREMENTS (DOSES)

Some medications are measured directly by their strengths—that is, they are measured in *units* (u) based upon their potency. A common medication measured in units is insulin. There are special insulin syringes calibrated to these units. In surgery, several antibiotics, including penicillin and bacitracin, are also measured in units. These medications are used in antibiotic irrigation solutions during surgical procedures (see Chapter 5). Other medications measured in units are those that affect coagulation. One is heparin, an anticoagulant administered intravenously to the patient by anesthesia personnel during vascular cases. Heparin is also used diluted in saline on the back table. Another is topical thrombin, a hemostatic agent, which comes in different strengths and preparations and is used to stop bleeding (see Chapter 9).

Other measurements used to indicate quantity of medicine prescribed are the international unit (IU) and the milliunit (mU). The international unit is used to measure vitamins and chemicals. The milliunit, which is one-thousandths (.001 or 1/1000) of a unit, is used for dosages of oxytocin (Pitocin). Pitocin is used in childbirth to stimulate the uterus to contract (see Chapter 8). Another measurement of medications according to their strength is the *milliequivalent* (mEq.) A milliequivalent is equal to 1/1000 (0.001) of a chemical equivalent, a measurement associated with electrolytes. Concentrations of electrolytes are often expressed as milliequivalents per liter. Electrolytes are

Box 3-1 APPROXIMATE MEASUREMENT EQUIVALENTS

Weight

1 kilogram = 2.2 pounds
1 gram = 15 grains
1 ounce = 30 grams
1 grain = 60 milligrams

Volume

1 kiloliter = exactly 1000 liters
1 liter = approximately 1 quart
1 milliliter = 1 gram = 1 minim = 1 cubic centimeter
1 fluid ounce = 8 fluid drams = 30 milliliters
1 gallon = approximately 4 liters
1 pint = approximately 500 milliliters
1 quart = 2 pints = approximately 1000 milliliters
1 gallon = 4 quarts = approximately 4000 milliliters
1 teaspoon = 60 drops
1 minim = 1 drop

Length

1 meter = 39.37 inches = approximately 1 yard
1 yard = 3 feet = 36 inches
1 inch = 2.54 centimeters

IN SIGHT 3-2 The Apothecary and Household Systems of Weights and Measures

The apothecary system was the system of weights and measures used for writing medication orders in ancient Greece and Rome, and in Europe during the Middle Ages. It is rarely used today. The apothecary system is based upon everyday items (such as the weight of a grain of wheat) and uses lowercase Roman numerals. For example, 4 grains would be written as gr. $\dot{\overline{\text{IV}}}$. Some medications continue to use this system, as do pharmacists, so the basic units of measure of the apothecary system are given:

Volume—the *minim* (fluid)

Weight—the *grain*

A minim is approximately equal to one drop. (As drops vary according to the dropper used, this measurement is not always accurate. For accuracy, a calibrated dropper should be used.) Larger quantities are multiples of the minim:

60 minims = 1 fluid dram
8 fluid drams = 1 fluid ounce
1 pint = 16 fluid ounces
2 pints = 1 quart
4 quarts = 1 gallon

The grain was based upon the average weight of a grain of wheat. Larger quantities are multiples of the grain:

20 grains (xx) = 1 scruple
3 scruples = 1 dram
60 grains = 1 dram
12 ounces = 1 pound
8 drams = 1 ounce

Note that in the apothecary system, 12 ounces equals 1 pound rather than 16 ounces (as in avoirdupois weight).

Although household measurements are used primarily for administering over-the-counter (OTC) medications—and never in surgery—it's useful to see how they compare with more accurate standard measures:

1 teaspoon = 5 milliliters = 5 cubic centimeters = 1 fluid dram
1 tablespoon = 1/2 fluid ounce = 4 fluid drams = 15 milliliters = 15 cubic centimeters
2 tablespoons = 1 fluid ounce = 30 milliliters = 30 cubic centimeters

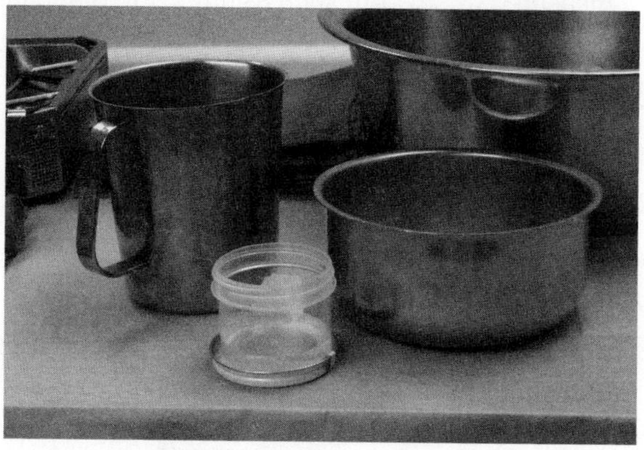

Figure 3-6 Measuring equipment in surgery.

essential for metabolic activities in the body and for normal function of body cells. A common electrolyte administered to the surgical patient is potassium chloride (KCl), which is necessary for the transmission of nerve impulses, control of heart rhythm, and fluid balance. Low potassium levels can pose a risk to the surgical patient undergoing general anesthesia. Potassium chloride is administered in milliequivalents preoperatively or by anesthesia personnel. See Table 3-7 for symbols of measurement.

Table 3-7 SYMBOLS OF MEASUREMENT

Metric System	
Meter	m
Liter	L
Cubic centimeter	cc
Millimeter	mm
Gram	g
Kilogram	kg
Milligram	mg
Milliliter	mL
Kiloliter	kL
Microgram	mcg, µg
Micron (micrometer)	µg
Unit	U
International unit	IU

Table 3-7 SYMBOLS OF MEASUREMENT—CONT'D

Milliunit	mU
Milliequivalent	mEq
Apothecary System	
Minim	m, min, ♏
Grain	gr
Dram	dr, ʒ
Fluid dram	fl dr, fʒ
Drop	gtt
Ounce	oz
Pint	pt
Quart	qt
Gallon	gal
Pound	lb
Scruple	scr, ℈
Household System	
Teaspoon	tsp
Tablespoon	tbsp
Ounce	oz
Pint	pt
Quart	qt
Gallon	gal
Inch	in
Yard	yd

Note: As discussed in Chapter 2, some symbols are not being used with medication orders in an effort to decrease medication errors. However, the surgical technologist should be familiar with symbols as hospital policies on their use vary.

KEY CONCEPTS

- Military time is used by hospitals and other medical institutions, and it uses a 24-hour scale without a.m. or p.m. designations.
- Surgical technologists may use fractions, decimals, and percentages, together with ratios and proportions, to solve problems and perform calculations and conversions.
- A fraction is a number that represents one or more equal parts of a whole and can be written as a quotient a/b.
- Fractions may be proper, improper, or expressed as mixed numbers.
- Decimals are numbers written by placing digits into value columns that are separated by a decimal point.
- Exponents are short cuts to showing multiplication of a number times itself.
- Percentages are special types of fractions that mean "per every hundred" and are shown by the symbol %.
- A ratio is a comparison of two numbers expressed as a:b, a/b, or $\frac{a}{b}$
- A proportion is a statement of equality between ratios expressed as a:b=c:d or a/b = c/d
- Two temperature scales are used in medicine, the Fahrenheit and the Celsius.
- Conversion from one temperature scale to the other can be accomplished by using one of the following formulas: $C = 5/9(F-32)$, or $F = 9/5C + 32$.
- The metric system is the international standard of weights and measures.
- In the metric system the base units are represented by length—meter, volume—liter, weight—gram.
- Other measurements include medications measured by strength such as units, international unit, milliunit, and milliequivalent.

Bibliography

Chernecky B, Graham I: *Drug calculations and drug administration*, Philadelphia, 2002, Saunders.

Olsen JL, Giangrasso AP, Shrimpton D, et al: *Medical dosage calculations*, ed 9, New Jersey, 2008, Pearson Prentice Hall.

Pickar GD, Abernethy AP: *Dosage calculations*, ed 8, New York, 2008, Thompson Delmar.

Snyder KC, Keegan C: *Pharmacology for the surgical technologist*, ed 2, St. Louis, 2006, Saunders/Elsevier.

Internet Resources

AAA Math: www.aaamath.com/meats2m.htm.

About.com, US Military, The Orderly Room: http://usmilitary.about.com/od/theorderlyroom/The_Orderly_Room.htm.

Space Archive, Military Time: www.spacearchive.info/military.htm.

LEARNING THE LANGUAGE (KEY TERMS)

Using your textbook and/or a medical dictionary, look up and write the definitions of each term.

Celsius scale
civilian time
decimal point
exponent
Fahrenheit scale
fraction
metric system
military time
percentage
proportion
ratio
relative value

MATH EVALUATION PRETEST

The following test includes the various mathematical skills explained in this chapter. Take the test and compare your answers with those given at the end. If you have difficulty with some of the questions, review that section in the chapter to improve your skills.

1. Write 5:10 am in military time. ____________________
2. Write 0010 in civilian time. ____________________
3. Write 1/10,000 as a decimal. ____________________
4. Write 3 5/8 as an improper fraction. ____________________
5. Write 50% as a fraction in lowest terms. ____________________
6. Write 35% as a decimal number. ____________________
7. Which decimal number is smaller, 0.151 or 0.251? __________
8. Write 7/10 ÷ 3/10 as a mixed number. ____________________
9. Write 5 3/4 ÷ 23 as a fraction and as a decimal. __________
10. Round 7.2235 to the nearest hundredth. ____________________
11. Write 3/8 as a decimal number. ____________________
12. Write an equivalent fraction for 5/9. ____________________
13. 2 3/4 + 3 1/8 = ____________________
14. 32 ÷ 0.5 = ____________________
15. 8.25 × 0.022 = ____________________
16. 0.655 − 0.011 = ____________________
17. Write 0.77 as a percent. ____________________
18. 2:3 = 10:x, x = ____________________
19. Write 96° F in Celsius. ____________________
20. Write 41° C in Fahrenheit. ____________________

REVIEW QUESTIONS

1. Explain the difference in calculating military and civilian times.
2. In the fraction 7/8:
  a) Which number represents the numerator?
  b) Which number represents the denominator?
  c) What type of fraction is this?
3. In the fractions 7/8 and 1/6, what is the least common denominator?
4. What is meant by "the order of operations?"
5. What is the place value of 3 in the number 22.0453?

Answers to Math Evaluation Pretest:
1) 0510, **2)** 12:10 am, **3)** 0.0001, **4)** 29/8, **5)** ½, **6)** 0.35, **7)** 0.151, **8)** 2 ⅓, **9)** 1/4, 0.25, **10)** 7.22, **11)** 0.375, **12)** 10/18, **13)** 5 ⅞, **14)** 64, **15)** 0.1815, **16)** 0.644, **17)** 77%, **18)** 15, **19)** 35.6, **20)** 105.8

6. What is the value of 5?
7. Complete the following sentences:
   a) The rule for division of fractions states "the number you are dividing by ________"
   b) Percentages are fractions that mean "per every ______"
   c) In a proportion, "the product of the means equals ______________"
8. Explain why the metric system is the preferred measurement system.

CRITICAL THINKING

1. Why is military time "safer" to use in the medical setting?
2. Dr. Kim is giving his patient propofol (Diprivan). The dosage is 2 mg per kilogram of patient's weight. The patient weighs 176 pounds. How much of the medication is given?
3. The procedure calls for 50 cc of 1% contrast media. You have 25 cc of 2% contrast media. How much saline and how much of the 2% solution are mixed for the proper amount and strength of the required contrast media?
4. The patient's body temperature is 39° C. What is this in Fahrenheit degrees? Will the patient's elective surgical procedure be performed? Why or why not?

CHAPTER 4 Medication Administration

OBJECTIVES *After completing this chapter, you should be able to:*

1. Describe the role of the surgical technologist in medication administration.
2. Explain the five "rights" of medication administration.
3. Describe the steps of medication identification.
4. Discuss aseptic techniques for delivery of medications to the sterile field.
5. State the procedure for labeling drugs on the sterile back table.
6. Identify supplies used in medication administration in surgery.

KEY TERMS

carpule
diluent
reconstitute

The role of the surgical technologist in medication administration varies from state to state and differs from facility to facility. As a surgical technologist, you should have firsthand knowledge of medication administration legislation in your state.

TECH TIP

Do not depend on hearsay or someone else's understanding or opinion regarding the limits of your practice. Use your computer competence and the easy availability of the Internet to read the pertinent legislative statutes for yourself. Ask for assistance at your facility's medical library or from the reference librarian at any public library. Remember, professional surgical technologists should be highly knowledgeable regarding their own practice.

Institutional policies and procedures regarding medication handling and administration should be clearly understood as well. All staff members have a duty to know and adhere to established medication policies and procedures. Handling medications is a critical function in the surgical technologist's job description. Several different types of medications are obtained and passed to the surgeon routinely during a procedure, and the surgical technologist must be knowledgeable regarding such drugs.

{NOTE} *The limits of legal authority for the surgical technologist to perform the indicated roles described in this text are controlled by each state through its statutes, case law, regulatory law, attorney general opinions, and medical licensing boards. Discussion of these sources of law is beyond the scope of this text.*

Except as otherwise noted, this book describes the general practice of surgical technology in the United States, not the legal authority for such practice. It is the surgical technologist's responsibility to consult the limitations in his or her area on acts described in this book.

SURGICAL TECHNOLOGIST'S ROLES IN MEDICATION ADMINISTRATION

Administration of drugs from the sterile field is a team effort. Each team member has a particular role in the process (Box 4-1). Most commonly, medications used from the sterile field are obtained by the *circulator* (a non-sterile team member) and delivered to the *scrub person* (a sterile team member). The scrub person is responsible for passing the medication to the surgeon for administration during the surgical procedure. Each team member is responsible for accurately identifying all medications used from the sterile field during a surgical procedure.

CIRCULATING ROLE

The surgical technologist in the circulating role obtains medications as specified on the surgeon's preference card, delivers those medications to the sterile field as needed, and documents the medications used from the sterile field during an operation. The circulator must be sure that the medication obtained is the exact drug and strength specified on the preference card. The circulator must also inspect the container for integrity and expiration date. The circulator must maintain strict sterile technique when transferring medications to the scrub person. All medications must be properly identified, both by the scrub and by the circulator. The circulator is responsible for documenting all medications used from the sterile field according to institutional policy.

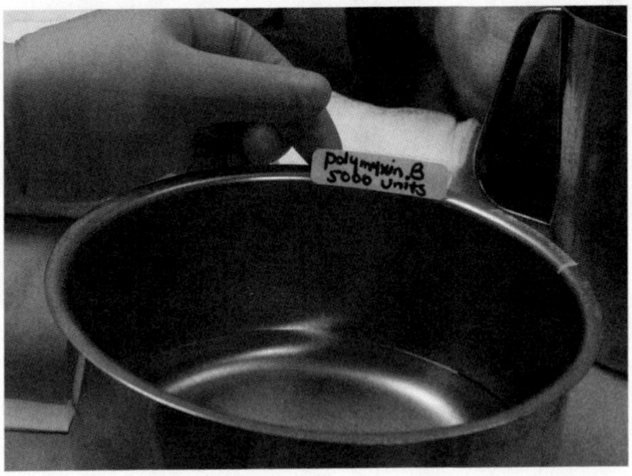

Figure 4-1 The scrubbed surgical technologist labels medications immediately.

SCRUB ROLE

The surgical technologist in the scrub role correctly identifies and accepts medications from the circulator, immediately labels (Fig. 4-1) those medications, and passes medications to the surgeon as requested. Accurate identification and immediate labeling of all drugs accepted onto the sterile field is crucial. If medications are not clearly identified, they should be discarded immediately and a new dose should be obtained. This practice is essential to avoid possible drug administration error. The surgical technologist must clearly state the name and strength of a medication when passing it to the surgeon.

THE FIVE "RIGHTS" OF MEDICATION ADMINISTRATION

To help prevent medication errors, the five "rights" of medication administration have been established (Box 4-2). Team members must work together to ensure that the right drug is given in the right dose, by the right route, to the right patient, and at the right time. It is also

BOX 4-1 THE SURGICAL TECHNOLOGIST'S ROLES IN MEDICATION ADMINISTRATION

Circulator Role	Scrubbed Surgical Technologist Role
Obtain correct medication.	Identify medication.
Deliver medication to the sterile field using aseptic technique.	Accept medication into the sterile field.
Document all medications used from sterile field.	Label the medication immediately.
	Pass the medication to the surgeon as requested.
	Say the drug name and strength aloud when passing.

BOX 4-2 FIVE "RIGHTS" OF MEDICATION ADMINISTRATION

- Right drug—**What** drug is required?
- Right dose—**How much** of the drug is required in **what concentration?**
- Right route—**How** will the drug be administered?
- Right patient—**Who** will receive the drug?
- Right time—**When** will the drug be administered?

important to ensure that all medications given are accurately documented.

RIGHT DRUG

Drugs that are routinely needed on the sterile field during a procedure should be clearly specified on the surgeon's preference card (Fig. 4-2). The information is initially obtained directly from the surgeon and entered on the preference card by a member of the surgery department staff (surgical technologists, registered nurses). The information stated on the preference card must be accurate, including correct spelling and strength. Handwritten preference cards must be written legibly to avoid confusion. Preference cards should be updated as needed to reflect any changes in routine medications. Additional drugs are obtained in response to verbal orders by the surgeon during the procedure.

When any medication is delivered to the sterile back table, it must be carefully identified by both the circulator and scrub, and labeled immediately and accurately by the scrubbed surgical technologist. All medication containers must be labeled including delivery container (such as a syringe) and intermediate containers (often a medicine cup or basin). Careful, mindful attention must be consistently practiced in the identification and labeling of drugs to prevent medication errors.

CAUTION

When accepting a medication, especially an antibiotic or an iodine-based contrast medium, the scrubbed surgical technologist should ask the circulator if the patient has any medication allergies. This team effort helps ensure that the patient does not get a medication to which he or she is allergic.

The scrub person must always state the name and strength of the drug aloud as he or she hands it to the surgeon; this practice serves as confirmation that the medication is correct. The name of the drug should be spoken aloud even though the syringe (or other delivery container) is labeled. Utilizing two processes, audible and visual, provides an additional level of patient safety. All empty medication vials and bottles should be kept in

Surgeon: Dr. Ferguson	**Procedure:** Excision skin lesions (local)
Glove size: $7\frac{1}{2}$ **Skin prep:** Betadine	**Position of patient:** According to lesions **Drapes:** Towels–drape sheets If face, split sheet and turban drape
Sutures and needles	**Instruments and equipment**
Ties: **Peritoneum:** **Fascia:** **Sub-cu:** 5-0 Dermalon P-3 > have in room **Skin:** 6-0 mild chromic SH-1 > do not open **Retention:** **Other:**	**Basic:** Small dissecting set **Special:** 4×8 Raytec sponges cautery pencil c̄ needle tip #11 knife blade 5cc syringe #18 g. and #25 g. needles $1\frac{1}{2}$"
Dressings: Steri-strips $\frac{1}{4}$"	**Local anesthetic:** 1% lidocaine c̄ epinephrine 1:100,000

Figure 4-2 A surgeon's preference card showing medication needed for procedure.

the room during the procedure as evidence that the proper medication has been delivered to the field.

RIGHT DOSE

The actual dose of a medication is a factor of both its amount (volume) and its strength (concentration). You might see, for instance, an order for 30 mL (amount) of 0.5% (strength) lidocaine with epinephrine 1:100,000 on a surgeon's preference card. This information must be clearly specified and clearly understood. It's especially important when the drug must be mixed or diluted on the sterile back table. Suppose, for example, a surgeon requests 0.5 mL of 1% phenylephrine (Neo-Synephrine) diluted in 20 mL of saline. Further suppose that 1% phenylephrine is available in 1 mL vials. If the entire 1 mL vial (instead of the 0.5 mL specified) is mixed with the correct amount (20 mL) of saline and dispensed to the sterile field, the dosage of phenylephrine administered will be *twice* the desired dose.

Written protocols may be instituted and posted to eliminate common confusions about some medications. Heparin (a systemic anticoagulant) is an excellent example of a medication that is available in a number of different strengths in the same volume (see Chapter 9). During insertion of a venous access port, different strengths of heparin may be needed from the sterile back table: 100 units per milliliter and 10 units per milliliter may be used, each concentration with a specific purpose. Given the 10-fold difference in heparin concentration, immediate labeling is crucial (Fig. 4-3). In addition, the scrubbed surgical technologist must understand the reasons or purposes for the various strengths of heparin required to know which concentration to hand at the appropriate time. In this case, a department routine or protocol for heparin dosages in venous access procedures may be established and posted to minimize the potential for error.

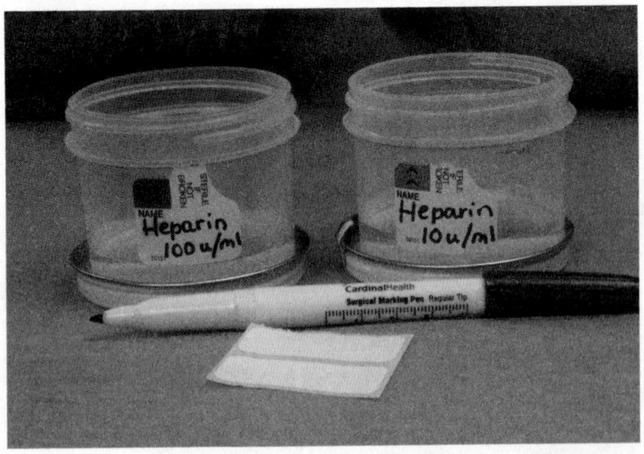

Figure 4-3 When different strengths of heparin are needed from the sterile back table, immediate and clear labeling is crucial.

The surgical technologist serves a key role in the prevention of administration of the wrong dosage of a medication from the sterile field. In addition to ensuring correct identification and labeling, the scrubbed surgical technologist provides the final safety check by stating out loud and clearly the name and strength of the medication as it is handed to the surgeon.

RIGHT ROUTE

Most medications administered in surgery are given intravenously, usually by the anesthesia provider. However, many other medications may be injected or applied topically by the surgeon at the surgical site. Different administration routes may require different preparations and concentrations of a medication. The preference card should clearly state administration route or form, so that the proper form of the drug for a particular route may be obtained. For example, the preference card for cystoscopy may state that 1% lidocaine jelly is needed for local anesthesia. Although the preference card should clearly state "for topical application," it may also be safely assumed that properly educated surgical team members know that jelly, a semisolid form of the drug, is intended for topical application, not injection. In a situation of a novice practitioner or a person with a knowledge deficit, careful reading of the medication label will reveal that this form of lidocaine is intended for topical use only. This situation also provides an excellent example of the importance of always reading the medication label carefully. When in doubt, always clarify the information stated on the preference card.

Another common example demonstrating the use of the right form of a drug for the right route is 1% lidocaine with epinephrine 1:100,000 for local anesthesia for procedures such as breast biopsy. Again, the administration route may not be stated clearly on the preference card, because the drug specified is formulated for injection. If for some unusual reason, a team member does not know that a local anesthetic agent is *injected* for breast biopsy, careful reading of the medication label will provide the necessary information.

RIGHT PATIENT

All surgical patients must be accurately identified before being transported into the operating room. Tools such as the Joint Commission's Universal Protocol and the

World Health Organization

SURGICAL SAFETY CHECKLIST (FIRST EDITION)

Before induction of anaesthesia ▸▸▸▸▸▸▸▸▸ Before skin incision ▸▸▸▸▸▸▸▸▸▸▸▸▸▸ Before patient leaves operating room

SIGN IN

- ☐ PATIENT HAS CONFIRMED
  - IDENTITY
  - SITE
  - PROCEDURE
  - CONSENT
- ☐ SITE MARKED/NOT APPLICABLE
- ☐ ANAESTHESIA SAFETY CHECK COMPLETED
- ☐ PULSE OXIMETER ON PATIENT AND FUNCTIONING

DOES PATIENT HAVE A:

KNOWN ALLERGY?
- ☐ NO
- ☐ YES

DIFFICULT AIRWAY/ASPIRATION RISK?
- ☐ NO
- ☐ YES, AND EQUIPMENT/ASSISTANCE AVAILABLE

RISK OF >500ML BLOOD LOSS (7ML/KG IN CHILDREN)?
- ☐ NO
- ☐ YES, AND ADEQUATE INTRAVENOUS ACCESS AND FLUIDS PLANNED

TIME OUT

- ☐ CONFIRM ALL TEAM MEMBERS HAVE INTRODUCED THEMSELVES BY NAME AND ROLE
- ☐ SURGEON, ANAESTHESIA PROFESSIONAL AND NURSE VERBALLY CONFIRM
  - PATIENT
  - SITE
  - PROCEDURE

ANTICIPATED CRITICAL EVENTS
- ☐ SURGEON REVIEWS: WHAT ARE THE CRITICAL OR UNEXPECTED STEPS, OPERATIVE DURATION, ANTICIPATED BLOOD LOSS?
- ☐ ANAESTHESIA TEAM REVIEWS: ARE THERE ANY PATIENT-SPECIFIC CONCERNS?
- ☐ NURSING TEAM REVIEWS: HAS STERILITY (INCLUDING INDICATOR RESULTS) BEEN CONFIRMED? ARE THERE EQUIPMENT ISSUES OR ANY CONCERNS?

HAS ANTIBIOTIC PROPHYLAXIS BEEN GIVEN WITHIN THE LAST 60 MINUTES?
- ☐ YES
- ☐ NOT APPLICABLE

IS ESSENTIAL IMAGING DISPLAYED?
- ☐ YES
- ☐ NOT APPLICABLE

SIGN OUT

NURSE VERBALLY CONFIRMS WITH THE TEAM:
- ☐ THE NAME OF THE PROCEDURE RECORDED
- ☐ THAT INSTRUMENT, SPONGE AND NEEDLE COUNTS ARE CORRECT (OR NOT APPLICABLE)
- ☐ HOW THE SPECIMEN IS LABELLED (INCLUDING PATIENT NAME)
- ☐ WHETHER THERE ARE ANY EQUIPMENT PROBLEMS TO BE ADDRESSED
- ☐ SURGEON, ANAESTHESIA PROFESSIONAL AND NURSE REVIEW THE KEY CONCERNS FOR RECOVERY AND MANAGEMENT OF THIS PATIENT

THIS CHECKLIST IS NOT INTENDED TO BE COMPREHENSIVE. ADDITIONS AND MODIFICATIONS TO FIT LOCAL PRACTICE ARE ENCOURAGED.

Figure 4-4 The World Health Organization's Surgical Safety Checklist. *(© WHO, 2010, available at www.who.int/patientsafety/safesurgery/tools_resources/SSSL_Checklist_finalJun08.pdf.)*

World Health Organization's Surgical Safety Checklist (Fig. 4-4) are used in the operating room to ensure that the correct surgical procedure will be performed on the correct patient. This process also includes relevant information about the patient such as a history of drug allergies or hypersensitivity to a particular drug. The surgical procedure and operating surgeon are verified, and the preference card containing medication orders for that specific procedure is kept available in the operating room for reference. In addition, a surgical safety "time out" is conducted just prior to the incision to further verify that the intended surgical procedure is being performed on the correct patient. Diligence and care taken to properly identify the patient will help ensure that the correct patient receives the medications intended for administration during a surgical procedure.

RIGHT TIME

In surgery, the surgeon (or as delegated to the surgical first assistant) administers all medications at the surgical site. This practice prevents the vast majority of medication *timing* errors during surgery (for drugs administered from the sterile back table). The purpose of the drug, when stated on the preference card, often indicates the timing of administration. If, for example, 1% lidocaine with epinephrine 1:100,000 is listed on the preference card for a local anesthetic, it will be administered prior to incision. In addition, it may be administered periodically throughout the procedure as needed (PRN) for patient comfort. If 0.5% bupivacaine with epinephrine 1:100,000 is listed on the preference card for postoperative pain control, it will usually be administered at the time of wound closure. Some routine medications (e.g., contrast media for cholangiography, antibiotics for irrigation, heparinized saline) are obtained and labeled during case setup and passed to the surgeon at the appropriate time. Other medications may be obtained, labeled, passed to the surgeon from the sterile back table, and administered by the surgeon as soon as requested.

RIGHT DOCUMENTATION

Traditionally, there are five "rights" of medication administration: right drug, right dose, right route, right patient, and right time. But, it is also crucial that medications given from the sterile table be accurately recorded in the operative record. The circulator will document all medications delivered to the field, and the scrubbed surgical technologist will verbally provide a final total of the amount of each medication administered for the circulator to note in the record. When a medication is repeatedly administered during a procedure, such as a local anesthetic, the scrubbed surgical technologist must also maintain an accurate ongoing total of the amount of medication being used throughout the procedure.

TECH TIP

Use a sterile marking pen on the field to keep a written tally of the amount of medications used during the procedure.

MEDICATION IDENTIFICATION

Both the scrub and the circulator are responsible for correctly identifying medications delivered to and used from the sterile field. This dual responsibility minimizes the potential for errors in medication administration, as does following a logical series of steps (Box 4-3) to properly identify drugs. The first step in medication identification is to carefully read the label on the medicine container (Fig. 4-5). The team member obtaining the drug reads the label initially and checks the container for cracks or discolored contents. If there is any doubt as to the integrity of the container, the medication should not be used. Rather, it should be returned to the pharmacy with a note indicating the specific concern. The medication label contains important information about the drug, as Table 4-1 shows. The most crucial information is the drug name (both generic and trade), the strength, the amount, and the expiration date. Special handling instructions (such as refrigeration, or keeping medication from direct light), the drug form and intended administration route are also key pieces of drug information contained on the label (for more detail see Chapter 2). The circulator reads vital

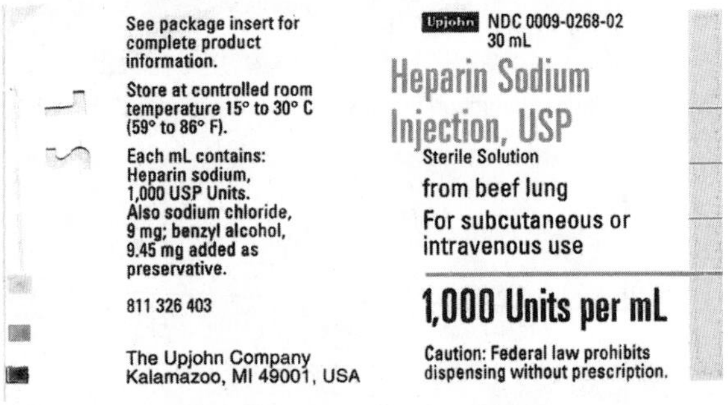

Figure 4-5 A label for heparin sodium. *(From Morris DG:* Calculate with confidence, *ed 3, St. Louis, 2002, Mosby.)*

BOX 4-3 STEPS FOR MEDICATION IDENTIFICATION

Circulator reads label.
Circulator reads label aloud to scrub.
Circulator shows label to scrub.
Scrub states medication information aloud.
Scrub accepts medication.
Scrub labels medication containers immediately.

Table 4-1 SAMPLE INFORMATION CONTAINED ON A MEDICATION LABEL

Type of Information	Example
Name (brand and generic)	Bupivacaine HCl (Sensorcaine)
Strength	0.5%
Amount	50 mL
Expiration date	01/2014
Administration route	Injection
Manufacturer	Astrazeneca
Storage directions	Store at room temperature
Warnings or precautions	Federal law prohibits dispensing without prescription
Lot number	1234567
Schedule	(C-I to C-V)*

**Only if drug is a controlled substance.*

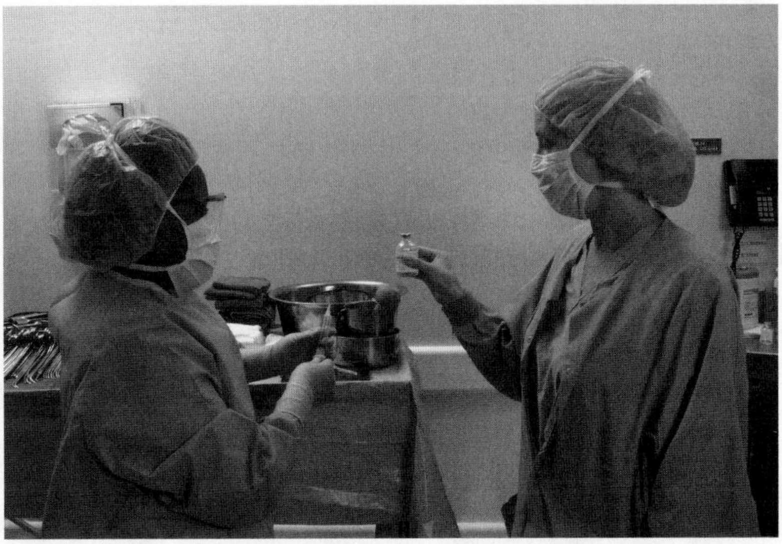

Figure 4-6 The circulator shows a drug label to the scrub.

label information aloud just prior to delivery to the sterile field, and shows the label to the scrub person (Fig. 4-6). Finally, the scrub repeats the label information aloud to confirm the correct drug. The drug should be delivered to the sterile field only after the steps described have been completed. Alternately, both scrub and circulator may read the information aloud together prior to delivery of the medication to the sterile field.

CAUTION

All medications delivered to the sterile field must be labeled immediately.

DELIVERY TO THE STERILE FIELD

Principles of asepsis (sterile technique) must be followed when delivering and receiving medications into the sterile field. Medications frequently used from the sterile back table are packaged in different types of containers including vials and ampules (Fig. 4-7) and aseptic delivery method varies by type of container. One of the most common containers is a glass or plastic vial with a rubber stopper encased in a metal cap. The metal cap is peeled away, so that the circulator can draw up the drug (if in liquid form) with a syringe and hypodermic needle and then empty the contents of the syringe into a sterile medicine cup held by the scrub (Fig. 4-8). The circulator should handle only the outside of the vial and should not touch the rubber stopper unless it is being removed.

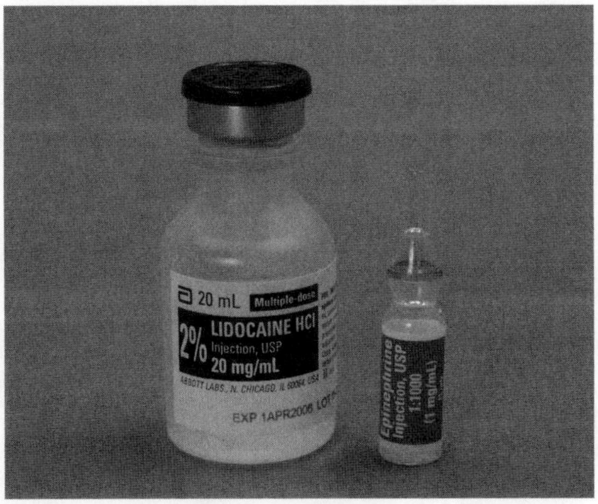

Figure 4-7 Medication vial and ampule.

Alternatively, the circulator may hold the vial in an inverted position while the scrub withdraws the drug from the vial with a syringe and needle (Fig. 4-9). The scrubbed surgical technologist should first draw some air into the syringe, then puncture the rubber stopper with the needle and inject air into the vial, which will allow the contents of the vial to enter the syringe rapidly. In addition, the hypodermic needle used to puncture the vial should be a larger needle, such as an 18-gauge, to permit rapid filling of the syringe. After the medication is in the syringe, the 18-gauge needle is removed and replaced with the correct gauge needle for injection (such as a 25-gauge).

If a drug is in powder form in a vial, the circulator must **reconstitute** it, that is, mix it with an appropriate liquid, such as saline (NaCl) solution. The resulting

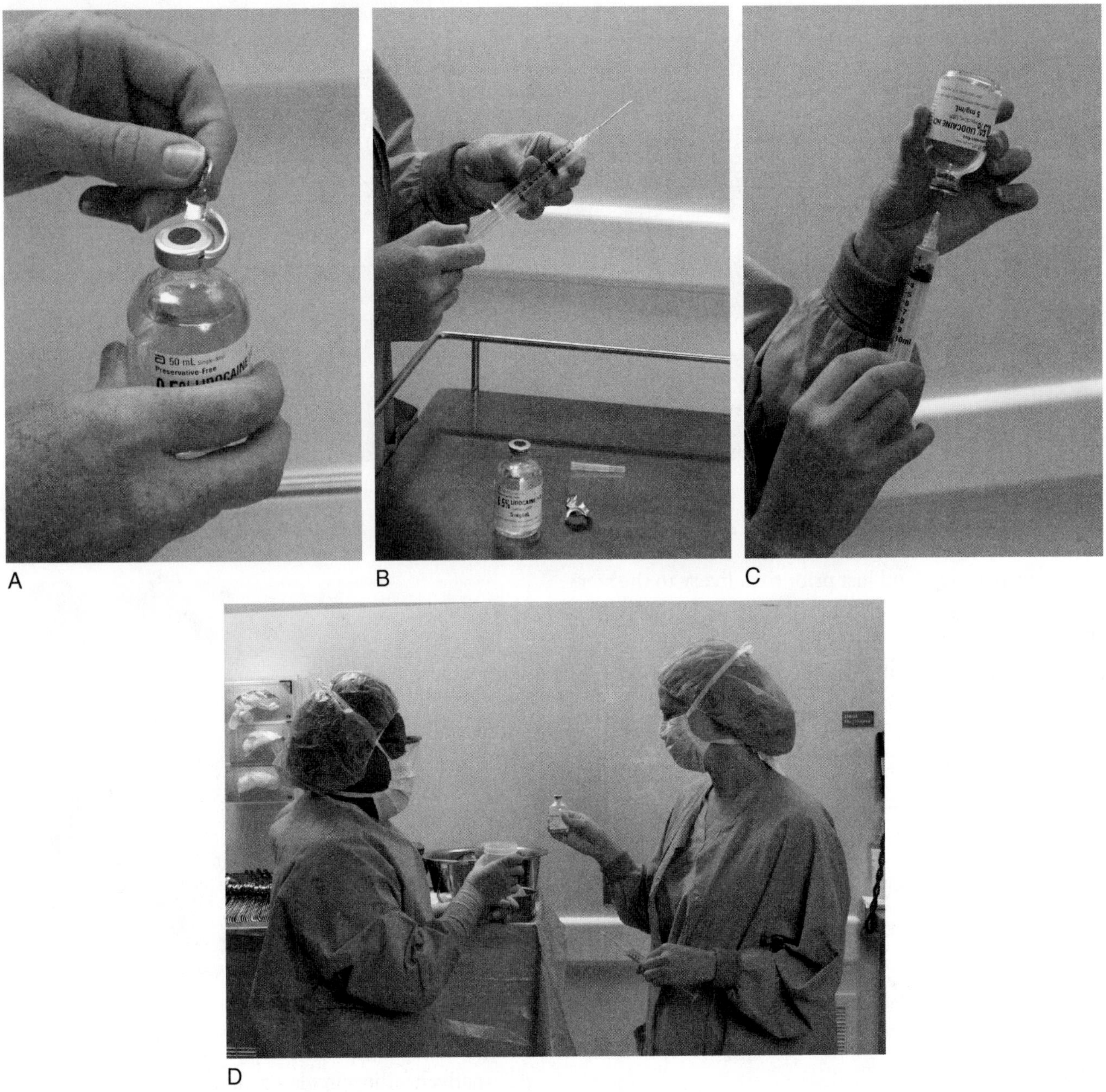

Figure 4-8 **Drawing medication from a vial. A,** Peel off the metal cap and remove plastic cover. **B,** Aspirate air into a syringe. **C,** Inject air into the vial to displace the medication, drawing medication into the syringe. **D,** Show the label to the scrub.

liquid is withdrawn from the vial with a syringe and delivered to the sterile field as described earlier. If a syringe is used to draw up and inject the reconstituting agent and to withdraw the mixture, care must be taken not to touch the sides of the plunger (Fig. 4-10). If unsterile hands touch the plunger, the plunger contaminates the inside of the barrel as it moves down the barrel when injecting. If the drug mixture is then drawn into the syringe barrel, it too becomes contaminated.

In some cases, the rubber top of a vial may be removed aseptically and the solution poured directly into a medicine cup (Fig. 4-11). If the stopper is removed for pouring, care must be taken to avoid contact with the lip of the vial, which must remain sterile. Sterile disposable spouts are commercially available to facilitate sterile delivery of medications contained in vials and in bags of intravenous solution. Medications may be added to a bag of intravenous solution, such as a

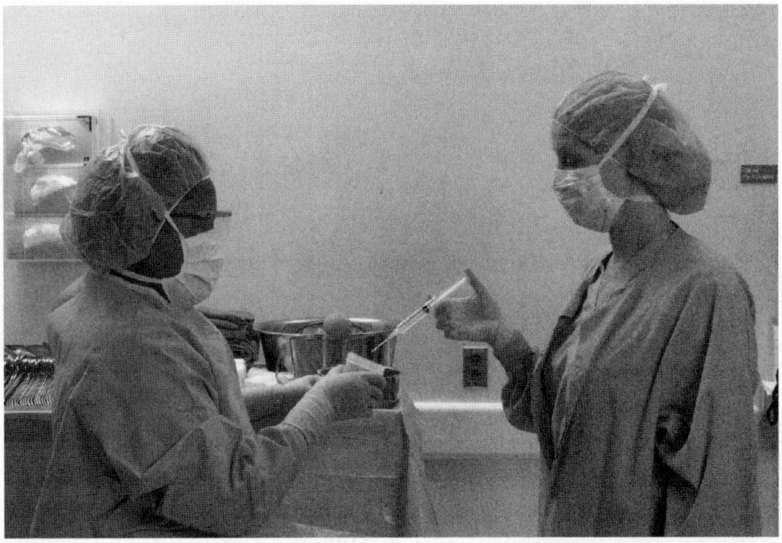

E

Figure 4-8—cont'd **E,** Squirt the medication into a medicine cup held by the scrub person.

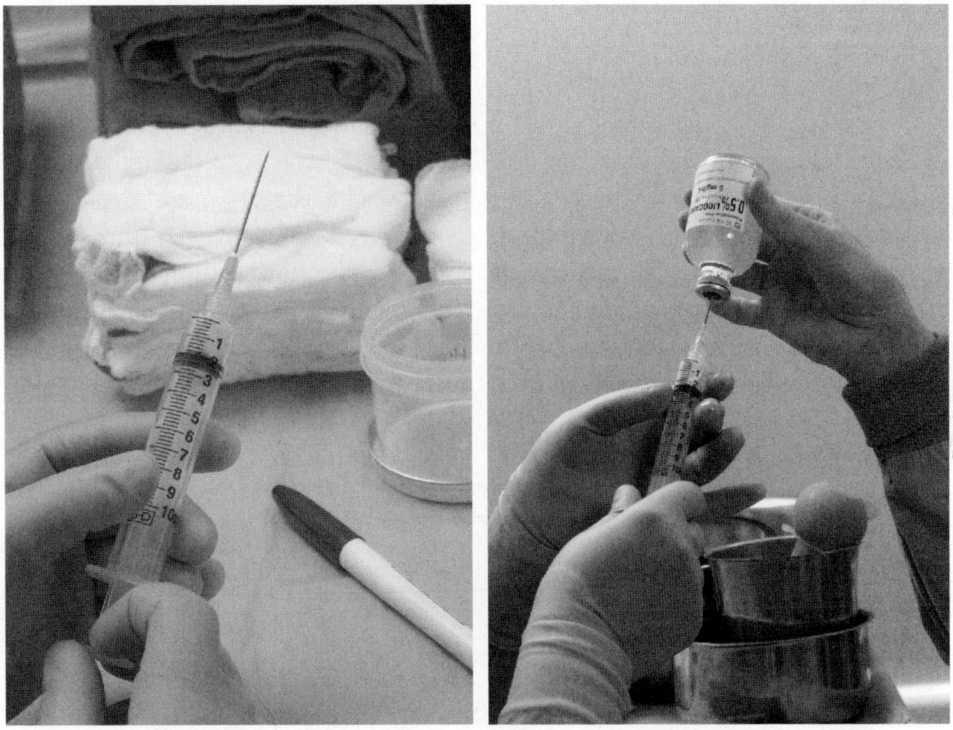

A B

Figure 4-9 The scrubbed surgical technologist may draw up medication from a vial held by the circulator. **A,** Air is drawn into the syringe. **B,** Air is injected into the vial to facilitate removal of medication.

gram of an antibiotic into 1000 mL of normal saline, and disposable spouts called bag decanters may be used to deliver the solution to the sterile field aseptically (Fig. 4-12).

Some medication vials and ampules are available in sterile packages, which can be opened directly onto the sterile field. The scrub is responsible for showing the medication label and expiration date to the circulator prior to opening the vial and drawing up the contents.

Some medications are available in an ampule, a sealed glass container with a narrowed neck. The top of an ampule is broken off at the neck and a sterile needle attached

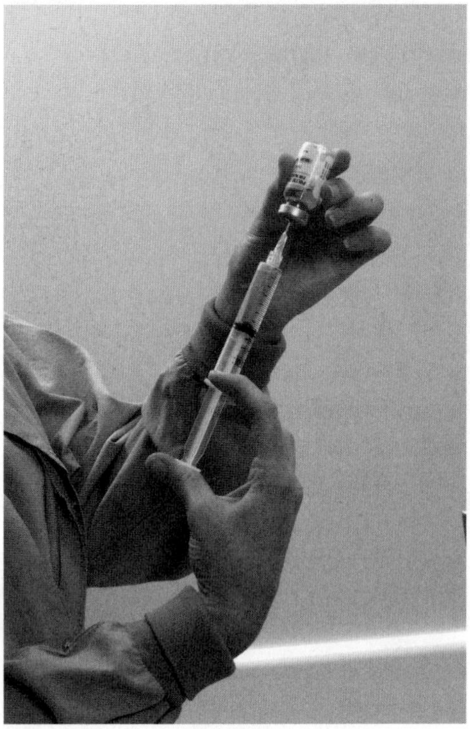

Figure 4-10 Unsterile hands must not touch the syringe plunger.

to a syringe is inserted to aspirate and withdraw the medication. Special care should be used when breaking the glass ampule, because glass may cut unprotected hands (Fig. 4-13). Some ampules come with a plastic protective cap that is used to prevent injury during opening. If the ampule does not come with a protective device, a gauze sponge may be placed over the narrowed area of the ampule for protection. A glass ampule should be broken away from the body to help prevent injury from the broken edge. Some glass ampules also come packaged sterile for use on the back table, such as the liquid component used to make polymethylmethacrylate (bone cement). Once again, care must be taken to protect the gloved hands. After the ampule is broken, the item used to protect the hands should be discarded from the sterile field to avoid accidental transfer of glass particles into the surgical wound.

While not technically considered a medication, saline irrigation is often delivered to the sterile field from a pour bottle. The bottle cap should be lifted straight up and off (Fig. 4-14), and the entire contents poured immediately. Unused portions should not be saved for later use, as sterility cannot be assured. If the bottle is recapped, its contents are considered unsterile because of potential contamination of the bottle lip during replacement of the cap.

To avoid potential contamination, the circulator must take care not to lean over the sterile field when delivering medications or solutions. The scrub should hold containers away from the sterile table or place containers at the table edge.

Several different types of containers are available to store medications and solutions on the sterile back table (Fig. 4-15). Medicine cups, pitchers, basins, or syringes may be used, depending on the volume of medication needed.

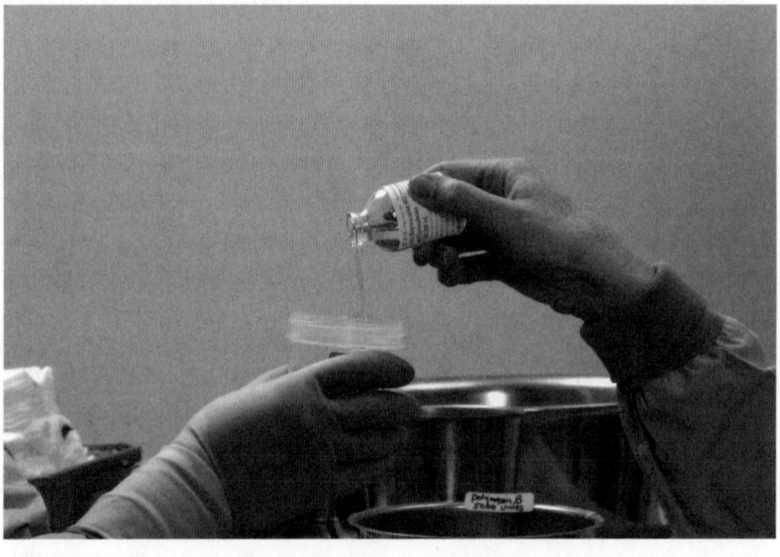

Figure 4-11 Medications may be carefully poured from an open vial into a medicine cup or other container.

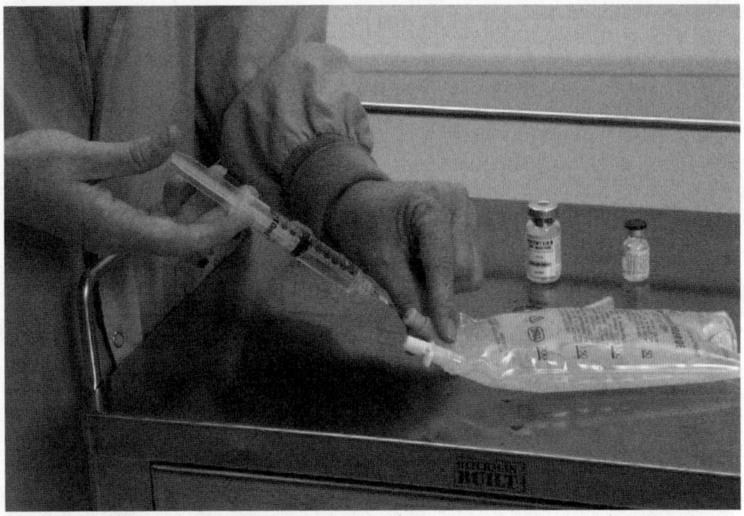

A

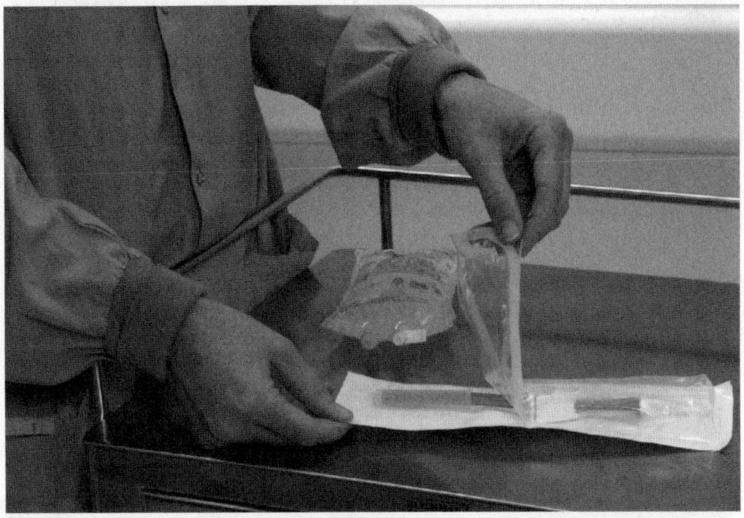

B

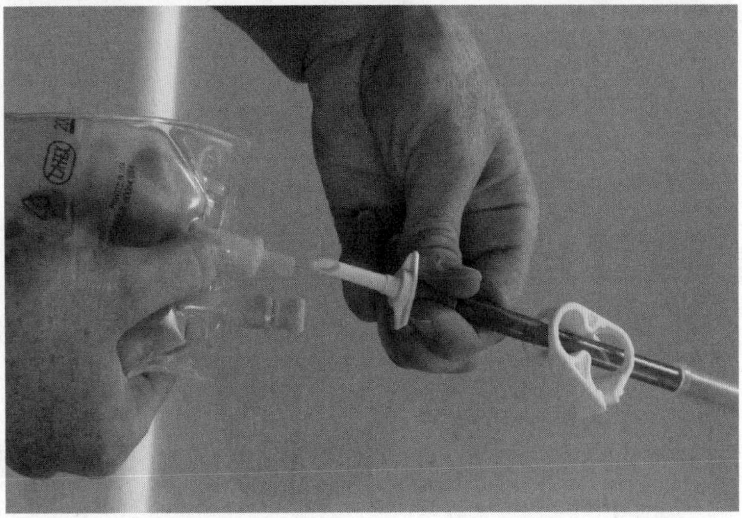

C

Figure 4-12 A sterile, disposable pour spout (decanter) is used to deliver medication contained in a bag of intravenous fluid. The metal cap and plastic cover are removed from the medication vial. **A,** The medication is injected into an injection port on the bag. **B,** The bag decanter is opened. **C,** The bag decanter is grasped by the hub and the prong is inserted into the injection port on the bag.

continued

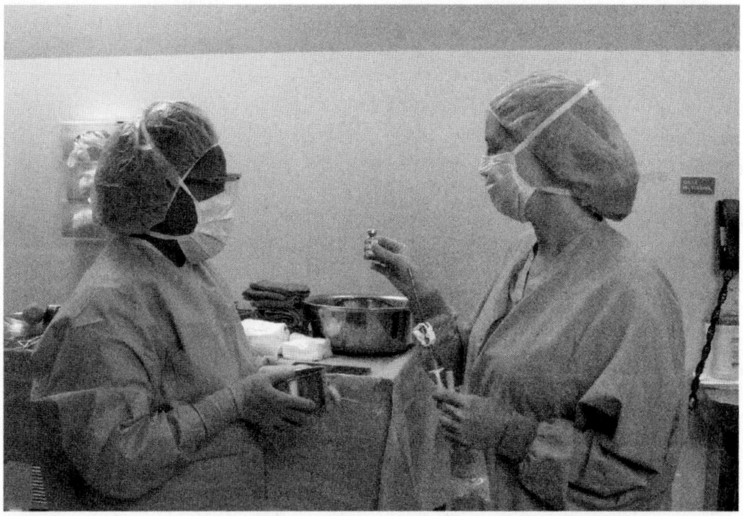

D

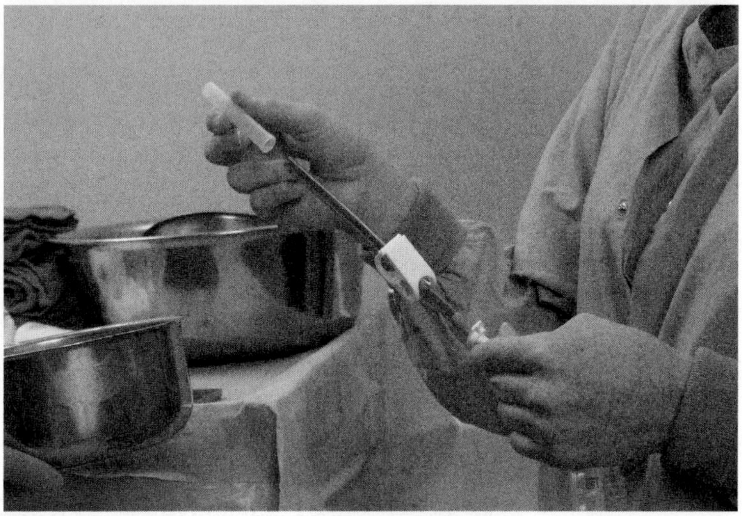

E

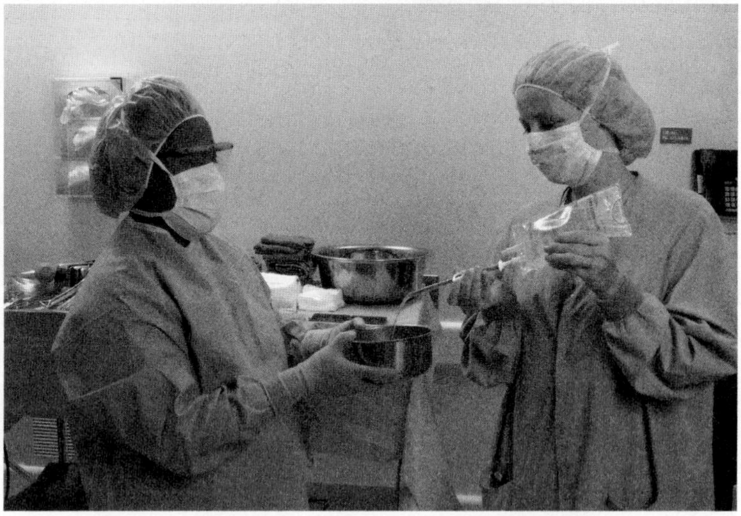

F

Figure 4-12—cont'd **D,** The label is shown to the scrubbed surgical technologist. **E,** The protective cover on the decanter pour spout is removed. **F,** The bag and decanter are inverted to pour medication into a container held by the scrubbed surgical technologist.

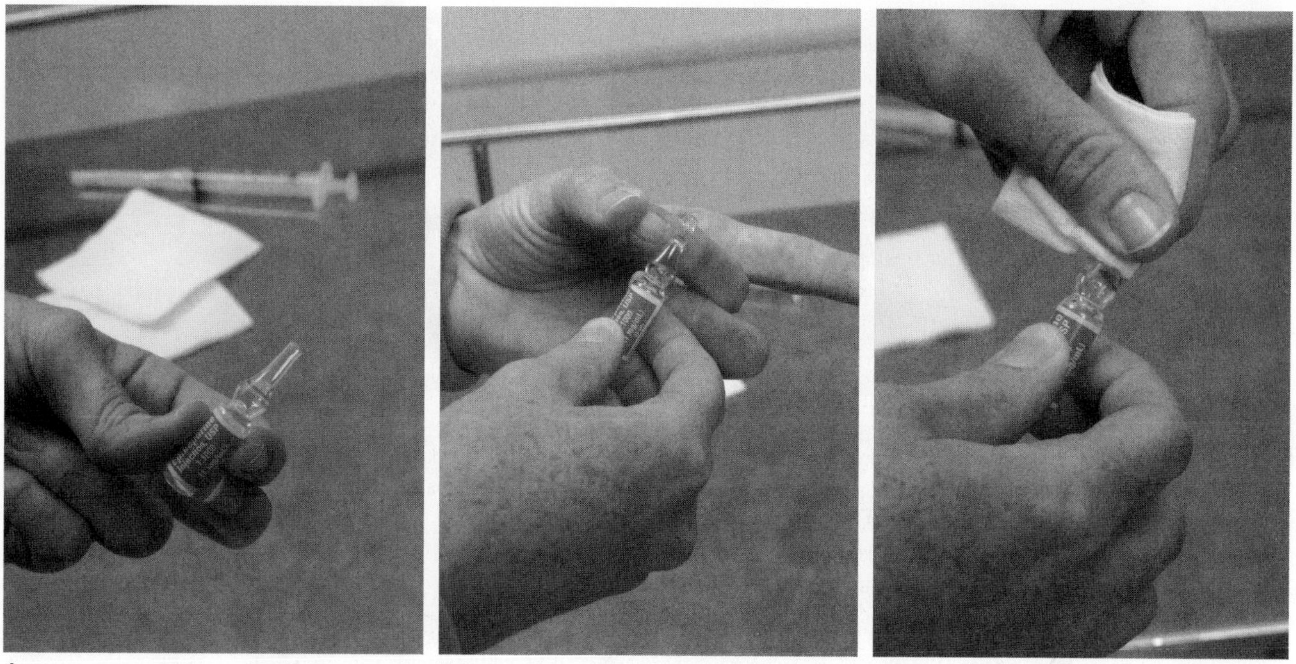

A B C

Figure 4-13 **Caution must be taken to protect the hands when breaking a glass ampule. A,** Grasp ampule firmly. **B,** Tap ampule to get entire contents into lower portion of ampule. **C,** Using protective mechanism, break ampule at narrowed area.

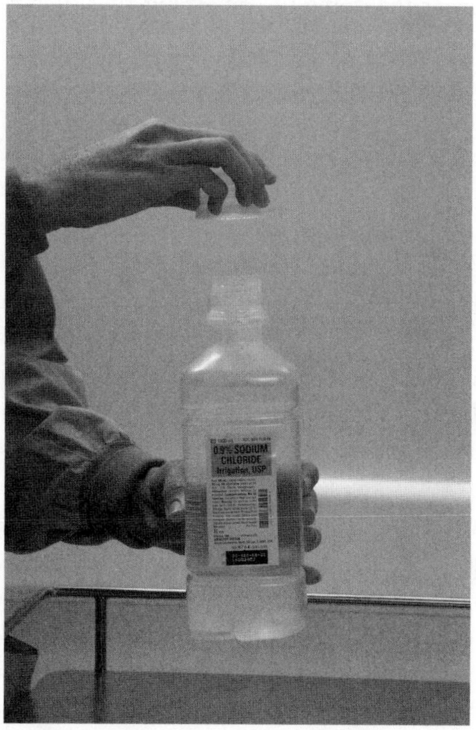

Figure 4-14 The cap of a pour bottle must be lifted straight up and off.

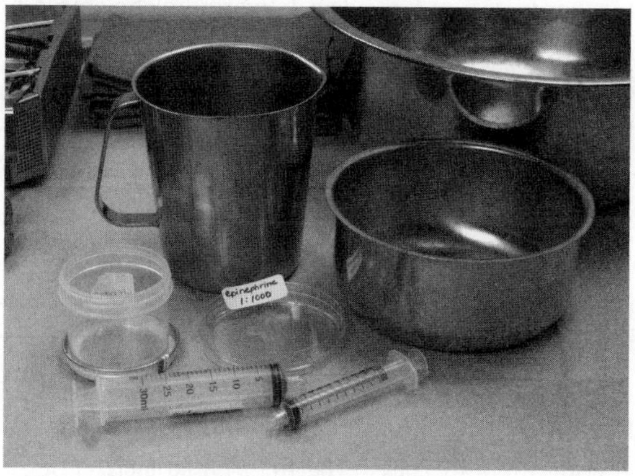

Figure 4-15 A variety of medication containers, such as pitchers, basins, medicine cups, petri dishes, or syringes, may be used on the sterile back table.

⚠ CAUTION

Medications intended for topical administration (such as thrombin or epinephrine 1:1000) should *never* be kept in a syringe on the back table. Syringes are used to inject medications. Some topical medications are *fatal* if injected. Use a labeled shallow container, such as a Petri dish, to store topical medications. The use of a shallow container will make it

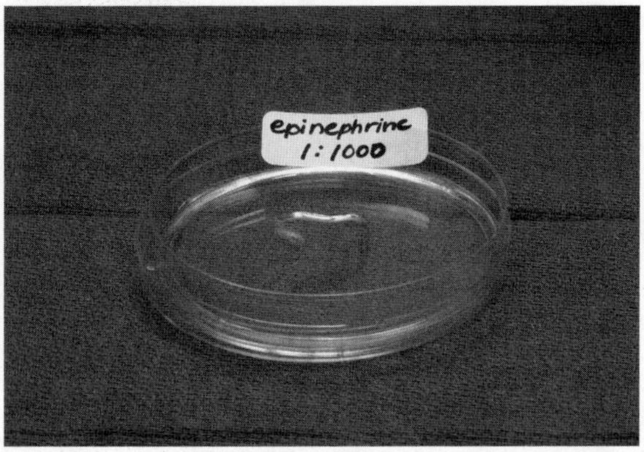

Figure 4-16 A medication intended for topical application, such as epinephrine 1:1000, should be kept in a shallow container, such as a Petri dish, rather than a syringe. For example, Gelfoam pledgets are dipped into topical epinephrine (1:1000) for hemostasis in the middle ear.

more difficult to accidentally draw up a topical medication into a syringe. In addition, a shallow container provides easy access to the medication when needed, for example, when dipping pieces of Gelfoam into the medication for topical application (Fig. 4-16).

MEDICATION LABELING ON THE STERILE BACK TABLE

Once a medication has been delivered to the sterile back table, it is no longer in its original container, so it must be labeled immediately. Most drugs used from the sterile field are clear in color; thus, they are easily confused if not clearly marked. There are different methods of labeling medications on the sterile back table, but the most important point is that each medication must be labeled—in the intermediate storage container (such as pitcher or medicine cup) and in any delivery vehicle (such as a syringe). The Joint Commission National Patient Safety Goal 3, Requirement D, requires that all medication containers in the sterile field be labeled. The most accurate medication labeling method is the use of preprinted medication labels available from sterile supply manufacturers. If preprinted labels are not available, a sterile skin marking pen may be used to write on blank labels (Fig. 4-17). If blank labels are not available, sterile skin adhesive strips may be used. Regardless of the labeling method employed, proper identification of all medications in the sterile field is an absolutely crucial step in preventing medication administration errors.

Occasionally, the scrubbed surgical technologist may be replaced during a procedure (e.g., for shift change or

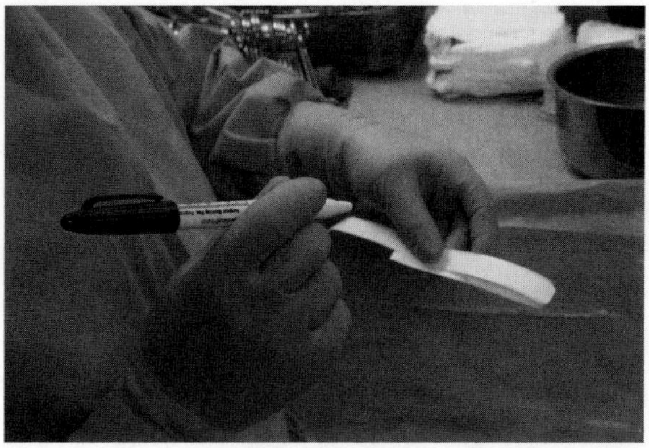

Figure 4-17 A marking pen may be used to complete a label for a medication on the sterile back table.

lunch relief). All medications must be plainly labeled and reported to the new scrub. If there is any doubt as to the identity of a solution, it must be discarded and new medication must be obtained.

There is no acceptable excuse for the presence of unlabeled (unidentified) medications on the sterile back table. Improper or inadequate labeling of drugs may be considered negligent. Negligence is defined in the Miller-Keane *Encyclopedia and Dictionary of Medicine, Nursing and Allied Health* as "failure to do something that a reasonable person of ordinary prudence would do in a situation or the doing of something that such a person would not do." By this definition, it is "reasonable" to expect that the correct medication will be obtained, identified, and passed to the surgeon and that a "prudent" person will perform these duties. This means that reason and prudence are everyone's responsibility, whatever the situation. This isn't always easy. The rapid pace of events in surgery often pressures team members to accomplish difficult tasks in a hurry. However, the process of medication identification should never be compromised nor should staff become complacent about routine medications. If a question or doubt arises regarding a medication, it must be clarified and resolved immediately. If the medication seems wrong or the dose appears to be incorrect, verify it with the physician before using it. It is better to be certain about the drug—even if it means provoking the surgeon—than to make an error and thus cause harm to the patient.

Special caution is required when handling controlled substances in surgery. Local policies regarding handling of controlled substances must be in compliance with federal law (see Chapter 2); thus, they must be understood and followed by all staff members. For example, cocaine is a schedule C-II drug frequently used for topical anesthesia in surgery. If needed for a particular procedure, cocaine is obtained immediately prior to use and is never left unattended. Any cocaine remaining at the end of the procedure must be rendered useless—usually by dilution with large amounts of water—and then discarded. The dilution and disposal of any controlled substance should be witnessed by at least two team members.

TECH TIP

Do not be embarrassed to admit ignorance or confusion, and always admit an outright error. Honesty and integrity are vital characteristics in health care professionals. If you make a medication error, acknowledge it at once so that corrective measures may be taken. Notify the surgeon immediately. Then follow institutional policy. Usually, when a medication error occurs, the unit supervisor is notified and an incident or occurrence report is completed. Above all, immediate action is taken to correct the error. The surgical technologist's primary focus in medication administration is patient safety.

HANDLING MEDICATIONS

When medications have been delivered to the sterile field and labeled, some additional handling may be necessary. Occasionally, the surgeon may order that two medications be mixed for concurrent administration. For example, an anti-inflammatory agent and a long-acting local anesthetic agent may be mixed for injection into a joint at the conclusion of an arthroscopy. Some medications may be diluted prior to use, such as Hypaque, which may be diluted with equal parts of injectable saline as ordered on the preference card. It is vital that the surgical technologist read the preference card carefully and use basic math skills (see Chapter 3) to assure the correct mixture or dilution of medications at the sterile back table. All containers (such as medicine cups) must be labeled for the original medications, and a separate container must be clearly labeled indicating the mixture or diluted medication. The administration container, usually a syringe, must be labeled with complete information on the mixture or dilution. The final check for accuracy is performed when the scrubbed surgical technologist states the complete mixing or dilution information when handing the medication to the surgeon.

Other medications may require reconstitution prior to use (Insight 4-1). An example is topical thrombin, which is available in a sterile kit with a pump spray bottle. The kit contains a vial of thrombin, a vial of **diluent** (an inert diluting agent; saline), and a spray bottle. The scrub draws the diluent into a syringe and injects it into the thrombin vial. The mixture is shaken until the thrombin is dissolved and transferred to the pump spray bottle for administration to large oozing surfaces such as the liver.

SUPPLIES

Syringes and hypodermic needles are used frequently in surgery to draw up, measure, and administer medications. Disposable syringes are made of plastic, but reusable glass syringes may be indicated for specific situations. The most common sizes of syringes routinely used in surgery range from 1 mL to 60 mL. A syringe has three basic parts: the barrel (or outer portion), the plunger (inside portion), and the tip. The barrel of the syringe is marked or calibrated to indicate the amount of medication contained in the syringe. The amount of medication in the syringe is measured from the innermost edge of the rubber tip on the end of the plunger. Some syringes have a finger-control attachment on the barrel and plunger to provide ease of motion and more

IN SIGHT 4-1 Reconstituting

Medications are not the only agents that may need to be reconstituted for a surgical procedure. Orthobiological implants (Restore), derived from porcine small-intestine submucosa that has been processed, disinfected, and sterilized, are designed as a tissue scaffold that is resorbable by the body. The implant helps to reinforce weakened or damaged soft tissue and is a less invasive alternative to allograft. Examples of surgical procedures that may use an orthobiological implant are rotator cuff repair and Achilles tendon repair. The implant must be kept refrigerated until needed and then soaked for 7 to 10 minutes (or reconstituted) in sterile saline/buffer or water prior to use.

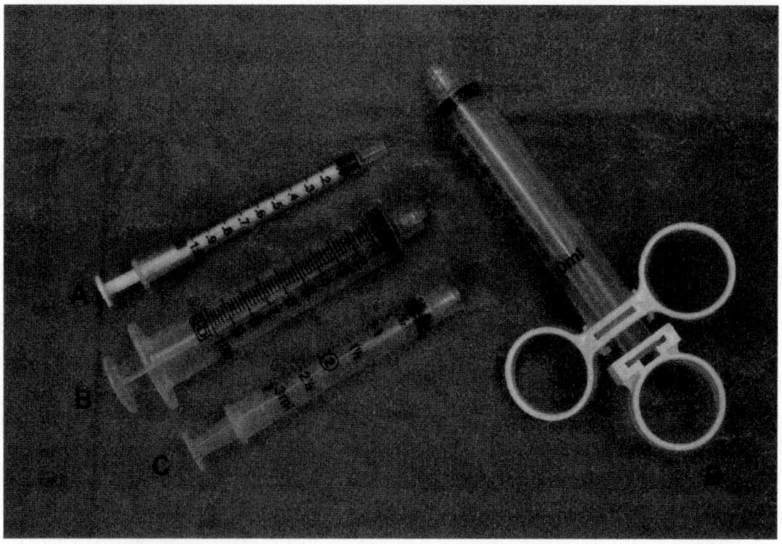

Figure 4-18 **Types of syringes. A,** A 1-mL plain-tip tuberculin syringe. **B,** A 10-mL Luer-loc syringe. **C,** A 3-mL Luer-loc syringe. **D,** A 10-mL finger-control Luer-loc syringe.

precise control when injecting (Fig. 4-18). The most common type of syringe tip used in surgery is the Luer-loc tip, which has a screw-type locking mechanism used to securely attach a hypodermic needle. Plain-tip or "slip-tip" syringes are also available, but these are used for specific purposes. For example, a plain-tip syringe may be attached to a spinal needle for subclavian venipuncture during a venous access procedure. Various sizes of syringes are used for various purposes, so consult the surgeon's preference card for specific information. Generally, 1-mL (called a TB or tuberculin syringe) and 3-mL syringes are used to inflate the tiny balloon on the end of an embolectomy catheter. By far the most common syringe size used in the operating room is a 10-mL syringe. That size syringe is used for a number of purposes, including inflating the cuff on a tracheostomy tube and injection of a local anesthetic agent throughout a surgical procedure. Thirty-mL syringes are most frequently used to inject saline irrigation and contrast media into the common bile duct, inflate a 30-mL balloon on a Foley catheter, or administer heparinized saline through an arterial irrigation catheter.

Special syringes are available for particular purposes. For example, a Tubex syringe has a metal or plastic device used to accommodate a **carpule** of medication for injection (such as lidocaine or heparin). A carpule is a glass tube with a rubber cap that is penetrated by a special needle attached to the Tubex syringe (Fig. 4-19). Another type of special syringe is a dual-syringe device used to deliver two medications simultaneously, such as those used to form a fibrin sealant.

Hypodermic needles are used to draw up and administer drugs. A hypodermic needle has three basic parts: the hub (which fits onto a syringe), the shaft, and the tip (the beveled end of the shaft). Needles vary in diameter (gauge) and length (measured in inches). The larger the gauge of a needle, the smaller the diameter of the lumen (inside channel). So, an 18-gauge needle has a much larger lumen than a 25-gauge needle. Most needles used in surgery are disposable and are color-coded by size at the plastic hub for ease in identification. Sizes of hypodermic needles routinely used in surgery range from 27-gauge needles (used in ophthalmology) to larger 18-gauge needles (used to draw up medications). The most common needle length used in surgery is $1^1/_2$ inches. Shorter, $^5/_8$-inch needles may be used for superficial

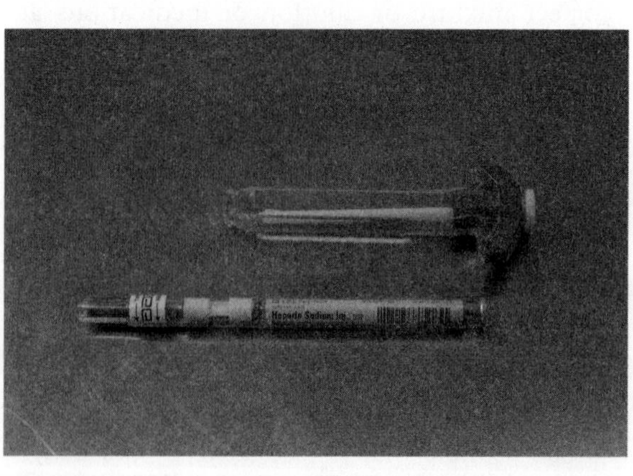

Figure 4-19 A Tubex syringe, glass carpule, and needle.

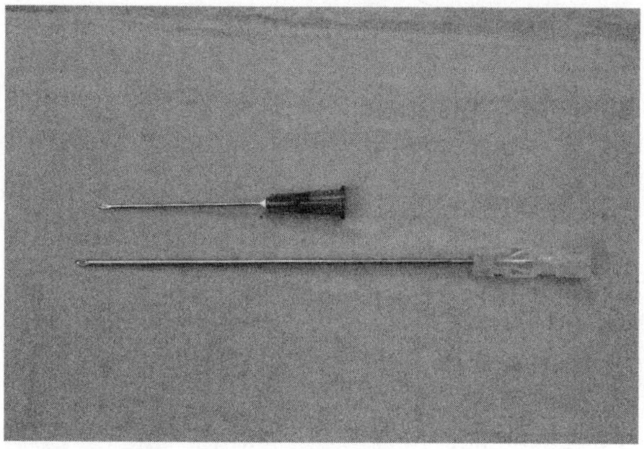

Figure 4-20 Hypodermic needles, $1^1/_2$-inch and 3-inch.

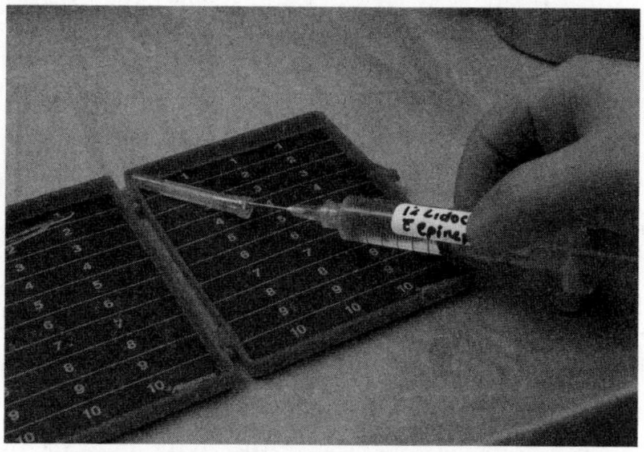

Figure 4-21 If a needle must be recapped for protection for reuse during an operation, such as the periodic injection of local anesthetic for patient comfort, use a one-handed recapping technique.

injections, whereas longer needles (3-inch), called spinal needles, may be used for specific purposes, such as aspiration of cysts (Fig. 4-20).

CAUTION

Standard precautions state that used needles must never be recapped, because most needle puncture injuries are the result of attempting to recap a used needle. However, it is also dangerous to leave an unsheathed hypodermic needle exposed on the sterile table during a surgical procedure. If a needle must be recapped for protection between repeated uses during a surgical procedure, you should use a one-handed technique (Fig. 4-21) or a recapping device intended for that purpose.

ADVANCED PRACTICES FOR THE SURGICAL FIRST ASSISTANT

CHAPTER 4—Medication Administration

Key Terms

- **bioavailability**
- **efficacy**
- **half-life**
- **potency**
- **systemic effect**

MEDICATION ADMINISTRATION FROM THE STERILE FIELD

Intraoperative administration of medications to the surgical patient presents a unique situation unlike any other medical environment, especially for the advanced practitioner functioning as a surgical first assistant. Different personnel administer medications to the patient through several routes, often at the same time. Although the surgical first assistant might not perform the actual administration of medications, it is important that he or she be aware of the effects any medication can have on the patient.

Personnel who fulfill the role of the surgical first assistant will have different educational and clinical backgrounds ranging from medical school to physician's assisting, nursing, and surgical technology. These different backgrounds and employment disciplines dictate different regulatory agencies under which each professional practices in regard to administration of medications. State statutes will supersede any other regulatory agency in regard to limitations of practice; however, when there is no statute regulating specific personnel, it is usually the individual facility that regulates the practice. All personnel practicing as surgical first assistants should be aware of the policies or bylaws regulating their practice. For example, the surgical first assistant functioning as an independent practitioner may be regulated by the medical staff bylaws of the facility. However, the surgical first assistant employed by the facility may be regulated by that facility's policies and procedures.

The process of administering medications at the sterile field requires a team effort. Medications will pass through at least two other people, the circulator and the scrub person, before being delivered to the surgeon. The medication will almost always be in a container different from its original; usually a syringe, medicine cup, basin, or pitcher on the field. To prevent medication errors, strict policies and procedures have been developed for delivery of medications onto the sterile field (as described in this chapter). The surgeon and the surgical first assistant may be the last line of defense to avoid medication errors; therefore, each should be aware of and follow all of these procedures. The person who administers the medication *always* has the right to question the procedure and decide if the medication will be given or a new medication obtained. It is always in the best interest of the patient to discard any questionable medication. (See Box A: Guidelines for Administering Medications at the Sterile Field).

{NOTE} *When medications are administered from the sterile field, it is important to communicate to the anesthesia provider the name of the agent and amount given. For example, when a local anesthetic agent that contains epinephrine is administered, the anesthesia provider should be notified immediately and verbally advised as to the amount of the medication ultimately injected (which is also noted on the operative record). This is important because epinephrine acts as a vasoconstrictor and can affect the patient's blood pressure.*

DRUG RESPONSE RELATIONSHIPS

All medications have **systemic effects** on the patient. It is important for the surgical first assistant to be aware of these effects as well as the duration and safe dosages of medications. This pharmacological principle is known as the dose-time-effect relationship. Drug effects are a result of the dose administered and the time from absorption to elimination. Medication dosage, time the medication is absorbed by the body, and the duration of action are all interrelated and interdependent. The duration of a medication's effect is based on the **half-life** of the medicine. Elimination half-life ($T_{1/2}$), also called biological half-life, is the time it takes for 50% of a drug to be cleared from the bloodstream. Each drug has a unique half-life dependent on its characteristics. Certain conditions such as decreased liver or renal function will alter the half-life of medications. It is important to note that a medication may go through many of its half-lives before it no longer has a therapeutic effect on the body. This must be recognized when calculating subsequent doses of the same medication to maintain a therapeutic level of its desired effects. Some half-lives are of short duration, such as those used in general anesthesia (a few minutes). Others may have a half-life of several days, such as those used to treat hypothyroidism. Therefore, drugs with long half-lives are dosed less frequently than those with short half-lives. Essentially, drugs with short half-lives are said to leave the body quickly—in 4 to 8 hours. Drugs with long half-lives are said to leave the body more slowly—in more than 24 hours, and there is a greater risk for accumulation of these medications in the bloodstream and toxicity. A common example in the surgical setting is the administration of sodium heparin to achieve anticoagulation during vascular surgery. It has a relatively short half-life of approximately 60 to 90 minutes and so would have to be administered frequently to maintain its initial effect. (See Table A: Half-life of Sodium Heparin).

Other terms related to drug effects are **efficacy** and **potency**. Drug efficacy is the degree to which a drug is able to produce its desired effects. Potency is the relative concentration required to produce that effect, as in how much of the drug is needed.

Bioavailability is the extent to which an administered amount of a drug reaches the site of action and is available to produce the drug effects. This is influenced by drug absorption and distribution to the site of action. Bioavailability is important in pharmacokinetics as it must be taken into consideration when calculating medication doses, especially those administered via non-intravenous routes. For intravenous administration, the bioavailability of the drug is considered to be 100%.

BOX A Guidelines for Administering Medications from the Sterile Field

- Always be aware of the process of delivering medications to the sterile field
- Always read the label on the device you receive which contains the medication
- Always confirm name and strength of the medication with the scrub person
- Always inform anesthesia personnel when administering medications
- Always be aware of any patient allergies
- Always be aware of the amount of the medication administered
- Never administer medications that are discolored or contain sediment
- Never administer medications that are contaminated with other materials from the sterile field
- Never administer a medication from any unlabeled container
- Never administer a medication when there is any doubt about its identification or strength

Table A Half-life of Sodium Heparin, 5000 u

Time from Dosage (in hours)	Remaining Serum Amount in Body (in units)
1	2500
2	1250
3	625
4	312
5	156

Advanced Practices Bibliography

Fulcher E, Fulcher R, Soto C: *Pharmacology principles and applications*, ed 2, 2009, Saunders/Elsevier.

Jensen SC, Peppers MP: *Pharmacology and drug administration for imaging technologists*, ed 2, St. Louis, 2006, Mosby/Elsevier.

Moscou K, Snipe K: *Pharmacology for pharmacy technicians*, St. Louis, 2009, Mosby/Elsevier.

Wissmann J, ed.: *Pharmacology for nursing*, Version 4.0, U.S. 2006, Assessment Technologies Institute.

Advanced Practices Internet Resources

Answers.com, Bioavailability: *www.answers.com/topic/bioavailability*
The Joint Commission: *www.jointcommission.org*
RxMed: *www.rxmed.com* (select Drug and Illness Information, "H," Heparin)
U.S. Drug Enforcement Administration: *www.dea.gov*

Advanced Practices: Learning the Language (Key Terms)

Using your textbook or a standard medical dictionary, look up and write the definitions of each term.

- bioavailability
- efficacy
- half-life
- potency
- systemic effect

Advanced Practices: Review Questions

1. All of the following statements are true concerning patient effects from medication administration EXCEPT:
A. All medications have a systemic effect
B. Topical medications affect only the localized area
C. Liver function influences medication effects
D. The time a medication is given influences its effect

2. When there is no state statute or federal law regulating an individual profession, what organization regulates health care workers in regard to medication administration?
A. OSHA
B. Joint Commission
C. Health care facilities
D. Health department

3. The duration of a medication's effect is based on the medication's
A. Dosage
B. Strength
C. Half-life
D. Administration route

4. The bioavailability of an intravenous medication is considered to be what percent?
A. 15
B. 25
C. 50
D. 100

5. Explain why it is important to notify the anesthesia provider when a medication is administered at the sterile field.

6. Explain the pharmacological principle known as the dose-time-effect relationship.

7. Which medication has the greater opportunity to become toxic in the body, drugs to treat hypothyroidism or heparin? Why?

8. List the guidelines for administering medications from the sterile field.

KEY CONCEPTS

- The role of the scrubbed surgical technologist in medication administration is to identify, accept, label, and clearly state the medication when passing it to the surgeon.
- Each facility's established policies and procedures must always be understood and scrupulously followed.
- In addition, the surgical technologist must be aware of state regulations regarding specific practices.
- Consistent application of the five "rights" of medication administration will reduce the potential for drug errors.
- The surgical technologist in the scrub role must never accept a medication without properly identifying it.
- Aseptic technique must be used when delivering or accepting drugs into the sterile field.
- Accurate and immediate labeling of drugs on the sterile back table is required to minimize potential for errors.

Bibliography

Fulcher E, Fulcher R, Soto C: *Pharmacology principles and applications*, ed 2, 2009, Saunders/Elsevier.

Moscou K, Snipe K: *Pharmacology for pharmacy technicians*, St. Louis, 2009, Mosby/Elsevier.

LEARNING THE LANGUAGE (KEY TERMS)

Using your textbook or a standard medical dictionary, look up and write the definitions of each term.

carpule

diluent

reconstitute

REVIEW QUESTIONS

1. What is the role of the surgical technologist in medication administration when serving as the scrub person? As the circulator?
2. Give examples of applications of the five "rights" of medication administration in surgery.
3. Which steps would you use to correctly identify medications that are going to be used from the sterile back table during a surgical procedure?
4. How do the principles of sterile technique apply to medication delivery to the sterile field?
5. How would you label drugs on your sterile back table?
6. What items are used to facilitate medication administration from the sterile back table?

CRITICAL THINKING

Scenario

It is 0725 and the patient has just been brought into the operating room. The circulator is in a hurry because the patient has come into the room late and the surgeon is in the department. The circulator asks you to put the medication containers at the edge of the sterile back table so she can pour the solutions as soon as she has time and you can continue setting up for the procedure.

1. Is this safe practice? Justify your answer.
2. List a better alternative to her request.

UNIT 2

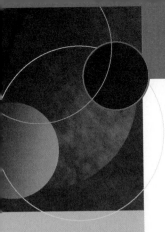

APPLIED SURGICAL PHARMACOLOGY

Many medications are used in surgery each day. This unit provides an introduction to the medications you will frequently encounter as a surgical technologist. We'll look at antibiotics, diagnostic agents, diuretics, hormones, fluids, and antineoplastic chemotherapy agents. We'll also examine medications that affect blood coagulation and medications used as ophthalmic agents. To understand these agents, you'll need to be familiar with basic anatomy and physiology, so we'll review some of those principles as well. Once you know the generic and brand names of common surgical medications and their categories, you'll be better able to recognize their purposes, action, administration, routes, and proper handling in order to provide safe patient care. Note that the generic name of the medication is given first with a brand name in parenthesis behind it. It is important for you to recognize generic names because medications may have more than one brand name.

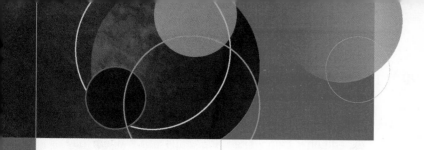

CHAPTER 5 Antibiotics

OBJECTIVES *After completing this chapter, you should be able to:*

1. Define terminology related to antimicrobial therapy.
2. Discuss the purpose of antibiotic therapy in surgery.
3. Describe various ways in which antimicrobials work.
4. Discuss antibiotic resistance.
5. List categories of antibiotics used in surgery and give examples of each.
6. Identify the category of various antibiotics.
7. Use drug resources to gather pertinent information on antibiotics.

KEY TERMS

antibiotic resistance
bactericidal
bacteriostatic
culture and sensitivity (C&S)
endogenous
eukaryotes
exogenous
Gram staining
methicillin-resistant *Staphylococcus aureus* (MRSA)
morphology
nephrotoxicity
ototoxicity
polymicrobic infections
prokaryotes
prophylaxis
selective toxicity
vancomycin-resistant enterococci (VRE)

Before the discovery of antimicrobial agents, surgical patients often died from infections of various kinds. Surgical procedures, such as amputations, were quite dangerous in themselves. The most common danger, however, was a postoperative wound infection. Even if patients survived surgery, the resulting wound infection was often fatal. Infection in the wound was so common that the physicians believed purulent drainage (called laudable pus) was a natural part of wound healing. Today, however, many antimicrobial agents are available. They are used (1) to prevent and (2) to treat infections caused by pathogenic (disease-causing) microorganisms. The term *antimicrobial* applies to several categories of agents: These include antivirals, antibacterials, antiprotozoals, antifungals, antiparasitics, and drugs such as sulfa and mercury (see Insight 5-1). In surgery, however,

IN SIGHT 5-1 Medicinals Used During Lewis and Clark's Expedition

In May of 1804, President Jefferson sent Meriwether Lewis and William Clark on an expedition to explore the land west of St. Louis to the Pacific Ocean. One of the primary medications of the journey was mercurial salts. At this time, antibiotics had yet to be discovered, but the medicinal properties of mercury were well known. Mercurials were used for the treatment of venereal diseases and also as powerful laxatives. Lewis and Clark's expedition took along Dr. Benjamin Rush's famous mercury pills, called "Thunderclappers." Archeologists looking for the expedition's camp sites and trails use modern day survey and excavating techniques to analyze and sample soil. They have discovered traces of this mercury in latrine trenches in Montana. The fact that mercury, which passed through the human digestive system more than 200 years ago, can still be detected speaks to the potency of this medication.

the only antimicrobial agents routinely used are antibacterials, commonly referred to as *antibiotics.*

Antibiotics take their name from the Greek words *anti,* which means "against" and *bios,* which means "life." They are natural chemicals (or *metabolites*) produced by microorganisms that inhibit the growth of other microorganisms. These natural substances include fungi (and molds, a type of fungi) and bacteria. They may be altered in the chemical laboratory to produce semisynthetic antibiotics, and those completely synthesized in the laboratory are called synthetics. About 85% of the antibiotics currently available are produced by actinomycetes—a family of bacteria that resemble fungi because of their filamentous projections. Other antibiotics, such as the penicillins and streptomycin, are derived from fungi. Cephalosporins are produced from the mold *Cephalosporium*, found in the ocean near sewage outflow. Artificial means have been used to produce other medications, which result in families of antibiotics. Each antibiotic in a family is similar to the original chemical, but can be used to treat different types of infections because it has different properties.

Between 30% and 50% of antibiotics prescribed in the United States are for **prophylaxis**—that is, prevention—of infections. For the surgical patient, antibiotics may be prescribed preoperatively, intraoperatively, or postoperatively. Postoperative wound infections (most commonly referred to as surgical site infection or SSI) are potential complications of every surgical intervention because any such procedure penetrates the body's first line of defense: the skin. SSIs may range from minor to serious; they may even be deadly, depending on several factors. Antibiotics do not take the place of aseptic technique. Rather, antibiotics are adjuncts that assist the patient's own defenses to prevent—or diminish the severity of—postoperative SSIs.

Further measures, which include the appropriate use of antibiotics, are being implemented to help prevent SSIs and improve surgical patient safety. The Joint Commission has developed a national quality partnership called the Surgical Care Improvement Project (SCIP). This focuses on reducing SSIs and one of its goals is to increase compliance for measures related to use of antibiotics such as the selection of the antibiotic; the time an antibiotic is received before the incision; the time an antibiotic is discontinued after surgery; and the identification of the person responsible for these actions and for verifying antibiotic names, times of administration, and documentation. The SCIP also includes measures to prevent venous thromboembolism (VTE), a dangerous postoperative complication. For more information go to www.jointcommission.org and type SCIP in the seach window.

Another measure that includes antibiotics and surgical patient safety has been developed by the World Health Organization (WHO). This is an international tool used in operating rooms called the Surgical Patient Checklist. It has three sections: before the induction of anesthesia, before the skin incision, and before the patient leaves the operating room. Under each section is a list of tasks to be accomplished and verified. In the second section there is a task relating to antibiotic prophylaxis (see Chapter 4, Figure 4-4).

MICROBIOLOGY REVIEW

SSIs are caused by the introduction of pathogenic microorganisms into a susceptible host (Fig. 5-1) via a route of transmission. The pathogen must have a source, a means of transmission, and a host to cause an infection. The source of pathogenic microorganisms may be **endogenous** or **exogenous**. That is, the infectious microbe may come from the patient's own bacteria (endogenous)

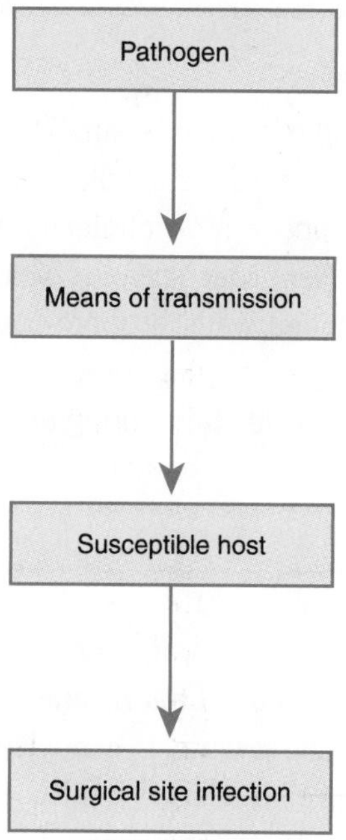

Figure 5-1 **Infection cycle.** Source of pathogenic microbe plus transmission route plus susceptible host equals infection.

or from outside the patient (exogenous). For example, among the most common causative agents of SSIs are bacteria known as *Staphylococcus aureus,* which are normally present on the patient's skin (endogenous source) and may be carried into the surgical site during the course of the operation. Exogenous sources of pathogenic microbes include surgical personnel and the environment. An example of an exogenous source of infectious microbes is various bacteria carried under artificial fingernails worn by sterile team members. Such microbes are introduced into the surgical site by glove tears commonly associated with long fingernails.

CAUTION

Long and/or artificial nails are prohibited in surgery, and team members who wear them are failing to follow policies established to prevent postoperative SSIs.

Another example of an exogenous source of pathogens is improperly cleaned or sterilized instruments, which may carry microbes into the wound. Regardless of the source, many other factors influence the surgical patient's susceptibility to an infection, including general health, nutritional status, operative site, and duration of the surgical procedure.

If an SSI occurs, treatment requires identification of the causative microorganism and selection of an appropriate antimicrobial agent. Pathogenic microorganisms causing SSIs are identified by several methods. Common methods used to identify pathogens include **culture and sensitivity (C&S)** and **Gram staining**. Culture and sensitivity is the process of growing microbes in culture to determine the infecting pathogen and the exposure of the pathogen to various antibiotics to determine which agent will best inhibit the pathogen's growth. To perform C&S, a fluid or tissue specimen is obtained with a swab from the infection site and placed in one or more culture tubes for transport to the microbiology laboratory. Note that separate culture tubes are available for aerobic (in oxygen) and anaerobic (lacking oxygen) testing. In the laboratory, the culture swab is used to spread the fluid sample onto nutrient agar and differential (distinguishing) media in Petri dishes called *plates.* This process is called *inoculation.* The inoculated plates are incubated for 24 to 48 hours, after which they can be examined for microbial growth. Miniaturized reaction containers allow laboratory personnel to identify causative microbes faster and easier. Once the microbe has been isolated, it is grown in a pure culture and exposed to different antibiotics. This process of successive exposure to antibiotics to determine which agent is most effective against it is called *sensitivity testing.* The conventional Kirby-Bauer disk diffusion method of sensitivity testing takes longer than the newer rapid antibiotic susceptibility test (RAST).

When the causative microorganism is identified and tested for antibiotic sensitivity, the appropriate therapy can be initiated. Often, however, a broad-spectrum antibiotic is prescribed to begin treatment while awaiting the results of C&S testing. Occasionally during a surgical procedure such as an incision and drainage (I&D), a sample of abscess fluid may be subjected to an immediate Gram stain process (Insight 5-2).

A Gram stain is a rapid identification test that assists the physician in prescribing an initial course of antibiotic therapy based on the probable pathogen causing the infection. Gram staining is a way of distinguishing types of bacteria. In combination with **morphology** (the study of shapes), it can be used to identify many common bacteria. Bacteria occur in many shapes, most of which may be placed in three major groups: spirilla (spiral shaped), bacilli (rod or oblong shaped), and cocci (round or spherical). Table 5-1 lists some common microorganisms classified by Gram stain and morphology.

To be effective, an antimicrobial agent must have **selective toxicity**, that is, it must act against pathogenic microorganisms without harming host cells. Antibiotics must target structures and functions in pathogenic

IN SIGHT 5-2 Gram Staining

Gram staining is a differential staining procedure, which means it is used to distinguish between two types of bacteria. The Gram stain procedure was developed in 1884 and is still widely used today. A specimen containing the pathogenic microorganism to be identified is swabbed onto a slide and fixed. Crystal violet is applied first, staining all cells a bluish-purple. Gram iodine is then applied to the slide as a mordant—an agent that increases the cell's affinity for the primary stain. The slide is then rinsed with acetone or alcohol, decolorizing the cells. Next, safranin—a red counterstain—is applied. Only cells that were decolorized pick up the red counterstain. The cell walls of gram-positive bacteria do not decolorize, remaining purple. Gram-negative bacteria lose the purple stain during decolorization, so they appear red or reddish-pink after application of safranin.

Table 5-1 PATHOGENIC MICROORGANISMS BY GRAM STAINING AND MORPHOLOGY

Gram-Positive (stain purple)	Gram-Negative (stain pink)
Cocci (round)	
Staphylococcus aureus	*Neisseria meningitidis*
Staphylococcus epidermidis	
Streptococcus pneumoniae	
Streptococcus pyogenes	
Enterococci	
Bacilli (rods)	
Mycobacterium tuberculosis	*Klebsiella pneumoniae*
Listeria monocytogenes	*Bacteroides*
Actinomyces israelii	*Escherichia coli*
	Pseudomonas aeruginosa
	Proteus
	Salmonella
	Serratia
	Haemophilus influenzae

microorganisms that differ from those of host cells. To understand how antimicrobials work, then, we need to know what differences exist between pathogen and host cell structure.

Bacteria are one-celled organisms that don't have a fully developed nucleus. This means they are classified as **prokaryotes**. (A karyote is a nucleus. A *pro*karyote is an early, or "pre" nucleus.) Multicellular organisms, including fungi, plants, and animals, are classified as **eukaryotes** ("true" karyotes). Both prokaryotic and eukaryotic cells have a plasma membrane that encloses the cell and preserves its integrity. Thus it both protects the cell and regulates the movement of materials in and out of the cell. Prokaryotes differ from eukaryotes because they have a cell wall in addition to the plasma membrane. This cell wall provides a potential location for antibiotic therapy (Fig. 5-2).

Prokaryotic cells also differ from eukaryotic cells in the structures responsible for protein synthesis—the *ribosomes.* These tiny structures assemble or synthesize proteins from amino acids. Both prokaryotes and eukaryotes have ribosomes, but prokaryotic ribosomes are smaller than eukaryotic ribosomes. This size difference offers another avenue of action for antibiotics. That is, antibiotics that bind to the smaller bacterial ribosomes do not bind to the larger ribosomes of the eukaryotic host cells.

ANTIMICROBIAL ACTION

MECHANISMS AND TYPES

The actual goal of antibiotic administration is to assist the patient's immune system to subdue the infection, so antibiotic therapy does not have to kill all of the infecting microorganisms. Antimicrobial agents may work against pathogenic microorganisms by five different mechanisms, as summarized in Box 5-1. Some agents, such as cephalosporins, penicillins, vancomycin, and bacitracin, keep bacteria from synthesizing adequate cell walls. They can stop cell walls from forming or inhibit the synthesis process so the walls are too weak to

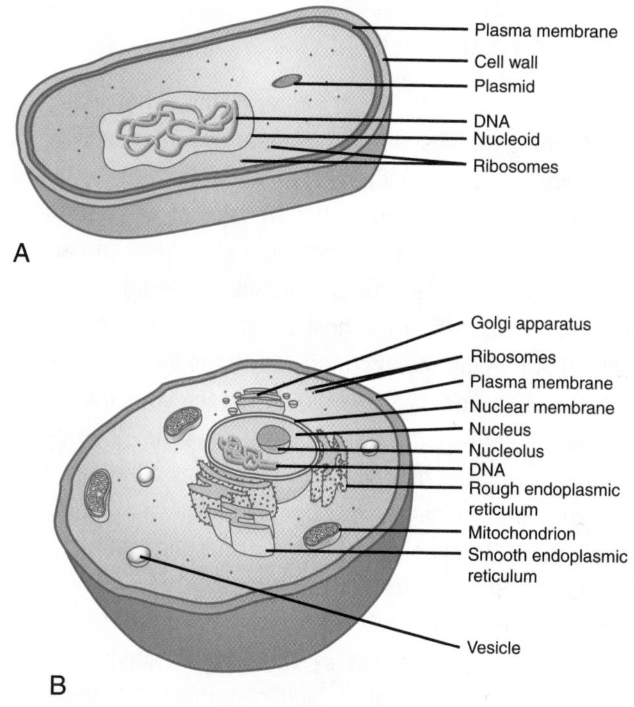

Figure 5-2 Eukaryotic cells are encased in a plasma membrane whereas prokaryotic cells have a cell wall in addition to a plasma membrane: **A,** Prokaryotic cell; **B,** eukaryotic cell.

maintain vital functions. Antibiotics such as aminoglycosides, erythromycins, and tetracyclines interfere with protein synthesis. This means they bind to prokaryotic ribosomes, thus preventing the assembly of critical proteins. Polymyxins and some antifungal agents work by disrupting the bacterial cell membrane, causing leakage of materials necessary for cell function. A few agents, such as fluoroquinolones and some antivirals, inhibit production of the nucleic acids (RNA or DNA) that are necessary for bacterial replication. Still other agents interfere with bacterial cell metabolism. Sulfonamides, for example, take the place of a vital substance needed to produce folic acid.

We classify antimicrobial agents as **bactericidal** or **bacteriostatic**. Bactericidal agents kill bacteria. These include agents such as the aminoglycosides, cephalosporins, and penicillins. Bacteriostatic agents inhibit bacterial growth, relying on the host's own immune system to take over once the pathogenic microorganism is suppressed. Bacteriostatic agents include the erythromycins and tetracyclines. Antimicrobial agents are also classified by their *spectrum* of activity. A *broad-spectrum* antibiotic has a wide range of activity—usually effective against both gram-negative and gram-positive bacteria. *Narrow-spectrum* antibiotics have a smaller range of activity—often effective against only one category of microorganisms, gram-negative or gram-positive. *Limited-spectrum* antibiotics are effective against just one species of microorganism.

ANTIBIOTIC RESISTANCE

Microorganisms multiply rapidly, can mutate, and adapt to new environments and hosts. Unfortunately, certain of these pathogenic microorganisms have also developed an alarming capacity to resist anti-infectives and new "superbugs" exist that are resistant to current antibiotics (Insight 5-3). **Antibiotic resistance** is the ability of some strains of pathogenic microbes to prevent or overcome the activity of antimicrobial agents. Antibiotic resistance mechanisms generally fit into four major categories:

- The microorganism may manufacture microbial enzymes that inactivate the antibiotic.
- The cell membrane may be altered to prevent the antibiotic from entering the cell.
- The target area, such as ribosome, may be altered so that the agent is no longer effective.
- The microorganism may add a substance to the antibiotic, which inhibits its ability to reach its desired binding site.

For example, some bacteria produce an enzyme known as penicillinase. This enzyme breaks down part of the chemical structure of penicillin, making the drug ineffective (Fig. 5-3). Penicillinase is produced by a number of microbes, including two common strains of staphylococci. Thus these microorganisms have become resistant to treatment with penicillin. When antibiotic resistance appears as a bacterial trait, pharmaceutical manufacturers attempt to develop new forms of the antibiotic or to overcome the bacterial resistance

Box 5-1 METHODS OF ANTIMICROBIAL ACTION

Inhibit cell-wall synthesis
Interfere with protein synthesis
Alter cell membrane function
Inhibit production of nucleic acids (RNA or DNA)
Interfere with cell metabolism

INSIGHT 5-3 Developing and Sharing Antibiotic Resistance

Microorganisms grow and divide rapidly, so genetic material (DNA) is constantly replicated (copied). When a microorganism develops a characteristic, such as resistance to an antibiotic, that characteristic is passed to every daughter cell through the DNA. Bacteria obtain antibiotic resistance by mutation (i.e., changes in the sequence of DNA). There are at least four known methods: random mutation, transformation, transduction, and conjugation. Some random mutations are beneficial to the cell, whereas others may be lethal. The addition or deletion of a single nucleotide (the building blocks of DNA) may confer resistance to an antibiotic, a trait crucial to bacterial survival. These changes can cause the production of an enzyme to break down the antibiotic, alter the structure of targeted antibiotic binding sites, or make the bacterial membrane impervious to the agent. Widespread use of antibiotics may actually promote the development and survival of antibiotic-resistant strains of bacteria. Transformation is the transfer of free DNA (probably leaked from destroyed bacteria) into another bacterium. The new DNA is incorporated into the host, transforming the host and subsequent daughter cells by displaying new characteristics, such as antibiotic resistance. Transduction is the transfer of DNA from one bacterium to another bacterium by a viral carrier, known as a *phage* (a virus that infects bacteria). When the virus replicates in the host bacterium, some of the host DNA may be incorporated within the viral capsule (the coat surrounding the virus). When the virus infects another bacterium, the previous host DNA may then be combined with the new host DNA, providing a trait such as antibiotic resistance. Conjugation, or joining together, is another means of transmitting antibiotic resistance. Some types of bacteria have the ability to join and thus share DNA in segments called plasmids. Microorganisms are adept at changing to survive. As scientists develop agents to kill microbial pathogens, these microorganisms change to resist the antimicrobial agent and pass the trait to the next generation. Antimicrobial resistance is one of the most challenging pharmacological problems in medicine today.

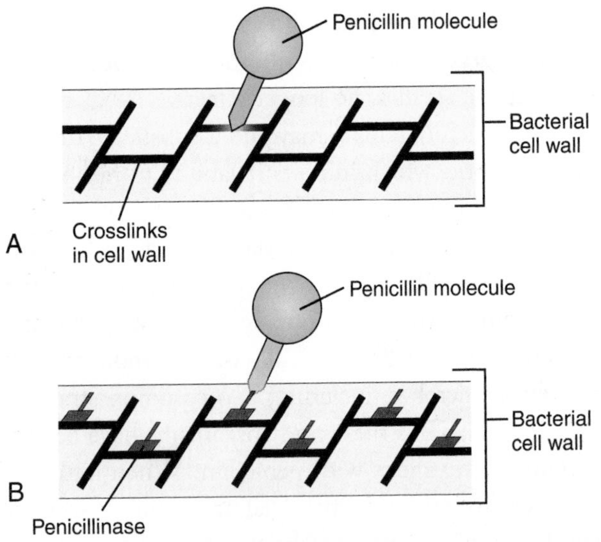

Figure 5-3 Penicillinase inactivates penicillin. A, Penicillin breaks down crosslinks in bacterial cell wall. **B,** Penicillinase breaks down a portion of penicillin structure, inactivating it.

mechanism. For example, methicillin (which is not broken down by penicillinase) was developed to treat some of the gram-positive pathogenic microbes. However, a strain of *S. aureus* developed a resistance to it. This strain is known as **methicillin-resistant *Staphylococcus aureus* (MRSA)**. Methicillin is no longer in clinical use, having been replaced by other penicillins (such as flucloxacillin, dicloxacillin, and oxacillin). However, the term continues to be used to represent *S. aureus* strains resistant to all penicillins. This resistant strain of bacteria is difficult to treat with available agents.

Other pathogens are becoming resistant to more than one antibiotic. Scientists have identified a plasmid (a segment of bacterial DNA) that confers resistance to six antibiotics. Multiple antibiotic resistance is found in a number of pathogens including a strain of the tubercle bacillus (TB), the pathogen that causes tuberculosis. This strain of TB resists several powerful antibiotics, including streptomycin and rifampicin. Similarly, one group of enteric (digestive tract) bacteria has developed resistance to vancomycin. These bacteria are known as **vancomycin-resistant enterococci (VRE)**. Additional strains of antimicrobial-resistant pathogenic microorganisms are being continually identified.

The major cause of concern in antibiotic resistance is that microbes are capable of developing resistance mechanisms to prevent or inactivate agents much faster than scientists can develop new agents. This is no longer a "drug for every bug." It is generally accepted that there will be increasing morbidity and mortality due to infections with resistant microbes for a significant time to come.

The rapid development of resistant pathogens is linked to the misuse of antimicrobial agents. Misuse includes the widespread practice of inappropriate prescribing; as prescribing antibiotics for colds, which are viral infections (not treatable with antibiotics). When normal host bacteria are frequently exposed to antibiotics, they have many opportunities to develop resistance; this means an antibiotic may be ineffective against a subsequent bacterial infection because the resistant trait has pervaded the host's bacterial population. Similarly, when patients do not take necessary antibiotics as prescribed—regularly and in the right dose—they give pathogens a chance to develop resistance. Weaker pathogens may be destroyed, but stronger, mutated strains may survive and reproduce. Another type of misuse is found with antibiotics in the food chain. They are used in agriculture, animal husbandry, even fish farms. These antibiotics find their way into the human body via food and water, and can lead to resistance. For example, a person can become sensitized to a medication through indirect exposure such as by eating beef or chicken from animals given antimicrobials.

ANTIBIOTIC AGENTS

Many antibiotics are available to treat a wide variety of infectious processes. In this text, however, we focus on the few categories of antibiotics commonly used in surgical procedures (Box 5-2). Antibiotics are usually administered intravenously both before and during a surgical procedure for prophylaxis against SSIs. Antibiotics may also be administered topically, often in the form of irrigating solutions or as ointments. Antibiotics are prescribed for postoperative use, to be administered intravenously or orally, to prevent or treat infection. Here, we look at some common categories of antibiotics, together with their origins, mechanisms of action, surgical uses, and bacterial resistance mechanisms against the agent.

CAUTION

Always label your medications on the sterile field. Antibiotics are generally clear liquids and can be easily confused when multiples are used during a procedure.

MAKE IT SIMPLE

Label your antibiotics with the name and strength; this makes it easier for you to remember the specifics of your medications when handing them up to the surgeon.

AMINOGLYCOSIDES

Aminoglycosides, which are derived from various strains of *Actinomyces* bacteria, interfere with protein synthesis by binding to bacterial (prokaryotic) ribosomes. They are bactericidal and relatively narrow in spectrum. Generally active only against aerobic, gram-negative bacteria, aminoglycosides also provide some activity against some gram-positive bacteria such as *Staphylococcus* species, including some methicillin-resistant strains. Otherwise, they are not very active against gram-positive organisms. All aminoglycosides are contraindicated if the patient has a history of hypersensitivity or toxic reactions to any aminoglycoside. Major adverse effects include **nephrotoxicity** and **ototoxicity**; that is, these drugs can damage kidney cells (nephrons) and cause hearing loss. Irreversible deafness, renal failure, and death have been reported after extensive irrigation of surgical fields with aminoglycosides.

Aminoglycosides are poorly absorbed orally, but are almost completely absorbed when applied topically during surgical procedures. Intramuscular and intravenous injections are the most common administration routes for aminoglycosides. However, they may be given orally (preoperatively) when used to reduce the bacteria in the bowel prior to colorectal surgery.

Box 5-2 MAJOR GROUPS OF ANTIBIOTICS

Aminoglycosides
Cephalosporins
Fluoroquinolones
Macrolides
Oxazolidinones
Penicillins
Tetracyclines

Table 5-2 AMINOGLYCOSIDES

Generic Name	Trade Name
Amikacin	Amikin
Gentamicin	Garamycin
Streptomycin	
Tobramycin	Nebcin
Neomycin	Neobiotic
Kanamycin	Kantrex

Aminoglycosides are indicated for short-term treatment of serious infections due to susceptible organisms. Such infections include bacterial septicemia as well as infections of the respiratory tract, bones and joints, central nervous system (meningitis), skin, and soft tissue. Aminoglycosides may also be prescribed for intra-abdominal infections.

Among the drugs in the aminoglycoside category are amikacin (Amikin), gentamicin (Garamycin), streptomycin, tobramycin (Nebcin), neomycin (Neobiotic), and kanamycin (Kantrex), as listed in Table 5-2. Amikacin is often effective even when strains of susceptible organisms are resistant to other aminoglycosides. Gentamicin is available in cream and ointment, ophthalmic solution and ointment, and solution for injection. Streptomycin is used in combination with other agents to treat infections caused by *Mycobacterium tuberculosis* (the tubercle bacillus) and is administered intramuscularly only. Neomycin is too toxic for systemic use, so it is applied topically only.

Bacterial resistance to aminoglycosides is conferred by the production of enzymes that modify the chemical structure of the agent, inactivating it.

CEPHALOSPORINS

Cephalosporins are broad-spectrum antibiotics derived from the fungus *Cephalosporium acremonium.* Cephalosporins are bactericidal, targeting cell-wall synthesis. That is, they block an enzyme needed to strengthen the bacterial cell wall, causing cell lysis (rupture). Cephalosporins are classified into five generations based on different ranges of activity. Each newer generation has greater gram-negative antimicrobial properties and has a longer half-life. This means doses are needed less frequently. The generations are:

First-generation cephalosporins are active against many gram-positive and some gram-negative microbes.

Second-generation cephalosporins are effective on a wider variety of gram-negative, but fewer gram-positive organisms.

Third-generation cephalosporins have a wider range of activity against gram-negative microbes than second-generation agents, but are less effective on gram-positive organisms. They may be used in treating some hospital-acquired infections.

Fourth-generation cephalosporins have an expanded spectrum on both gram-positive and gram-negative microorganisms. Many can cross the blood-brain barrier and are effective against meningitis. They are also used against *Pseudomonas aeruginosa.*

Fifth-generation cephalosporins are on the fast track for approval by the U.S. Food and Drug Administration (FDA) (although the terminology is not universally used at this time). One medication, ceftobiprole (Zeftera, Zevtera), reportedly has powerful antipseudomonal characteristics, potent activity against MRSA and some strains of *Streptococcus* pneumoniae that are resistant to penicillin and according to trials, appears to be less susceptible to development of resistance.

{NOTE} *There are several other fourth-generation cephalosporins listed in the literature; some are not marketed in the United States and have little information available. There are also medications classified under cephalosporins that have progressed far enough in clinical trials and testing to be named, but have not been assigned to a specific generation.*

Cephalosporins are used as prophylaxis in a variety of surgical procedures and are often indicated when patients are allergic to penicillins (although some cross-reactivity is possible). Administration is oral, intramuscular, or intravenous, depending on the particular cephalosporin. Some cephalosporins may be used as topical irrigation solutions in surgery. Bacterial resistance to cephalosporins is conferred by the production of an enzyme (cephalosporinase) that changes the chemical structure of the agent, inactivating it. Table 5-3 lists some of these cephalosporins by generation.

MACROLIDES

Macrolides, which include the erythromycins, are a group of broad-spectrum agents that inhibit bacterial protein synthesis by binding to the prokaryotic ribosomal subunit. Bacteriostatic for most bacteria, macrolides are bactericidal for several gram-positive bacteria such as

Table 5-3 CEPHALOSPORINS

Generic Name	Trade Name
FIRST GENERATION	
Cefazolin	Ancef, Kefzol
Cefadroxil	Duricef, Ultracef
Cefapirin	Cefadryl
Cephalexin	Keflex, Keflet
Cephalothin	Keflin
Cephradine	Anspor, Velosef
SECOND GENERATION	
Cefoxitin	Mefoxin
Cefprozil	Cefzil
Cefaclor	Ceclor, Keflor, Raniclor
Cefmetazole	Zefazone
Cefotetan	Cefotan
Cefuroxime	Ceftin, Zinacef, Zinnat
THIRD GENERATION	
Cefotaxime	Claforan
Cefixime	Suprax
Cefoperazone	Cefobid
Ceftazidime	Fortum, Fortaz
Ceftizoxime	Cefizox
Ceftriaxone	Rocephin
FOURTH GENERATION	
Cefepime	Cepimax, Maxcef, Maxipime
FIFTH GENERATION	
Ceftobiprole*	Zeftera, Zevtera

**Not approved by the U.S. Food and Drug Administration at this time; is available in Canada, Switzerland, and the Ukraine.*

Legionella. This cidal activity is explained by the fact that these antibiotics can penetrate the cell walls of gram-positive organisms. Macrolides may be obtained from isolates of *Streptococcus erythreus* or may be synthesized in the laboratory. Macrolides are only partially metabolized and are excreted almost unchanged

Table 5-4 MACROLIDES

Generic Name	Trade Name
Erythromycin	E-Mycin, ERYC
Erythromycin Ethylsuccinate	EES, EryPed
Azithromycin	Zithromax
Clarithromycin	Biaxin

in bile. Most macrolides are administered orally; however, erythromycin is available in topical ointment and solution, as well as in an ophthalmic ointment for local infections and for newborns to prevent gonococcal infections. Bacterial resistance is primarily due to changes in bacterial cell-wall permeability, such as some strains of *Pseudomonas,* which have developed resistance to erythromycin. Macrolide antibiotics include erythromycin (E-Mycin, ERYC), erythromycin ethylsuccinate (EES, EryPed), azithromycin (Zithromax), and clarithromycin (Biaxin), as listed in Table 5-4.

PENICILLINS

Penicillin was the first of the true antibiotics (Insight 5-4). Originally extracted from the mold *Penicillium,* this antibiotic is now available in many natural and semisynthetic forms effective against a wide variety of gram-positive and gram-negative microbes. Penicillins are bactericidal; they block an enzyme needed to strengthen the bacterial cell wall, so the cell eventually ruptures. Four basic categories of penicillins are available: natural penicillins, penicillinase-resistant penicillins, aminopenicillins, and broad-spectrum penicillins. Penicillins may be given orally or by intramuscular or intravenous injection, depending on the agent. Penicillins are often used preoperatively for prophylaxis against surgical site infections. They may be prescribed before dental or other medical procedures to prevent bacterial infection to the heart (endocarditis) in patients with prosthetic heart valves. Allergic reactions to penicillin are common, with cross-reactivity among penicillins and some of the cephalosporins. Some species of bacteria have become resistant to penicillin by producing *penicillinase,* an enzyme that breaks down the drug molecule, inactivating it. Table 5-5 lists some of the penicillins by category.

Natural penicillins include penicillin G, penicillin V, and benzathine penicillin G. Advantages of natural penicillins are low cost and low toxicity. Natural penicillins

IN SIGHT 5-4 Yesterday and Today: Vaccines and the Discovery of Penicillin

Penicillin, discovered by Alexander Fleming in 1928, was the first of the "wonder drugs" known as antibiotics. It revolutionized medicine by fighting bacterial infections, which, at that time, could be deadly complications to any type of wound. A chain of events led to the development of this wonder drug. Prominent in these events were men who would lay the foundations for modern-day bacteriology and immunology.

The first event took place in 1796, more than a hundred years before Fleming's discovery, when Edward Jenner discovered a way to prevent smallpox. An English country doctor, Jenner had observed that dairy maids who contracted a mild infection known as cowpox did not come down with smallpox. So he injected patients with pus from cowpox sores. These injections immunized his patients against smallpox. He knew nothing about the viruses that caused the disease and even less about the antibodies his inoculations stimulated. But his work was the first step toward understanding the disease-causing mechanisms of certain microorganisms. The next step was taken in the 1850s when a French chemist named Louis Pasteur began work with microscopic organisms called bacteria (or germs). By 1870, he proved that disease in silkworms was caused by germs. He then reasoned that germs could also cause disease in animals, including humans. But as Pasteur was not a physician, he kept his research centered on animals. Next, he worked with chicken cholera. When he accidentally infected some chickens with an old strain of cholera, he found that the inoculated chickens did not develop the full-blown disease. In fact, the chickens recovered from their mild infection and subsequently proved immune to cholera. Pasteur was familiar with Jenner's work, so he deduced that old or weakened germs could be used to protect people from contracting a particular disease. Pasteur called his inoculum a "vaccine," and went on to develop other vaccines for anthrax and rabies.

Another event took place when a highly respected Scottish surgeon named Joseph Lister became interested in Pasteur's work. He reasoned that germs could get into surgical wounds and cause postoperative problems—pus, swelling of tissue, fevers, and (all too often) death. Lister added a surgical link to the chain by using chemicals to kill germs in the operating room. His methods—which included spraying the room with carbolic acid—yielded impressive results. Lister's germ-killing chemicals were the first antiseptics. In the meantime, the chain of events strengthened as a German physician, Robert Koch, worked on the role played by bacteria in disease. It was he who proved that specific germs causing diseases in animals caused them in humans as well. In 1876, Koch identified the germ that causes anthrax, showing that it affects cattle, sheep, and people, too. Then, in 1882, he isolated the tuberculosis germ, a common killer of that time.

In 1893, an influential British Army Medical School physician named Almroth Wright forged another link in the chain when he began the search for a typhoid vaccine. He was concerned that this disease was a serious threat to soldiers in the field. Spread by unsanitary conditions that contaminated water, milk, or food, typhoid killed 10% to 30% of its victims at that time. Wright took six years to produce a successful vaccine. Then the army authorities refused to use it on a large scale. As a result, thousands of British troops contracted typhoid during the Boer War (1899–1902), and more troops died of this disease than from battle wounds. Shocked and bitterly chagrined, Wright resigned from the Medical School and joined the faculty at St. Mary's Hospital in London. There he created a department to study germs, immunity, and vaccines. In 1910, Wright hired a new research worker—Alexander Fleming.

To develop vaccines, Fleming and the staff of Wright's "Inoculation Department" took blood and pus samples from patients with ulcers, boils, and sores. They kept their samples in Petri dishes filled with agar (a gelatin made from seaweed). Fleming was particularly interested in a pus-producing bacterium called *Staphylococcus,* which is commonly found on the skin. He prepared many microscopic slides from these germ samples. One day, Fleming noticed a mold growing on one of his samples. Molds are simple, nonflowering organisms from the fungi family; they can float freely in the air and this one had blown onto his Petri dish by accident. But this "spoiled" sample was special: *Around the area*

INSIGHT 5-4 Yesterday and Today: Vaccines and the Discovery of Penicillin—Cont'd

of the mold was a wide, clean area—no staphylococci. Even beyond this clean area, the staphylococci were dissolving. Clearly, something from the mold was killing the disease-causing germs. Fleming found out the killer mold was a common one, often found on ripened cheese, stale bread, and rotting fruit. It was from the group of molds called *penicillia,* so Fleming named his discovery "penicillin." However, when he announced his discovery to the rest of the department, no one was impressed. Even Wright showed little enthusiasm. Fortunately, Fleming continued his research, growing more of the mold and testing it on a variety of bacteria. Some were not affected, but a number of them were destroyed. Among those affected were the germs that cause pneumonia, scarlet fever, meningitis, diphtheria, and gonorrhea. Then Fleming took the next step. He went on to test the mold on human blood and found it did not kill white blood cells. He successfully used it topically on a lab assistant to cure an eye infection. But Fleming was no chemist, so he had problems extracting and purifying the mold. This left him believing the new medicine was good for topical use only. When he presented a paper on penicillin to a medical audience in 1929, he was met with indifference. Fleming's interest waned and his work was directed along other paths.

Ten years later, a team of Oxford medical researchers picked up where Fleming left off. The Oxford team took samples of penicillin to the United States, sought backing, and found manufacturers for the new antibiotic. The mass production of this wonder drug in the United States was to save millions of Allied soldiers' lives during World War II. And after the war, penicillin and its "wonder-full" derivatives were to change the history of medicine forever.

display a relatively narrow spectrum of action, primarily against gram-positive microbes.

Penicillinase-resistant penicillins are semisynthetics that include flucloxacillin, cloxacillin, dicloxacillin, nafcillin, and oxacillin. This class of penicillins was developed to be effective against strains of bacteria that produce penicillinase. However, some bacteria have developed a means of resistance against penicillinase-resistant penicillins. MRSA is actually resistant to all penicillinase-resistant penicillins.

Aminopenicillins have been chemically altered by adding an amino group, which makes them effective against gram-negative species, but they are not penicillinase resistant. These semisynthetics include ampicillin, amoxicillin, and bacampicillin.

Broad-spectrum penicillins include mezlocillin, piperacillin, and ticarcillin. Broad-spectrum penicillins are semisynthetics that have been chemically altered to be effective against strains of gram-negative microbes.

TETRACYCLINES

Tetracyclines were the first broad-spectrum antibiotics, originally obtained from cultures of *Streptomyces.* Bacteriostatic in action against many gram-positive and gram-negative bacteria, tetracyclines bind to the bacterial ribosomal subunit, interfering with protein synthesis. They also exhibit some action on bacterial cell membranes, causing leakage. Many common bacteria have developed resistance to tetracyclines, so their use is now limited. They are used primarily to treat acne and rickettsial infections. Resistance factors are carried in plasmids (pieces of bacterial DNA), which are widely distributed among many bacteria. Tetracycline antibiotics are listed in Table 5-6.

Tetracycline hydrochloride is administered orally, as no parenteral form is available. Minocycline may be administered intravenously if the oral route is not feasible. Oxytetracycline (Terramycin) may be administered intramuscularly if the oral route is not feasible; it is also available in an ophthalmic ointment combined with polymyxin B sulfate. Doxycycline may be administered orally or intravenously. Chlortetracycline hydrochloride is available only in ophthalmic and topical ointment. In septoplasty or tympanoplasty, packing strips may be saturated with chlortetracycline hydrochloride and used as dressings.

OXAZOLIDINONES

Oxazolidinones are an entirely new class of synthetic antibiotics. The only available agent in this class is linezolid (Zyvox). Zyvox inhibits bacterial protein synthesis by an entirely different mechanism of action from other

Table 5-5 PENICILLINS

Generic Name	Trade Name
NATURAL PENICILLINS	
Penicillin G	Pentids, Pfizerpen
Benzathine penicillin G	Bicillin L-A, Permapen
Penicillin V	Pen-Vee K, V-cillin K
PENICILLINASE-RESISTANT PENICILLINS	
Flucloxacillin	Flopen, Floxapen
Cloxacillin	Cloxapen
Dicloxacillin	Dycill, Pathocil
Nafcillin	Nafcil, Unipen
Oxacillin	Bactocill
AMINOPENICILLINS (NOT PENICILLINASE-RESISTANT)	
Ampicillin	Omnipen
Amoxicillin	Amoxil, Polymox
Bacampicillin	Penglobe, Spectrobid
BROAD-SPECTRUM PENICILLINS	
Mezlocillin	Mezlin
Piperacillin	Pipracil
Ticarcillin	Ticar

Table 5-6 TETRACYCLINES

Generic Name	Trade Name
Tetracycline Hydrochloride	Achromycin-V, Sumycin
Minocycline	Minocin
Oxytetracycline	Terramycin
Doxycycline	Vibramycin
Chlortetracycline Hydrochloride	Aureomycin

agents, targeting a specific ribosomal subunit. It is administered intravenously or orally and is used to treat infections caused by MRSA, VRE, and some streptococci. It is bacteriostatic against enterococci and staphylococci, and bactericidal against the majority of streptococci.

Table 5-7 OXAZOLIDINONES AND FLUOROQUINOLONES

Generic Name	Trade Name
OXAZOLIDINONE	
Linezolid	Zyvox
FLUOROQUINOLONES	
First Generation	
Cinoxacin	Cinobac
Second Generation	
Ciprofloxacin	Cipro
Ofloxacin	Floxin
Norfloxacin	Noroxin
Enoxacin	Penetrex
Third Generation	
Levofloxacin	Levaquin
Fourth Generation	
Trovafloxacin	Trovan

Resistance to linezolid is conferred by altering the site of action (ribosomal subunit) (Table 5-7).

FLUOROQUINOLONES

Fluoroquinolones are a category of antibiotics that inhibit DNA-gyrase, a protein necessary for bacterial replication. They are classified as first, second, third, and fourth generation. Fluoroquinolone antibiotics have a relatively low toxicity and a broad spectrum of activity against both gram-positive and gram-negative aerobes, including *Pseudomonas.* They are given orally or intravenously for systemic infections or for urinary tract infections (UTIs), and are also formulated for ophthalmic use. Agents include cinoxacin (Cinobac), ciprofloxacin (Cipro), ofloxacin (Floxin), norfloxacin (Noroxin), enoxacin (Penetrex), levofloxacin (Levaquin), and trovafloxacin (Trovan). See Table 5-7.

MISCELLANEOUS ANTIBIOTICS

Many other antibiotics are available for prophylaxis and treatment of infections caused by susceptible microorganisms, as listed in Table 5-8. Miscellaneous agents presented in this chapter include sulfonamides, several individual agents, and three combination agents.

Table 5-8 INDIVIDUAL AND COMBINATION AGENTS

Generic Name	Trade Name
SULFONAMIDES	
Silver sulfadiazine	Silvadene
Sulfisoxazole	Gantrisin
Sulfamethoxazole	Gantanol
Sulfasalazine	Azulfidine
Sulfacetamide sodium	Sodium Sulamyd
Sulfamethoxazole with trimethoprim	Bactrim, Septra
INDIVIDUAL AGENTS	
Aztreonam	Azactam
Chloramphenicol	Chloromycetin
Clindamycin	Cleocin
Imipenem	Primaxin
Metronidazole	Flagyl
Polymyxin B sulfate	Aerosporin
Vancomycin	Vanocin
COMBINATION AGENTS	
	Coly-Mycin S
	Cortisporin
	Neosporin

Sulfonamides

Sulfonamides are not really antibiotics; they are antimicrobials, more commonly known as sulfa drugs. Sulfonamides are laboratory-synthesized chemicals that interfere with cell metabolism by inhibiting bacterial synthesis of folic acid. Introduced in 1935 by Gerhard Domagk, sulfonamides are the oldest of the chemotherapeutic agents. They are in limited use today (owing to increasing microbial resistance) but are still prescribed for nonobstructive UTIs, severe burns, and superficial eye infections. Sulfonamides are administered orally, topically, and occasionally intravenously. Resistance is conferred by altering bacterial cell-wall permeability, thus preventing the agent from entering the bacterium. Examples of sulfonamides include silver sulfadiazine, sulfisoxazole, sulfamethoxazole, sulfasalazine, and sulfacetamide sodium. Sulfamethoxazole is also combined with trimethoprim (another antibacterial) and is available as Bactrim and Septra (see Table 5-8).

Individual Agents

Aztreonam (Azactam) is the first drug in a new class of antibacterials called monobactams. Aztreonam is the totally synthetic form of an antibiotic originally isolated from *Chromobacterium violaceum.* It inhibits bacterial cell-wall synthesis and has a wide spectrum of cidal activity against gram-negative aerobic pathogens. It is available for intramuscular or intravenous injection.

Chloramphenicol (Chloromycetin) is the synthetic form of an antibiotic originally isolated from *Streptomyces venezuelae,* and is structurally different from all other antibiotics. It is bacteriostatic, inhibiting protein synthesis, with a wide range of activity against gram-positive and gram-negative microbes. Chloramphenicol has potential for serious toxicity, so it is used only when less hazardous antibiotics are ineffective. Adverse effects include bone marrow depression and various blood disorders; consequently, chloramphenicol is inappropriate for prophylaxis. Chloramphenicol may be taken orally or injected intravenously; it is also available as a topical ointment, an otic solution, and as an ophthalmic solution and ointment.

Clindamycin (Cleocin) is the synthetic analogue of the natural antibiotic lincomycin. It is active against gram-positive and anaerobic bacteria. It inhibits protein synthesis by binding to the bacterial ribosomes. Used to treat infections in patients who are allergic to penicillin, clindamycin may be administered orally or intravenously. Its high affinity for bone makes it effective in the treatment of osteomyelitis. In addition, clindamycin may be used to treat serious respiratory, pelvic, and intra-abdominal infections caused by anaerobic bacteria. Resistance is obtained by changes in the ribosomal structure, which prevents the agent from binding.

Imipenem (Primaxin) has the widest spectrum of activity of all antibiotics currently available. It works by inhibiting bacterial cell-wall synthesis and is available in forms suitable for intramuscular and intravenous administration. Primaxin is indicated only for serious infections, especially **polymicrobic infections** (caused by several different microbes) and infections caused by bacteria resistant to other antibiotics.

Metronidazole (Flagyl) is a synthetic antibiotic intended for intravenous administration. It is bactericidal against anaerobic gram-positive and gram-negative bacilli, inhibiting both DNA and RNA synthesis. Often used for prophylaxis in colorectal procedures when contamination from enteric anaerobic bacteria is possible, Flagyl is also used to treat postoperative SSIs caused by susceptible anaerobic bacteria. Bacterial resistance is accomplished by the production of enzymes and by changes in cell membrane permeability.

Bacitracin is an antibacterial polypeptide derived from the strain of bacterium *Bacillus subtilis* that interferes with bacterial cell-wall synthesis. It is effective against a wide range of gram-positive and a few gram-negative microorganisms. It has similar properties to penicillin and is effective against staphylococci and streptococci. Bacitracin is used in combination with other medications such as polymyxin B in a topical ointment form to treat ophthalmic and other types of infections. It is also used in doses of 50,000 units to 500 or 1000 mL of normal saline for antibiotic irrigation solution, or to soak mesh for hernia repair. Polymyxin B sulfate (Poly-Rx) is a bactericidal antibiotic effective against nearly all species of gram-negative bacilli. It works against bacteria by increasing the permeability of the cell membrane. Polymyxin B sulfate is available in powder form, which is reconstituted for topical, intravenous, or intramuscular administration. It is measured in units rather than milligrams. Resistance is rare.

Vancomycin (Vancocin) is a glycopeptide antibiotic derived from *Amycolatopsis orientalis* and used to treat infections caused by MRSA. It is bactericidal, only against gram-positive bacteria, blocking a reaction needed to form crosslinks in the cell wall. Vancomycin also alters cell-membrane permeability and interferes with RNA synthesis. It is administered intravenously and is active against staphylococci, streptococci, and enterococci. Bacterial resistance occurs by altering the bacterial binding site. Due to its toxicity, vancomycin use is restricted to the critically ill patient.

Silver preparations are antiseptics used on applicator sticks as silver nitrate to cauterize tissue; for example, on granulation tissue around a stoma. Silver sulfadiazine (Silvadene) comes as a cream and is used for the treatment and prevention of wound infections in patients with second- and third-degree burns. It is effective against a variety of bacteria and yeast.

Combination Agents

Several antibiotics are combined with other drugs and used to treat specific conditions. Coly-Mycin S Otic is a combination drug used topically to treat bacterial infections of the external auditory canal. It is often administered in surgery after myringotomy and insertion of pressure equalization (PE) tubes. Coly-Mycin contains two bactericidal antibiotics, colistin and neomycin, in combination with hydrocortisone (a corticosteroid used as an anti-inflammatory agent).

Cortisporin otic suspension is a drug used topically when an anti-inflammatory agent is needed in combination with an antibiotic. It contains neomycin and polymyxin B sulfate with hydrocortisone. Because Cortisporin is in suspension, it must be shaken prior to administration to distribute the drug particles evenly. It is not intended for injection. Cortisporin is also available combined with bacitracin in an ointment.

MAKE IT SIMPLE

Otic preparations are intended for use in the ear.
Ophthalmic preparations are intended for use in the eye.

Neosporin G.U. Irrigant is a combination of neomycin and polymyxin B sulfate. It is used as a topical bladder irrigant when the presence of an indwelling urinary catheter increases the risk of bladder infection.

ADVANCED PRACTICES FOR THE SURGICAL FIRST ASSISTANT

CHAPTER 5—Antibiotics

Key Terms

- HAI
- peak and trough
- sepsis
- superinfection
- surgical site infections (SSIs)

ANTIBIOTIC THERAPY

Advanced practitioners functioning as surgical first assistants will encounter the use of antibiotic therapy for the treatment and prevention of infections in the surgical patient. Preoperative, intraoperative, and postoperative care of the surgical patient has expanded from the hospital setting to include outpatient facilities, surgery centers, specialty clinics, nursing homes, and even long care facilities. Thus, the term for a hospital-acquired infection (nosocomial) has been expanded to healthcare-associated infection (**HAI**). HAI is defined by the Centers for Disease Control and Prevention (CDC) as a localized or systemic condition that results from an adverse reaction to infection (infectious agents or toxins), and was not present, or incubating, at the time of admission. So, an infection is considered a HAI if it is not related to the admitting diagnosis or develops within 48 hours after admission. This is described in the National Nosocomial Infection Surveillance System (NNIS) established by the CDC to track, investigate, and help prevent nosocomial infections. Antibiotics are administered for the treatment of **sepsis**, prevention of **surgical site infections (SSIs),** and for intra-operative wound irrigation. Because there are many classifications of antibiotics, the selection of the appropriate medication relies on several factors. For any specific infection, however, there is usually one antibiotic that research determines to be superior. Some of the factors for medication selection include patient allergy, inability of the antibiotic to reach the site of infection, patient susceptibility to the medication's toxicity, medication efficacy, and medication's spectrum. Although the physician selects the appropriate antibiotic, the surgical first assistant must have knowledge of antibiotic use and actions to ensure that the patient receives the correct dosage of antibiotic at the right time. The surgical first assistant acts as another line of defense against medication errors and adverse reactions caused by antibiotic therapy.

ANTIBIOTIC RESISTANCE

The main reason for the development of drug-resistant bacteria is the misuse of antimicrobial agents. This misuse includes inept prescribing and inappropriate use, failure to complete the full course of medication, administering antibacterial agents to treat viral infections (such as influenza), antibiotics in the food chain, and not following all guidelines established to prevent the spread of infections in patient care settings. Microbial resistance is bacteria's ability to overcome the bactericidal effects of an antibiotic. Resistance traits are encoded into the bacteria's genes and can be transmitted to other bacteria. Microorganisms have the ability to proliferate and mutate rapidly, and can adapt to new environments and hosts. Because of these abilities, microorganisms can "learn" to withstand the effects of antibiotics and new superbugs exist. Multidrug resistance is a serious problem that has spread out of the hospital environment and into the community. This acquired resistance can render currently effective antibiotics useless. In 2008, these resistant pathogens were dubbed the "ESKAPE" bacteria that include: *Enterococcus faecium*, *Staphylococcus aureus*, *Klebsiella pneumoniae*, *Acinetobacter baumannii*, *Pseudomonas aeruginosa*, and *Enterobacter* species. Added to this list are *Escherichia coli* and *M. tuberculosis*. Unfortunately, there is an ever-widening gap between the number of these deadly antibiotic-resistant microorganisms and new, effective drugs to treat them. Few of the right type of new antibiotics are completing the drug development requirements of the FDA, and added to this, companies are not spending the money to develop antibiotics that are used short-term and are expensive to produce. This is unlikely to change in the near future and the result is antibiotic development not keeping pace with microbial resistance.

A **superinfection** is an additional infection that appears during the course of antibiotic treatment of a primary infection. An example is a yeast infection that occurs during treatment of bacterial pneumonia with penicillin. Broad-spectrum antibiotics (such as tetracyclines and penicillins) kill off more normal flora and so set the stage for superinfections. They may occur if the antibiotic dosage was too large for the patient (i.e., patient's size/weight), or by the drug's inhibition or alteration of the normal flora within the body, which allows the secondary infection to occur.

NEW ANTIBIOTICS

A new class of antibiotics, called glycylcyclines, was developed in the 1990s to treat bacteria that had become resistant to tetracyclines. They were derived by making modifications to tetracyclines and have similar mechanisms of action and side effects. Currently there is one glycylcycline available for clinical use, tigecycline (Tygacil). Another antibiotic recently approved by the FDA is telavancin (Vibativ), a synthetic derivative of vancomycin. Like vancomycin, telavancin inhibits cell-wall synthesis and disrupts bacterial membranes. It is used in the treatment of complicated skin and skin structure infections. In 2007, the FDA approved doripenem (Doribax), an ultra–broad spectrum injectable antibiotic for the treatment of complex abdominal infections, UTIs including kidney infections that have progressed into the bloodstream, and pneumonia within the hospital setting. While these antibiotics were developed to treat the current drug-resistant microbes, they are potent medications that many patients can't tolerate.

PEAK AND TROUGH

Antibiotic medications rely on their ability to penetrate the bacteria cell wall and bind with sufficient concentration levels to be effective. The concentration levels depend on the half-life and elimination of the medication. When maintaining a therapeutic dosage of antibiotics, it is important to understand **peak and trough** levels. The time when the medication is at the highest plasma concentration is referred to as its peak level. This peak level depends on the absorption rate and the route of administration. Intravenous administered medications take much less time to reach peak levels than do oral medications. The point of time when the medication is at the lowest level of plasma concentration is referred to as the trough level. Ideally, to maintain a therapeutic response an antibiotic would be redosed before it reaches trough level.

ASSISTANT *ADVICE*

Check the dosage and timing of the antibiotic ordered for the patient. Be sure the next doses are available in the surgical suite if required during the procedure. Also check with the surgeon concerning any extra bolus of medication that may be needed, and have it available.

SEPSIS

Antibiotic therapy is essential for the treatment of sepsis. Sepsis is defined as a systemic inflammatory response to the presence of pus-forming bacteria or their toxins in the blood or tissues. It is a life-threatening syndrome that is the leading cause of death in intensive care units, usually resulting from an overwhelming infection. The patient's response to sepsis may be low and short term, to critical and long term or demise. Sepsis can be divided into several categories according to symptoms and certain criteria. Each category has an associated mortality rate (Table A). The clinical management of sepsis is a multifocal approach that includes resuscitation, organ system support, and control of the infection. The control of infection combines the use of antibiotics in addition to drainage or débridement of involved tissues. Septic patients will be on an antibiotic therapy and it is imperative that therapy be continued throughout the surgical procedure.

Table A Associated Mortality Rates of Sepsis

Definition	Symptoms and Criteria	Mortality Rate
Systemic inflammatory response syndrome (SIRS)	Two or more of the following: temperature $\leq 36°$ C or $\geq 38°$ C heart rate $\geq$ 90 bpm respirations $\geq$ 20 breaths/min or $Paco_2 < 32$mm of Hg WBC $\geq$ 12,000 or $\leq$ 4,000 or 10% immature cells	3%–17% depending on the number of symptoms
Sepsis	SIRS with the addition of an infection site confirmed by culture (positive blood cultures are not necessary)	16%
Severe sepsis	Sepsis plus organ dysfunction and tissue hypoperfusion or hypotension	20%
Septic shock	Hypotension induced by sepsis despite fluid bolus or organ and tissue hypoperfusion	46%*

** **Note:** Sources are quoting some studies that mortality rates may be as high as 70%.*

{NOTE} *The antibiotic ordered initially for infection treatment may have been selected because of the Gram stain and the source of the infection. The exact microorganism may not have been isolated prior to the time of surgery. Aerobic and anaerobic cultures will be taken during the procedure. The results of these cultures will help isolate the pathogens, and the antibiotic may be changed to target these specific microorganisms.*

PREOPERATIVE ANTIBIOTIC PROPHYLAXIS

The use of prophylactic antibiotics to prevent SSIs has proved beneficial in certain procedures. However, in other situations these antibiotics have no benefit to the patient. Prophylactic antibiotics may be beneficial when used before implant procedures and clean-contaminated (surgical wound classification category 3) surgical wounds (category IA). They have no benefit in clean surgical wounds (incised, non-infected) or contaminated wounds. They may be used on the patient with congenital or valvular heart disease or who has had rheumatic fever. This is to reduce the about of normal flora and thus decreasing the chance of endocarditis from bacteria. Another indication for preoperative antibiotics is neutropenia (low neutrophil counts) that could increase the risk for infection. The risk of side effects, creating superinfections, and adverse reactions must be carefully weighed against the advantages of administering prophylactic antibiotics in each patient. Infants and the elderly have metabolisms and excretion that differ from normal adult patients, so this puts them at higher risk for drug toxicity, because antibiotics can accumulate to toxic levels in their blood. Women who are pregnant or lactating pose problems with antibiotic therapy, because some drugs can cross the placenta and can enter into breast milk.

Errors that occur most during prophylactic antibiotic therapy concern the timing of administration and the duration of the therapy. In general, preoperative antibiotics should be administered within 30 minutes before incision and be continued not more than 24 hours postoperatively.

The administration of the initial dose of preoperative antibiotics presents a challenge to health care providers in today's fast-paced systems. Patients may arrive at the facility within one hour of their scheduled procedure. Most facilities will have a standard protocol for starting pre-operative antibiotics. The surgical first assistant must be familiar with the protocol and make sure that it is followed at all times. Many surgeons are requiring the administration of the antibiotic to the patent when he or she arrives in the surgical suite to ensure proper timing of anti-infective coverage. The choice of antibiotic will depend on the type, classification, and site of the procedure. The medication will cover against any natural flora in the surgical field. *Staphylococcus aureus* and *Staphylococcus epidermidis* cause most surgical wound infections. Administering a first-generation cephalosporin such as cefazolin can cover these microorganisms. Another indicator of antibiotic choice is any allergies the patient may have. In patients with an allergy to penicillin, the surgeon may prescribe clindamycin or, in some cases, vancomycin.

INTRAOPERATIVE ANTIBIOTIC WOUND IRRIGATION

Many surgeons choose to use an antibiotic agent in the irrigation fluid to help prevent surgical site infections. This usually will be the final irrigation before closure of the wound. The antibiotic of choice, such as Ancef, is mixed in the appropriate volume of irrigation fluid (usually 500 mL). To prevent the irrigation solution from cooling, this should not be mixed in advance. When the irrigation solution is placed into the wound it should remain a short period of time to allow the antibiotic to absorb into the tissues. (Refer to Chapter 11 for more information on irrigation fluids.)

CAUTION

Cool temperature irrigation fluid may adversely affect the patient's core body temperature.

ANTIVIRALS AND ANTIFUNGALS

Antibacterials (antibiotics) are the more commonly used antimicrobial agents in surgery. However, the surgical first assistant should have a basic knowledge of other types of antimicrobials. Two of these are antivirals and antifungals. The identification of viral infections, including those that affect the surgical team members, has brought about the development of new drugs. Antivirals are a class of drugs that specifically treat viral infections, and like antibiotics, specific antivirals are used to treat specific infections. They work by inhibiting the pathogen's ability to reproduce rather than destroying it. Viruses use the host's cells to replicate, and this makes it difficult to develop drugs that will harm the virus without harming the host. Viral infections include HIV, the herpes virus, hepatitis B and C, and influenza B and C. (Viral drugs used for treatment of HIV can be found in Chapter 2 under Federal Agencies). A breakthrough in using antivirals for cancer treatment has been established with the human papillomavirus vaccine (HPV) for cervical cancer. Many cancers could have a viral origin, but research is just now finding the few that have been implicated as actually causing human cancers.

Antifungals are drugs used to treat fungal infections such as athlete's foot, candidiasis (thrush), and types of dermatophyte infections such as ringworm. Both fungal and human cells are eukaryotes and similar on the molecular level. This makes it difficult to develop antifungals that will not harm the host cells. Antifungal drugs have the potential for serious side effects such as liver damage and anaphylaxis if not used properly.

Advanced Practices Bibliography

Baue AE, et al: Systemic inflammatory response syndrome (SIRS), multiple organ dysfunction syndrome (MODS), multiple organ failure (MOF): are we winning the battle? *Shock* 10(2), August 1998.

Rangel-Frausto MS, et al: The natural history of systemic inflammatory response syndrome (SIRS), *JAMA* 273(2), 1995.

Snyder K, Keegan C: *Pharmacology for the surgical technologist,* ed 2, St. Louis, 2009, Saunders/Elsevier.

Advanced Practices Internet Resources

Answers.com, antiviral drugs: *www.answers.com/topic/antiviral-drug*

Advanced Practices: Learning the Language (Key Terms)

Using your textbook or a standard medical dictionary, look up and write the definitions of each term.

- peak and trough
- sepsis
- SSI
- superinfection

Advanced Practices: Review Questions

1. List three factors to consider when choosing an appropriate antibiotic.

2. The time when a medication is at the highest plasma concentration is referred to as the ______________________________.

3. The decay and putrefaction of living tissue from an overwhelming infection is called

A. Dehydration
B. Sepsis
C. Sciatica
D. Antibiotic resistance

4. How long before a surgical procedure should preoperative prophylactic antibiotics be administered?

A. 10 minutes
B. 30 minutes
C. 1 hour
D. 2 hours

5. An antibiotic commonly used within the sterile field is ______________________________ .

KEY CONCEPTS

- Antibiotics are antimicrobial agents used in surgery for prophylaxis against wound infections. They are also given to treat postoperative surgical site infections. Despite meticulous aseptic technique, SSIs may arise when pathogenic microorganisms are transmitted to a susceptible host. When that happens, the causative microbe will be identified, and tested for antibiotic sensitivity before a definitive course of antibiotic therapy is selected.
- Antibiotics work against microbes in five major ways. The agent may inhibit bacterial cell-wall synthesis, impede protein synthesis, interfere with nucleic acid (RNA or DNA) synthesis, alter bacterial cell-wall function, or disrupt bacterial cell metabolism. Antibiotics may be bacteriostatic or bactericidal and may have a broad, narrow, or limited spectrum of activity. Some bacteria have developed resistance to some leading antibiotics, making treatment protocols difficult. Antibiotics may be administered orally, intramuscularly, intravenously, or topically, depending on the agent.
- Major categories of antibiotics include aminoglycosides, cephalosporins, fluoroquinolones, macrolides (erythromycins), oxazolidinones, penicillins, and tetracyclines. Several other categories of antibacterials are in use today, as well as several unique agents. Surgical technologists should become familiar with antibiotics used routinely during surgery.

Bibliography

Finn OJ, Edwards RP: Human Papillomavirus vaccine for cancer prevention, *N Engl J Med* 361(19):1899–1901, 2009.

Fulcher E, Fulcher R, Soto C: *Pharmacology principles and applications*, ed 2, 2009, Saunders/Elsevier.

Hopper T: *Mosby's pharmacy technician principles and practice*, St. Louis, 2004, Saunders.

Jensen SC, Peppers MP: *Pharmacology and drug administration for imaging technologists,* ed 2, St. Louis, 2006, Mosby/Elsevier.

Moscou K, Snipe K: *Pharmacology for pharmacy technicians*, St. Louis, 2009, Mosby/Elsevier.

Price P, Frey K: *Microbiology for surgical technologists*, Clifton Park, NY, 2003, Thomson-Delmar Learning.

Internet Resources

Antibiotics, Antibacterial Agents: http://users.rcn.com/jkimball.ma.ultranet/BiologyPages/A/Antibiotics.html.

Caring for the Men, The History of Civil War Medicine: www.civilwarhome.com/medicinehistory.htm.

Centers for Disease Control and Prevention: *Get Smart: Know When Antibiotics Work.* www.cdc.gov/getsmart.

Discovery Health: *How Do Antibiotics Work?* www.howstuffworks.com/question88.htm.

Drugdevelopment-technology.com: *Ceftobiprole - Injectable Anti-MRSA Cephalosporin Antibiotic.* www.drugdevelopment-technology.com/projects/ceftobiprole/.

Drugs.com: *Silvadene Cream 1%.* www.drugs.com/pdr/silvadene-cream-1.html.

Baci-IM. www.drugs.com/mtm/baci-IM-injection.html.

www.britannica.com/EBchecked/topic/4401/actinomycete.

Fischinger PJ: Prospects for reducing virus-associated human cancers by antiviral vaccines, *J Natl Cancer Inst Monogr* (12):109–114, 1992. www.ncbi.nlm.nih.gov/pubmed/1616793.

The Free Dictionary: *Bacitracin.* www.medical-dictionary.thefreedictionary.com/bacitracin.

Howard Hughes Medical Institute's BioInteractive: *Antibiotics Attack.* www.hhmi.org/biointeractive/Antibiotics_Attack/frameset.html.

Infectious Disease News: *Ceftobiprole Medocaril: The New Generation of Cephalosporins.* www.infectiousdiseasenews.com/article.aspx?id=3893.

Lewis and Clark Trail: *Medicine at the Turn of the Nineteenth Century.* www.lewisandclarktrail.com/medical.htm.

MedlinePlus: *Antibiotics.* www.nlm.nih.gov/medlineplus/antibiotics.html.

Neonatal conjunctivitis. www.nlm.nih.gov/medlineplus/ency/article/001606.htm.

Molecular Expressions, Antibiotics: http://micro.magnet.fsu.edu/micro/gallery/pharm/antibiotic/antibiotic.html.

University of Maryland Medical Center: *Antibiotics.* www.umm.edu/altmed/ConsDrugs/DrugCats/Antibiotics.html.

Wikipedia: *Antibiotic Resistance.* http://en.wikipedia.org/wiki/Antibiotic_resistance.

Dermatophyte. http://en.wikipedia.org/wiki/Dermatophyte.

Meticillin. http://en.wikipedia.org/wiki/Meticillin.

World Health Organization: *Patient Safety, Safe Surgery Saves Lives*, www.who.int/patientsafety/safesurgery/en/.

LEARNING THE LANGUAGE (KEY TERMS)

Using your textbook or a standard medical dictionary, look up and write the definitions of each term.

antibiotic resistance
bactericidal
bacteriostatic
culture and sensitivity (C&S)
endogenous
eukaryotes
exogenous
Gram staining
morphology
MRSA
nephrotoxicity
ototoxicity
polymicrobic infections
prokaryotes
prophylaxis
selective toxicity
VRE

REVIEW QUESTIONS

1. What does MRSA stand for? VRE? Why are these important in surgery?
2. Why are antibiotics administered in surgery?
3. Which test is used to identify the organism that causes TB?
4. What does a C&S reveal?
5. Why would a Gram stain be ordered during surgery?
6. How do antibiotics work?
7. What is the difference between bactericidal and bacteriostatic?
8. Why is antimicrobial resistance a problem in surgery?
9. How are antibiotics administered in surgery?
10. Have you served as a scrubbed surgical technologist or in a procedure when an antibiotic was administered? Which antibiotic was used? What category did the agent belong in? How was it administered?

CRITICAL THINKING

Scenario 1

Mrs. Chacon is a 55-year-old female admitted to surgery for insertion of a venous access catheter. The chart indicates that she has an allergy to cefazolin (Ancef) and the preference card lists a standing order for cephalothin (Keflin) 1 g mixed with 30 cc of NaCl for topical irrigation.

1. Is this medication order of concern? Explain why or why not.
2. How should you handle this situation to ensure the patient's safety?

Scenario 2

Mr. Fayed is a 33-year-old male who cut his hand while working in the garden 10 days ago. He was initially treated in the emergency room, where the wound was irrigated and closed. He was sent home with a prescription for piperacillin (Pipracil), which he has taken as instructed. The wound remains infected, so he is admitted to surgery for incision and drainage of the wound. Swabs are taken for routine and fungal C&S, because the surgeon suspects the infectious agent may be a soil-based fungus.

1. How is a fungus different from bacteria?
2. Why wouldn't the antibiotic work on a fungal infection?

CHAPTER 6

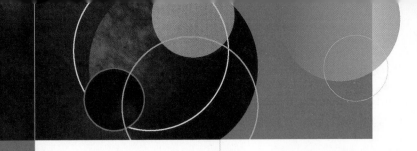

Diagnostic Agents

OBJECTIVES *After completing this chapter, you should be able to:*

1. Define contrast media, dyes, and staining agents.
2. Describe how contrast media are used in radiographic studies in surgery and give examples.
3. Describe how dyes are used in surgery and give examples.
4. Describe how staining agents are used in surgery and give examples.

KEY TERMS

contraindicated
dye
hypersensitivity
radiopaque
radiopaque contrast media (ROCM)
staining agent

Surgery is a discipline that depends on visualizing the anatomy and the physiological functioning of body organs and systems. It is very dependent on techniques that give insight into the position, activity, and health of these structures. Since the discovery of x-rays at the turn of the 19th century by Carl Roentgen, imaging (or radiographic testing) has played a central role in the management of patients, and this guidance is used for both diagnosis and treatment. Pharmacologic agents called **radiopaque contrast media (ROCM)** are used in certain diagnostic radiographic tests. To perform these tests, a contrast medium is injected into the circulatory system or instilled into a body cavity; then a radiograph is taken. Many contrast media contain iodine or barium, which are **radiopaque**, the opposite of *radiotransparent.* Radiopaque means the substance does not permit the x-rays to pass through. Thus anatomic structures that take up iodine or barium appear opaque on radiographic examination; this means that such pathologic conditions as tumors, stones, or blockages become visible. In surgery, these agents are often referred to *incorrectly* as dyes.

Dyes are solutions that color or mark tissue for identification. Dyes may be used to mark skin incisions, delineate normal tissue planes, or enhance visualization of certain anatomic structures during a surgical procedure. Dyes may be applied topically, injected into the bloodstream, or instilled into a body cavity.

Staining agents are used in surgery to help visually identify abnormal cells, most frequently in procedures on the cervix. Staining agents are chemicals in solution that react differently with abnormal cells from the way they react with normal cells.

CONTRAST MEDIA

Contrast media are high-density pharmacological agents used to visualize low-contrast body tissues that include vascular structures, the urinary bladder, kidneys, the gastrointestinal tract and the biliary tree. Several different contrast media are available for various diagnostic examinations (Table 6-1). Four common contrast media frequently used in surgery are discussed here as examples. As a surgical technologist, you must exercise caution when preparing these agents because they are clear in color and may easily be confused with other medications on the sterile back table. As per your facility policy, all containers and syringes (including those containing contrast media) must be clearly labeled to avoid administration errors. Most contrast media are sensitive to light, so they should be stored covered and away from direct lighting. However, these agents may be safely exposed to light when on the sterile back table during a procedure. This is because the duration of exposure is not sufficient to cause damage to the contrast media.

Many contrast media contain iodine; therefore, a thorough patient history of allergies or reactions to iodine must be obtained and noted in the chart (this includes shellfish allergies). The circulator will also check for a history of patient allergies or reactions to iodine during the preoperative assessment. If the patient has a positive history for iodine reaction, and use of contrast media is anticipated during the surgical procedure, the surgeon should be alerted prior to patient transport to the operating room.

Generally, the various intravascular ROCM work immediately when injected into veins and arteries, or instilled intravascularly into heart chambers to make heart and the major thoracic vessels visible. Urinary tract visibility is achieved with intravenous injection if the patient has normal renal function. Intravascular ROCM are excreted by the kidneys, usually within 24 hours.

MAKE IT SIMPLE

Contrast media is often referred to as x-ray dye in surgery. Don't become confused!

MAKE IT SIMPLE

A commonly used term you will see used in the surgical setting for a radiograph is *x-ray.*

OMNIPAQUE

Iohexol (Omnipaque) is a water-soluble, iodine-based radiographic contrast medium, containing approximately 45% iodine. Omnipaque is available in various strengths (140, 180, 240, 300, and 350), expressed as milligrams of iodine per milliliter (mg/mL). It comes in glass vials ranging in size from 10 mL to 250 mL. Omnipaque is absorbed from the site of administration into the bloodstream; it undergoes little or no metabolism and is excreted by the kidneys virtually unchanged. It is **contraindicated** (inappropriate) for use in patients with known **hypersensitivity** (those excessively sensitive) to iodine without proper premedication protocols.

{NOTE} *If the patient has a sensitivity to iodine, many facilities require a premedication protocol of prednisone and diphenhydramine (Benadryl) before using any ROCM containing iodine.*

Omnipaque may be injected intrathecally or intravascularly, or it may be instilled into a body cavity prior to radiographic examination. Intrathecal (into the lumbar subarachnoid space) injection of Omnipaque is used for myelography and contrast enhancement of computed tomography (CT) myelography to visualize the spinal cord and nerve roots (Fig. 6-1). For many years, myelography was the standard method used to diagnose a ruptured intervertebral disk. Because myelography involves the injection of contrast media and use of x-rays, it is considered an invasive diagnostic examination. In many instances, traditional myelography is being replaced by magnetic resonance imaging (MRI), a noninvasive diagnostic tool.

When injected into a blood vessel, Omnipaque will opacify that blood vessel—and all other vessels in the path of flow—on radiographic examination (angiography). Angiography is used to demonstrate blockages or anatomic abnormalities of the vascular system. Variations of angiography include angiocardiography, aortography, and peripheral arteriography. Angiography may be performed on vessels of the head, neck, abdomen, or kidneys, as well as on peripheral blood vessels. Omnipaque may be used for intraoperative angiography. For instance, it may be used to confirm removal of a

Table 6-1 CONTRAST MEDIA FOR RADIOGRAPHIC STUDIES

Name	Purpose
Amipaque	Myelography and CT
Angio-Conray	Arteriography
Barium sulfate	Gastrointestinal studies
Cardiografin	Angiography and aortography
Conray	Angiography, cholangiography, CT
Cystografin	Urography
Dionosil	Bronchography
Hypaque meglumine, 30%, and Hypaque sodium, 25%	Urography and CT
Hypaque meglumine, 60%, and Hypaque sodium, 50%	Urography, cerebral and peripheral angiography, aortography, venography, cholangiography, hysterosalpingography, and splenoportography
Hypaque 76	Angiocardiography, angiography, aortography, and selected renal arteriography
Isovue	Myelography, cerebral angiography, peripheral arteriography, venography, angiocardiography, left ventriculography, selective coronary angiography, aortography, selective visceral arteriography, urography, arthrography, and CT
Renografin	Cerebral angiography, peripheral arteriography and venography, cholangiography, splenoportography, arthrography, urography, and CT
Renovist	Aortography, angiocardiography, peripheral arteriography and venography, venacavography, and urography
Cholografin Meglumine	Cholangiography and cholecystography
Omnipaque	Angiography, excretory urography, myelography, body cavity procedures
Optiray	Arteriography and CT
Pantopaque	Myelography
Renovue	Excretory urography
Sinografin	Hysterosalpingography
Ultravist	Cholangiography, CT, angiography, carotid arteriography, peripheral angiography, urography
Visipaque	Cardiography, peripheral, visceral and cerebral arteriography, CT, excretory urography, peripheral venography

CT, *Computed tomography.*

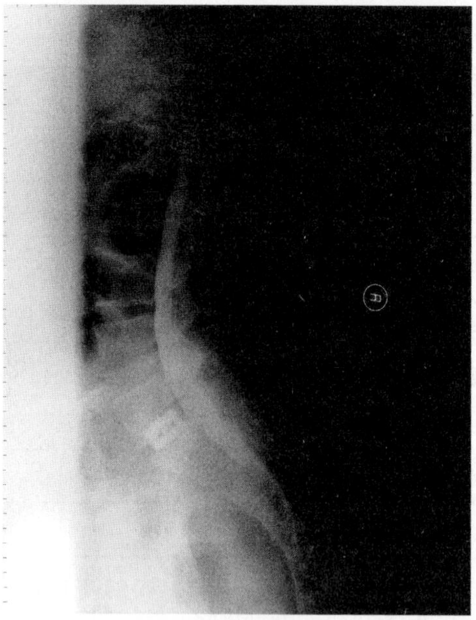

Figure 6-1 Normal myelogram.

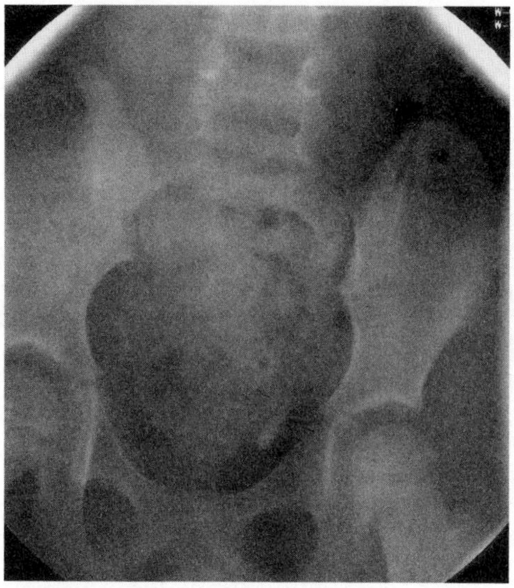

Figure 6-2 Retrograde urogram.

blockage in a peripheral vessel, such as after a femoral embolectomy or laser atherectomy.

Retrograde urography (Fig. 6-2) may be performed with intravascular injection of Omnipaque. The contrast medium will travel to the kidneys and a urogram may be taken to visualize renal structures or detect possible blockage. Omnipaque is also used for cholangiography.

HYPAQUE

Diatrizoate meglumine 30% and 60%, diatrizoate sodium 25% and 50% (Hypaque), and diatrizoate meglumine 66% with diatrizoate 10% (Hypaque 76) are water-soluble radiopaque contrast media. The percentage given in the names refers to the amount of meglumine or sodium per 100 mL of solution, not the amount of iodine. (Hypaque comes in other concentrations and forms, including a powder for oral administration.) It is supplied in glass vials of 50 mL and 100 mL. Hypaque is *not* intended for intrathecal administration. Common uses for Hypaque include excretory urography, angiography, cerebral angiography, peripheral arteriography, central venography, renal venography, and cholangiography.

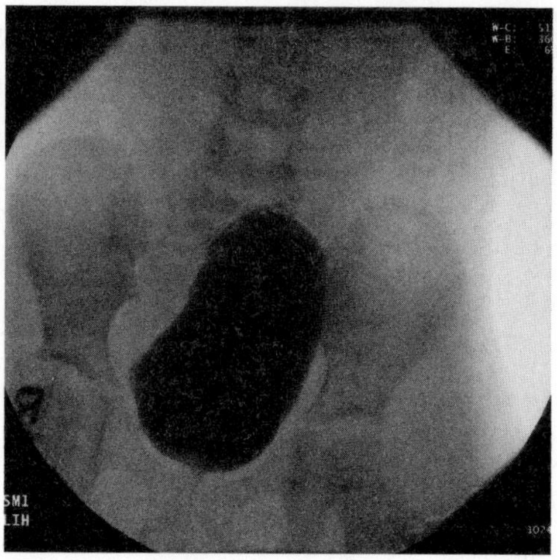

Figure 6-3 Cystogram showing distended bladder.

This type of contrast media (containing diatrizoate meglumine) can also be inserted directly into the urinary bladder via a catheter. The bladder is then filled (distended) with the contrast and a radiograph is taken (Fig. 6-3).

VISIPAQUE

Iodixanol (Visipaque) is a water-soluble radiopaque contrast media. It is available in concentrations of 270 and 320 mg of organically bound iodine per mL. It has many of the same properties as Omnipaque: it is absorbed into the bloodstream and excreted virtually unchanged by the kidneys. When injected into a blood vessel it opacifies that vessel and others in the path of flow for radiographic examination. However, Visipaque is not for intrathecal use. It is supplied in 50-mL vials, and 100-mL, 150-mL, and 200-mL glass and plastic bottles. It is used in cardiography; peripheral, visceral, and cerebral arteriography; contrast-enhanced computed tomography (CECT) of the head and body, cholangiography, excretory urography, and peripheral venography.

ISOVUE

Iopamidol (Isovue) is a water-soluble contrast media for intravascular, intrathecal, and body cavity administration for radiographic procedures. It is rapidly absorbed into the bloodstream and excreted predominantly via the kidneys. It should be used immediately after opening and any remaining in the bottle should be discarded. Isovue comes in concentrations of 200 mg/mL, 250 mg/mL, 300 mg/mL, and 370 mg/mL. It is used for lumbar and thoracocervical myelography, cerebral angiography, peripheral arteriography, venography, angiocardiography, left ventriculography, selective coronary angiography, cholangiography, aortography, selective visceral arteriography, urography, arthrography, computed tomography (CT) enhancement, and contrast-enhanced computed tomography (CECT) head and body imaging. Isovue is supplied in 20-mL, 30-mL, 50-mL, 75-mL, and 100-mL vials and 75-mL, 100-mL, 150-mL, 175-mL, and 200-mL bottles.

OPERATIVE CHOLANGIOGRAMS

Institutions use various contrast media in surgery for operative cholangiograms (open or laparoscopic) to determine the presence of stones in the common bile duct (Fig. 6-4). Often the contrast media is diluted at the sterile back table with equal parts of normal saline solution. A method of cholangiography involves attaching one 30-cc syringe filled with saline and one 30-cc syringe filled with contrast media solution to a three-way stopcock adapter, and this is connected to a cholangiogram catheter (Fig. 6-5). Saline is injected into the catheter to verify correct placement; then the contrast media is injected and a radiograph is taken. These syringes must be clearly identified to prevent inadvertent injection of saline prior to radiographic exposure. Although saline will not harm the patient, inadvertent injection prior to x-ray will negate the examination and require additional radiographic exposure and extended anesthesia time.

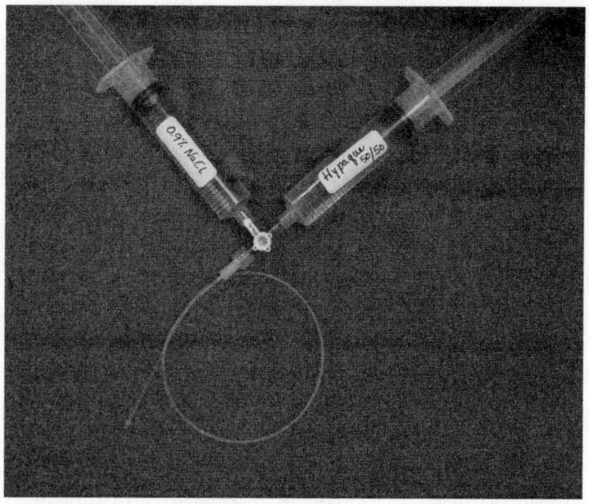

Figure 6-5 Cholangiogram catheter set for injection.

DYES

Dyes have varied uses in surgery. They are used to mark skin incisions and structural positioning of normal body anatomy, and for visual identification of organ injury or pathology. Four of the most common dyes used in surgery are discussed here, with examples of practical applications (Table 6-2).

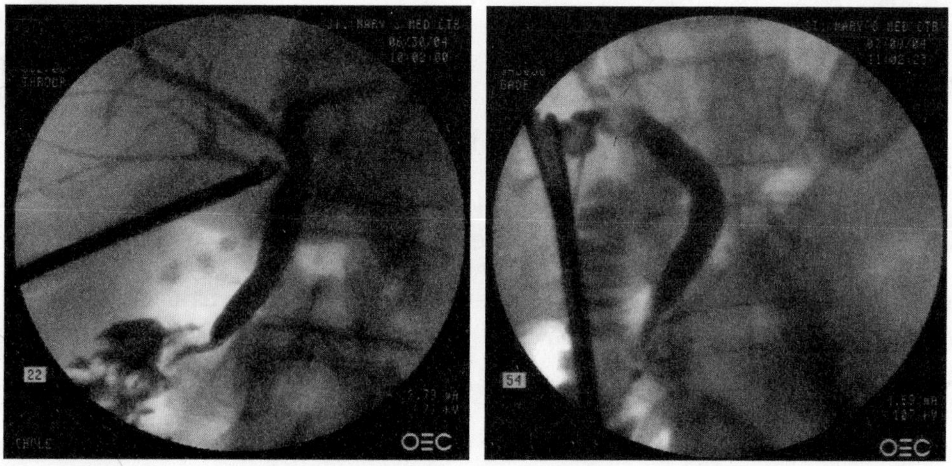

A B

Figure 6-4 **Cholangiogram: A,** normal; **B,** calculus.

Table 6-2 DYES USED IN SURGERY

Name	Purpose
Methylene blue	Cystoscopy: detect bladder injury Tubal dye studies: Verify patency of uterine tubes Bladder surgery or exploration: detect bladder injury
Lymphazurin	Delineation of lymphatic vessels for sentinel lymph node biopsy
Indigo carmine	Kidney or bladder procedures: detect injury to urinary structures Verify kidney function during any surgical procedure: colored urine will be excreted
Gentian violet	Skin marking

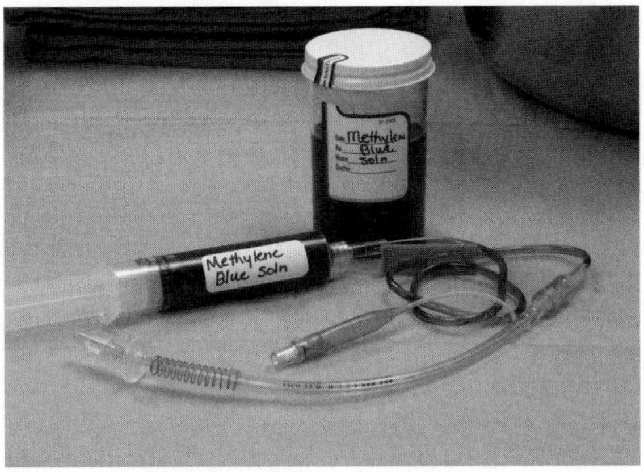

Figure 6-6 Cervical cannula with methylene blue solution for tubal dye study (TDS).

METHYLENE BLUE

Methylene blue USP is available in a 1% solution (10 mg/mL of water), packaged in 1-mL and 10-mL vials or 5-mL ampules. It is most often used in surgery during procedures on the urinary bladder or fallopian tubes. Methylene blue is added to a fluid, such as normal saline, to give a deep blue color to the solution. To detect possible injury, the solution is then instilled into the bladder through an indwelling urinary catheter. If the bladder has a leak or tear, blue solution will be obvious in the pelvis and will be visible as it flows out of the damaged area. Methylene blue can be given intravenously and is released into the urine. This allows the surgeon to check the urinary tract for leaks or fistulas.

In gynecology, a methylene blue solution is used to demonstrate patency of the fallopian tubes. During a procedure called tubal dye study (TDS), or chromotubation, a laparoscope is used to observe the fimbria (ends of the uterine tubes) while methylene blue solution is instilled into the uterus through a special cervical cannula (Fig. 6-6). Methylene blue solution enters the fallopian tubes and is observed exiting into the pelvic cavity, verifying patent tubes. If the tubes are blocked, often due to pelvic inflammatory disease, methylene blue solution will not be evident in the pelvis.

In endoscopic polypectomy, methylene blue can be injected into the submucosa under the polyp to determine tissue planes. It can also be used to verify complete removal of a polyp or to check for perforation.

Methylene blue may also be used immediately before the surgical procedure to outline, or mark, normal body anatomy or position, such as when a tissue flap or graft is measured, marked, "cut," and then transferred to fill a defect on the body (Insight 6-1). Methylene blue is commonly used to mark the planned skin

INSIGHT 6-1 Marking the Skin for Breast Surgery

In the surgical procedure reduction mammoplasty, measurements and markings are made for removing excess breast tissue and skin and transposing the nipples-areola complexes. The marks with a skin-marking pen are made immediately preoperatively by the surgeon with the patient standing or sitting upright, because this is the natural position of the breasts. It is important for the circulator not to remove these markings with the skin prep. Once the patient is positioned on the table and anesthetized, additional markings may be done with a 25-gauge needle dipped into methylene blue and used to "tattoo" breast tissue as additional guides for the surgeon during the procedure.

incisions for surgical procedures. The solution is poured into a medicine cup, and a sterile toothpick or 25-gauge needle is dipped into the solution and applied to the skin. More commonly, manufactured skin-marking pens are replacing this method.

ISOSULFAN BLUE (LYMPHAZURIN 1%)

Lymphazurin is a sterile, aqueous solution for the delineation of lymphatic vessels. It is administered subcutaneously and is selectively picked up by lymphatic vessels that drain the region of the injection site, making them a bright blue color. This makes the vessels easily discernible from the surrounding tissue. It is primarily excreted via the biliary route and should not be used on patients with known hypersensitivity to the medication or related compounds. Lymphazurin is supplied as 5-mL single-dose vials.

Lymphazurin is used as an adjunct to lymphography to diagnose primary and secondary lymphedema of the extremities, lymph node involvement by primary or secondary neoplasm, and lymph node response to therapeutic modalities. Lymphazurin is most commonly used in the surgical setting for sentinel node biopsy for breast tumors. Three to 5 mL of the medication is injected by the surgeon before the skin preparation. This allows approximately 5 minutes time before the first incision is made, allowing the medication to be carried by the lymphatic system. The surgeon follows the blue path of lymphatic drainage from the breast tumor to the first node of the axillary basin, or sentinel node, which is then dissected for pathological examination (Insight 6-2).

{NOTE} *Methylene blue is also used in lymphadenectomy procedures.*

INDIGO CARMINE

Indigo carmine is a blue dye that is usually given intravenously to color urine for verification of bladder integrity or kidney function. Each 5 mL of indigo carmine contains 40mg of indigotindisulfonate sodium in water. It is excreted by the kidneys, usually within 10 minutes after intravenous injection, retaining its color in urine. This process allows immediate identification of possible leaks or damage to the ureters or bladder, as well as demonstration of kidney function. Intravenous injection of indigo carmine during cystoscopy may be used to help identify the location of ureteral openings. Indigo carmine is packaged in 5-mL glass ampules and, when stored, should be protected from light.

IN SIGHT 6-2 Sentinel Lymph Node Biopsy

Sentinel lymph node biopsy is performed following a diagnosis of breast cancer. Within a few hours of the procedure, the patient is taken to the radiology and nuclear medicine departments. The radiologist places a localization wire into the tumor to pinpoint its location. Then the patient goes to nuclear medicine for a mapping of the lymphatic system. This is accomplished with a radioactive isotope (called a tracer), technetium-99, which is injected at or around the tumor site. The tracer enters the lymphatic system and travels to the regional basin and settles in the first, or sentinel, lymph node. The radiologist will use a gamma, or scintillation, camera to map this drainage path and a scan, such as a radiograph, is taken and sent to surgery. This is called lymphoscintigraphy.

The patient is taken to surgery where the surgeon injects 3 to 5cc of isosulfan blue (Lymphazurin 1%) or methylene blue approximately 5 minutes before the incision is made. The dye travels through the lymphatic system just as the tracer did. The surgeon may use a gamma probe, which is covered with a sterile sleeve, to find the radioactive "hot spots" and then mark the skin with a skin-marking pencil at the site of the sentinel node. The incision is made and the surgeon follows the Lymphazurin blue path to excise the node, which is sent to the pathology department for examination. If the pathology report comes back negative for cancer, the breast cancer is considered to have not spread, or metastasized, to the lymph nodes. If the report comes back showing cancer in the node, further lymph node dissection is carried out, with more specimen sent to pathology for diagnosis.

GENTIAN VIOLET

Gentian violet is a purple dye most frequently used in surgery to mark incision lines. Special sterile marking pens containing gentian violet are available from various manufacturers. These pens are particularly useful for plastic and reconstructive procedures involving complicated incisions such as Z-plasty (Fig. 6-7) or tissue flap or grafts. Sterile marking pens may be used to label containers of medications (Fig. 6-8). Gentian violet also belongs to a category of medications called antifungals. Topically, it works to treat types of fungal infections inside the mouth (thrush), the vagina (yeast infection), and of the skin.

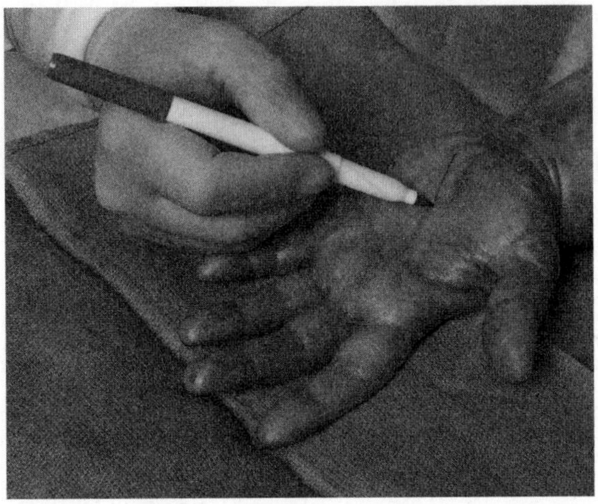

Figure 6-7 Use of a commercial marking pen to mark a skin incision.

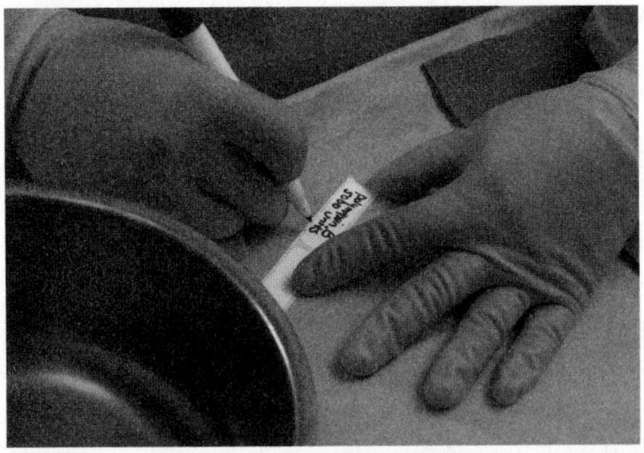

Figure 6-8 Marking medications on the back table.

STAINING AGENTS

Staining agents may be used in surgery to help identify abnormal tissue for biopsy or excision. Because of differences in cell metabolism between normal and abnormal cells, some chemicals applied to the suspect area react in a way that more clearly demonstrates the location of tissue changes. In surgery, staining techniques are most often used by gynecologists to locate areas of cervical dysplasia for biopsy or excisional conization.

LUGOL'S SOLUTION

Lugol's solution is a strong iodine mixture used to perform Schiller's test on cervical tissue. For Schiller's test, Lugol's solution is applied topically to the external cervical os with a sponge stick or large cotton-tipped applicator. Abnormal cells will not take up the brown iodine stain as readily as normal cells, visually demonstrating the area of cervical dysplasia to be biopsied. Lugol's solution is contraindicated for use in patients with a history of hypersensitivity to iodine. Lugol's solution is also used to treat overactive thyroid gland function, iodine deficiency, and to protect the thyroid gland from the effects of radiation as a result of radiation therapy treatments with radioactive iodine (see Chapter 8).

CAUTION

Lugol's iodine solution is packed in a container identical to Monsel's Paste (by Miltex, Inc.). It is important to always correctly identify medications with their labels and not take the type of container for granted.

ACETIC ACID

Acetic acid (commonly known as vinegar) may also be used to help identify areas of cervical dysplasia. Although it is not specifically a colored staining agent, acetic acid causes abnormal tissue to appear whiter than surrounding healthy tissue. Acetic acid may be used as a staining agent when laser is used to excise dysplasia. Laser energy is absorbed by different colors in the spectrum, and tissue stained brown with an iodine solution may interact less effectively with the laser.

Key Terms

- acute renal failure (ARF)
- diaphoresis
- hydration
- iodinated
- nephrotoxicity
- urticaria

RADIOPAQUE CONTRAST MEDIA (ROCM)

As previously defined in this chapter, radiopaque contrast media (ROCM) are high-density pharmacological substances administered to the patient in order to visualize low-contrast body tissues. The most often used ROCM are iodine and barium. Both of these substances have a higher atomic number and mass density than the lower-contrast tissues being examined. When one of these iodinated compounds fills a blood vessel or when barium fills a section of the gastrointestinal tract, these internal structures become visible on radiograph. Serum iodine concentrations must be within the range of 280 to 370 mg/mL for a normal x-ray film to show a vascular lumen. It must be injected intravascularly at a rate equal to or greater than the patient's blood flow. If the ROCM is injected too slowly, the cardiovascular system will dilute its iodine concentration before imaging can be achieved. Intravascular ROCM do not cross cellular membranes well and are distributed into the bloodstream where they enhance visibility of veins and arteries. When administered IV into the heart chambers, the ROCM will enhance visibility to the heart and major thoracic vessels. The urinary tract can be visualized within 15 minutes of a rapid IV injection and within 30 minutes of a slow IV infusion in patients with normal renal function. Urinary tract visibility will be delayed or not occur in patients with renal dysfunction or failure. Intravascular ROCM are excreted mainly by the kidneys. In normal renal function, up to 100% of the intravascular dose is excreted in 24 hours. A very small percentage may be passed through the intestines via the hepatic-biliary system. For patients with renal dysfunction, several days may be required to completely excrete the ROCM.

RISK FACTORS FOR IODINATED CONTRAST MEDIA

In recent years there has been a dramatic increase in the use of diagnostic agents in the surgical setting, especially **iodinated** contrast media used for radiologic imaging. The advanced practitioner performing as the surgical first assistant should be aware of patient risk factors before administration of these agents. Risk factors have been identified that may add to the susceptibility of an adverse reaction. An estimated one of every 20,000 to 40,000 patients receiving ROCM dies as a result of adverse effects. One factor is the route of administration. The risk of reaction from intravascular administration of contrast media occurs more often than extravascular administration (through the gastrointestinal tract). Reactions occurring through intravascular administration are usually mild and self-limiting, and those from extravascular administration are rare. However, either route can produce serious and, at times, life-threatening reactions. Other risk factors include advanced age and class IV congestive heart failure because these can increase the likelihood of renal failure following administration of the contrast media. Patients who have had a previous reaction to contrast materials are understandably at higher risk, although reactions do not re-occur in all patients. Patients with chronic renal insufficiency, asthma, and diabetes mellitus must have these diseases addressed and treated before the administration of any contrast media.

ADVERSE REACTIONS

As previously mentioned in the chapter, the identification of allergies is essential before administering any radiographic contrast agents. Symptoms for reactions are categorized according to their severity (Table A). It should be noted that reactions can occur 20 to 30 minutes after injection of the agent and up to 7 days after the procedure. In addition to allergic reactions, an adverse effect of special importance is nephrotoxicity resulting in **acute renal failure (ARF).** Renal insufficiency is caused by a dosage-related toxic injury to the renal tubules. Patients should be assessed for risk factors that may contribute to ARF (Table B). The assessment should also include renal function studies before contrast is administered by obtaining a blood urea nitrogen (BUN) and creatinine laboratory tests. These are the best indicators of renal function and the results must be available before the procedure. Current treatment to reduce **nephrotoxicity** is **hydration** to keep the kidneys flushing during the procedure and to minimize the volume of contrast media administered. ROCMs can also cause vasodilation with flushing experienced by some patients, and osmotic fluid shifts that can result in acute heart failure in patients with chronic congestive heart failure. High-osmotic ROCMs (those that dissociate into active particles in the bloodstream) can cause some anticoagulation to occur which may result in bleeding and bruising in the patient.

Table A Symptoms of Adverse Reactions for Contrast Media

Mild	Moderate	Severe
Scattered **urticaria**	Persistent vomiting	Cardiac arrhythmia
Nausea	Headache	Hypotension
Vomiting	Facial edema	Severe bronchospasm
Diaphoresis	Mild bronchospasm	Laryngeal edema
Coughing	Dyspnea	Seizures
Dizziness	Palpitations	Pulmonary edema

Table B Risk Factors for Contrast-Induced Nephropathy

Patient Factors	Procedural Factors
Pre-existing renal conditions	High volume of contrast administered
Diabetes	Failure to verify renal lab function tests
Dehydration	Failure to obtain medical history
Advanced age	Failure to aggressively hydrate
Nephrotoxic medications	Failure to space procedures at least 5 days apart
Congestive heart failure	Failure to get appropriate medications preoperatively
Liver disease	

MEDICATIONS

Current studies suggest the administration of acetylcysteine, an antioxidant, may reduce the incidence of contrast-induced ARF. Patients may be given acetylcysteine the day before, the day of, and two days after the procedure. Other medications used to reduce the incidence of adverse reactions to contrast media include methylprednisolone (Medrol) and prednisolone (Prednisolone), which are corticosteroids; diphenhydramine (Benadryl), which is an antihistamine used to treat allergic symptoms; hydroxyzine (Vistaril) to relieve itching, nausea, and vomiting caused by allergies; and histamine H_2 receptor blockers such as cimetidine (Tagamet), famotidine (Pepcid), or ranitidine (Zantac).

Many factors must be considered before any medications are given to the patient receiving contrast media for radiologic imaging. The surgical first assistant must assist the physician in providing the best patient care by identifying patient risk factors, understanding and minimizing adverse effects, and managing reactions of contrast agents.

NEW DIAGNOSTIC IMAGING PROCEDURES

New diagnostic approaches for whole body imaging are using quantum dots, or nanocrystals, as fluorescent and bioluminescent reporters (or tags) that are genetically encoded. These "glowing" tags can provide information for better understanding of human biology as well as help develop treatments for diseases such as cancer, infection, and cardiovascular disease.

One example of this new imaging technology used to diagnose cardiovascular disease and malfunction is an ultrasound contrast agent that consists of millions of tiny bubbles. These ultrasound microbubbles scatter light and allow the physician to see which part of the heart muscle is not functioning properly. The ultrasound component of this technology is highly sensitive and produces a characteristic transient effect for better diagnosis. Other applications include imaging systems to obtain and process information on the molecular and cellular levels of our bodies, models to track neurological damage and repair the central nervous system, and radiodiagnostic agents to label white blood cells without the need to remove and reinject blood into patients. Research is ongoing for these and many more applications using molecular imaging.

An example of a new process using an established dye is fluorescein. There are many fluorescein derivatives, and fluorescein sodium has been traditionally applied to the cornea to detect abrasions (see Chapter 10). This dye is used intravenously for angiography to diagnose and categorize vascular disorders of the eye such as macular degeneration, diabetic retinopathy, and intraocular tumors. Fluorescein is now being used during craniotomy to assist with guided resection of brain tumors.

Advanced Practices Bibliography

Jensen SC, Peppers MP: *Pharmacology and drug administration for imaging technologists,* ed 2, St. Louis, 2006, Mosby/Elsevier.

Mosby's medical dictionary, ed 8, St. Louis, 2009, Mosby/Elsevier.

Pickar GD, Abernathy AP: *Dosage calculations,* ed 8, New York, 2008, Thomson Delmar.

Advanced Practices Internet Resources

eMedicine from WebMD, Contrast Medium Reactions, Recognition and Treatment: *www.emedicine.com/radio/topic864.htm*

MedicineNet.com, Methylprednisone: *www.medicinenet.com/methylprednisolone/article/htm*

MedlinePlus, Drugs, Herbs and Supplements: *www.nlm.nih.gov/medlineplus/druginformation.html*

RxList,

Medrol: *www.rxlist.com/cgi/generic/methprd.htm*

Tagamet: *www.rxlist.com/cgi/generic/cimet/htm*

Advanced Practices: Learning the Language (Key Terms)

Using your textbook or a standard medical dictionary, look up and write the definitions of each term.

- ARF
- diaphoresis
- hydration
- iodinated
- nephrotoxicity
- urticaria

Advanced Practices: Review Questions

1. Which route of administration for iodinated contrast media is more likely to cause an adverse reaction?
   A. Oral
   B. Intravascular
   C. Extravascular
   D. Rectal
2. Name three risk factors that may contribute to acute renal failure after administration of contrast media.
3. Which is the current treatment to reduce nephrotoxicity after the administration of contrast media?
   A. Antibiotic therapy
   B. Administration of a vasodilator
   C. Hydration
   D. Dehydration
4. Name three symptoms of an adverse reaction to contrast media.
5. A new ultrasonic diagnostic contrast media used to study the heart consists of millions of ____.

KEY CONCEPTS

- Different agents, such as contrast media, dyes, and staining agents are used in surgery to facilitate diagnosis of various pathologic conditions.
- Contrast media are used to demonstrate anatomic structures or abnormalities under radiographic examination.
- Dyes are used to mark (color) tissue or structures for direct visualization.
- Staining agents are used to provide visual contrast between normal and abnormal tissue.

Bibliography

Jensen SC, Peppers MP: *Pharmacology and drug administration for imaging technologists*, ed 2, St. Louis, 2006, Mosby/Elsevier.

Mosby's medical dictionary, ed 8, St. Louis, 2009, Mosby.

Pickar GD, Abernathy AP: *Dosage calculations*, ed 8, New York, 2008, Thomson Delmar.

Internet Resources

American Journal of Roentgenology: Using CT and Cholangiography to Diagnose Biliary Tract Carcinoma Complicating Primary Sclerosing Cholangitis. www.ajronline.org/cgi/content/full/177/5/1095.

Blessing WD, Stolier AJ, Teng SC, et al: A comparison of methylene blue and lymphazurin in breast cancer sentinel node mapping, *Am J Surg* 184(4):341–345, 2002. www.ncbi.nlm.nih.gov/pubmed/12383897.

Drugs.com:

Hypaque. www.drugs.com/pro/hypaque.html.

Hypaque-76. www.drugs.com/pro/hypaque-76.html.

Isovue. www.drugs.com/pro/isovue.html.

Omnipaque Injection. www.drugs.com/pro/omnipaque-injection.html.

Geneva Foundation for Medical Education and Research: www.gfmer.ch/.../Cervical.../Aided_visual_.shtmlinspection.htm.

Imaging Technology News: *Bracco Offers Isovue Contrast Agent for X-Ray/CT.* www.itnonline.net/node/21911/.

MedicineOnline: *Medical Drugs, Hypaque.* www.medicineonline.com/drugs/H/Hypaque.com>...> DrugsbeginningwithH. www.medicineonline.com/drugs/H/1056/HYPAQUE-Sodium-Diatrizoate-Sodium-Injection-USP-50.html.

Medsafe, Isovue: www.medsafe.govt.nz/profs/datasheet/I/Isovueinj.htm.

Okuda T, Kataoka K, Taneda M: Metastatic brain tumor surgery using fluorescein sodium: technical note, *Minim Invasive Neurosurg* 50(6):382–384, 2007. www.ncbi.nlm.nih.gov/pubmed/18210365.

RxMed.com: www.rxmed.com.

San Jose State University: *Materials Engineering 297, Special Topics: Applications of Nano Materials,* Spring 2006. www.engr.sjsu.edu/MatE297?Busain_Bio_QD.doc.

Satoh K, Sakamoto N, Shinohe Y, et al: Indigo carmine-induced bradycardia in a patient during general anesthesia, *Anesth Analg* 92:276–277, 2001. www.anesthesia-analgesia.org/cgi/reprint/92/1/276.pdf.

LEARNING THE LANGUAGE (KEY TERMS)

Using your textbook or a standard medical dictionary, look up and write the definitions of each item.

contraindicated
contrast media
dye
hypersensitivity
radiopaque
staining agent

REVIEW QUESTIONS

1. What is the difference between contrast media and dyes?
2. Why should contrast media be labeled on the sterile back table?
3. How does isosulfan blue (Lymphazurin) help the surgeon find the sentinel node?
4. Why should the patient's medical history for allergies be considered before a contrast medium is administered?
5. How is methylene blue used in tubal dye studies (TDS)?

CRITICAL THINKING

1. List two ways to label your contrast media on the back table.
2. Explain the importance of sentinel lymph node biopsy for breast cancer diagnosis.
3. How do surgeons at your clinical facility mark incision sites?
4. Name a procedure that uses methylene blue placed into the bladder.

Scenario

Nancy Cho is scheduled for a cholecystectomy and a common bile duct exploration. Her diagnosis is cholecystitis and cholelithiasis. You have Hypaque 50% and normal saline 50 cc on the back table.

1. The patient's chart should be checked for allergies. What allergy in particular would impact her cholangiogram?
2. Both Omnipaque and normal saline are drawn up into 30 cc syringes. How are they properly identified on the field?
3. Which solution is injected first? Why?
4. Where are these solutions injected for the procedure?

CHAPTER 7

Diuretics

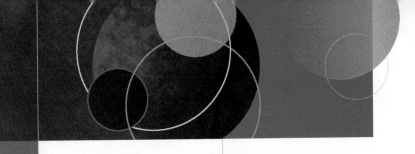

OBJECTIVES *After completing this chapter, you should be able to:*

1. State the general purpose of a diuretic.
2. Describe the physiology of the kidney.
3. Identify anatomic structures of the nephron.
4. List diseases that use diuretics for management.
5. Describe the impact of long-term diuretic therapy on the patient about to undergo a surgical procedure.
6. Discuss the type of patient who may come to surgery on long-term diuretic therapy.
7. Differentiate between the purposes for long-term and short-term use of diuretics.
8. List the two most common diuretics administered intraoperatively and their purpose.

KEY TERMS

congestive heart failure (CHF)
creatinine
diuresis
diuretic
dysrhythmia
electrolyte
glaucoma
homeostasis
hyperkalemia
hypertension
hypokalemia
nephron

Diuretics are medications administered to prevent reabsorption of sodium and water by the kidneys. As a result, the patient excretes large amounts of dilute urine. **Diuretics** are used in the management of several chronic medical conditions such as **hypertension**, **congestive heart failure (CHF)**, and **glaucoma**.

MAKE IT SIMPLE

A simple statement about the physiology of fluid and **electrolyte** balance is this principle: Where the fluid goes, so go the electrolytes.

Electrolytes are minerals that are dissolved in body fluids. They are particles that develop an electrical charge when dissolved in water. The major body electrolytes include sodium, potassium, calcium, chlorine, magnesium, bicarbonate, phosphate, and sulfate. Electrolytes are found inside and outside of cells and are acquired through food and water.

Most diuretics also cause excretion of electrolytes other than sodium (Na^+), including potassium (K^+) and calcium (Ca^{++}). Potassium may be seriously depleted in patients taking certain diuretics, a condition known as **hypokalemia**. If patients on long-term diuretic therapy require surgery, blood chemistry tests are performed to determine serum potassium levels (normal 3.5 to 5.0 mEq/L). Potassium levels that are either too low or too high may cause cardiac **dysrhythmias** under anesthesia (Insight 7-1). Patients with hypokalemia may require administration of intravenous potassium prior to nonemergency surgery. The necessity of preoperative potassium treatment may cause a delay in procedure start time or scheduled date, so operating room staff should be mindful of such possibilities. Long-term diuretic therapy is most frequently seen in elderly patients with systemic fluid management conditions.

Short-term use of diuretics is indicated when a condition requires a rapid but temporary reduction in fluid. An example of short-term use of diuretics is intravenous administration by the anesthesia provider during some surgical procedures. Diuretics may be used during surgery to reduce intraocular pressure, intracranial pressure, or to protect kidney function. During intraocular surgery such as retinal detachment, a diuretic may be given to prevent the accumulation of fluid due to the inflammatory response to tissue manipulation. Diuretics may be administered during craniotomy to prevent brain swelling, especially when the tissue has been damaged by traumatic injury. During vascular procedures on the aorta (especially those near the kidney) diuretics may be given to keep fluid flowing through the kidneys, thus providing a measure of continued kidney function. Note that the risk of hypokalemia is significantly reduced when diuretics are used for short-term treatment of such specific temporary conditions.

Diuretics lower blood pressure by increasing the elimination of fluids (water, sodium, and electrolytes) from the body: this decreases the blood volume. When

IN SIGHT 7-1 **Physiology Insight: The Importance of Potassium in Cardiac Function**

Potassium (K^+), a mineral element, is the primary intracellular electrolyte in the body. It plays a vital role in many body functions, such as nerve impulse conduction, acid-base balance, and promotion of carbohydrate and protein metabolism. Every body cell, especially muscle tissue, requires a high potassium content to function. It facilitates contraction of both skeletal and smooth muscles—including myocardial (heart muscle) contraction. Potassium levels in the body have a very narrow normal range (3.5 to 5.0 mEq/L) and even a slight deviation in either direction can cause problems. An excess of potassium (*hyper*kalemia) alters the normal polarized state of cardiac muscle fibers. This results in a decrease in the rate and force of the heart's contractions. Very high potassium levels can block conduction of cardiac impulses. This results in rapid heart rate (tachycardia) initially and, later, slow heart rate (bradycardia). If potassium levels are too low (*hypo*kalemia), the heart can develop an abnormal rhythm (dysrhythmia). Both hyperkalemia and hypokalemia can lead to muscle weakness and flaccid paralysis. Abnormal potassium levels can diminish excitability and conduction rate of the heart muscle and lead to cardiac arrest. The cause of abnormal levels is usually not dietary deficiency. Many foods contain potassium, including meats, milk, peanut butter, potatoes, bananas, apples, carrots, tomatoes, and dark-green leafy vegetables. Rather, hypokalemia can result from excessive vomiting and diarrhea, severe trauma such as burns, chronic renal disease, excessive doses of cortisone, or long-term diuretic therapy for chronic conditions such as hypertension (high blood pressure). Hyperkalemia results from renal dysfunction, such as the kidneys' inability to excrete excess amounts of potassium, or when there is decreased urine output or renal failure.

there is less blood volume circulating, there is less pressure on the blood vessels and the heart does not pump as forcefully or fast (referred to as cardiac output). This concept can be compared to a water balloon. When it is full (has a high volume of water) the pressure of the water pushing on the walls of the balloon is high. When some of the water is removed (lowering of the volume) the pressure is lessened (lower).

Although diuretics are not administered from the sterile back table, it is important that surgical technologists understand how the use of diuretics affects the surgical patient. There are two primary issues that the surgical team must consider.

1. Long-term diuretic therapy may cause the delay or rescheduling of a surgery, so the patient's potassium levels must be verified prior to opening the sterile field.
2. Short-term intraoperative use of diuretics requires the insertion of an indwelling urinary catheter in the patient before surgery. A urinary drainage bag with an accurate measuring device is often used to record urinary output at regular intervals.

To understand the action of diuretics, it is necessary to briefly review renal physiology. Consult your physiology textbook for additional information.

REVIEW OF RENAL PHYSIOLOGY

The primary function of the renal (urinary) system is to maintain **homeostasis**, the balancing of fluids and electrolytes in the body. This is done by filtering blood and removing excess water and dissolved substances, or *solutes,* such as sodium and potassium. The **nephron** (Fig. 7-1) is a microscopic filtering unit that removes water and waste solutes. Millions of nephrons are present within the kidneys. Blood is brought to the nephron through the afferent arteriole into Bowman's capsule, where filtration occurs. Filtration is the process of forcing fluids and solutes through a membrane by pressure. Filtered blood then returns to the circulatory system via the efferent arteriole. The remaining fluid, or *filtrate*—which contains all the substances present in blood, except formed elements and most proteins—then undergoes tubular reabsorption. Only specific amounts of needed substances, including water, are reabsorbed. Tubular reabsorption takes place in the proximal convoluted tubule and the ascending and descending limbs of the loop of the nephron (loop of Henle).

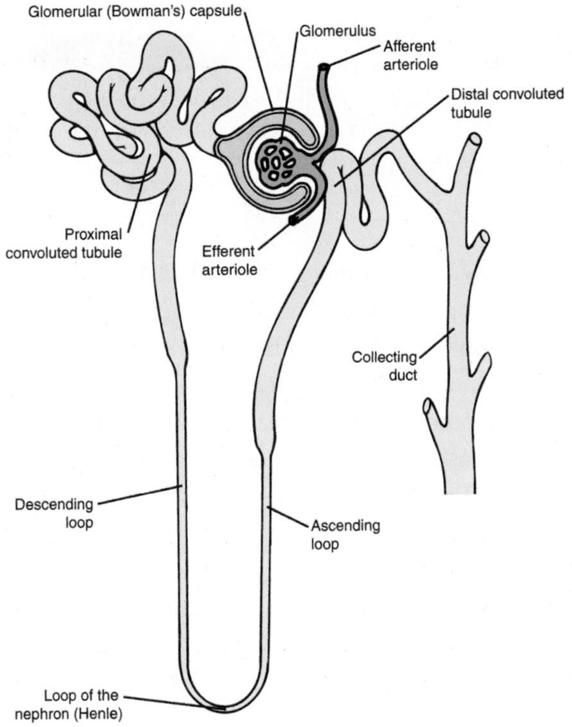

Figure 7-1 The nephron.

The filtrate next receives such materials as potassium, **creatinine**, and hydrogen ions from blood surrounding the tubule; this process is called tubular secretion. Tubular secretion, which takes place in the distal convoluted tubule, eliminates waste products and controls blood pH. Additional water is reabsorbed when filtrate proceeds to the collecting ducts. Filtrate is emptied from collecting ducts into the renal pelvis to the ureter and bladder and is excreted as urine.

DIURETICS

Most diuretics exert effects at different locations along the nephron. Diuretics cause elimination of excess fluid by preventing reabsorption of sodium and water, increasing urine output. Diuretics are classified by site of action and the mechanism by which the solute is altered (Table 7-1).

MAKE IT SIMPLE

Diuretics are classified by where and how they work.

LOOP DIURETICS

Loop diuretics are highly potent diuretics used to remove fluid arising from renal, hepatic, or cardiac dysfunction and to treat acute pulmonary edema. They inhibit the reabsorption of 20% to 30% of the

Table 7-1 DIURETICS BY CLASSIFICATION

Class	Generic Name	Trade Name
Loop diuretics	Bumetanide	Bumex
	Ethacrynic acid	Edecrin
	Furosemide	Lasix
	Torsemide	Demadex
Thiazide diuretics	Bendroflumethiazide	Naturetin
	Chlorothiazide	Diuril, SK-Chlorothiazide
	Hydrochlorothiazide	Esidrix, HydroDIURIL, Oretic
Potassium-sparing diuretics	Amiloride	Midamor
	Eplerenone	Inspra
	Spironolactone	Aldactone
	Triamterene	Dyrenium
Carbonic anhydrase inhibitors	Acetazolamide	Diamox
Osmotic diuretics	Mannitol	Osmitrol

sodium load. Hepatic dysfunction may be due to cirrhosis or liver failure. The most common cardiac dysfunction requiring treatment with diuretics is CHF (Insight 7-2). The oral form of high-ceiling diuretics may be used in treatment of hypertension. Loop diuretics work by decreasing the reabsorption of sodium (Na^+) and chloride (Cl^-) ions along the whole renal tubule, especially in the ascending loop of Henle. These diuretics exert a potent effect, because the site of action is so broad. Examples of loop diuretics are bumetanide (Bumex), ethacrynic acid (Edecrin), torsemide (Demadex), and furosemide (Lasix). Furosemide is the most commonly used agent in this category. In surgery, furosemide is particularly useful in intracranial procedures. Furosemide decreases intracranial pressure by quickly removing fluid that accumulates in response to the trauma of intracranial procedures or injuries. When furosemide is administered intravenously, onset of **diuresis** (eliminating large amounts of urine) can be expected within 5 to 15 minutes and will continue for approximately 2 hours. The usual initial dose of furosemide is 20 to 40 mg intravenously, to be given over a period of 1 to 2 minutes. A second dose may be administered 2 hours later. As all patients are not the same, dosages may vary.

THIAZIDE DIURETICS

Thiazide diuretics are low potency diuretics used to treat essential hypertension and mild chronic edema. They inhibit the reabsorption of 5% to 10% of the sodium load. Thiazides work by inhibiting the reabsorption of sodium (Na^+) and chloride (Cl^-) ions in the end of the ascending loop of the nephron and the beginning of the distal convoluted tubule. Examples of thiazide diuretics include bendroflumethiazide (Naturetin), chlorothiazide (Diuril, SK-Chlorothiazide), and hydrochlorothiazide (Esidrix, HydroDIURIL, Oretic).

POTASSIUM-SPARING DIURETICS

Potassium-sparing diuretics are low potency diuretics commonly used to treat edema and hypertension and to help restore potassium levels in hypokalemic patients. They inhibit only 1% to 3% of the sodium load. Potassium-sparing diuretics are usually administered in combination with other diuretics such as thiazides and loop diuretics to minimize potassium loss. Potassium-sparing diuretics prevent the reabsorption of sodium in the distal convoluted tubules by altering membrane permeability. This change in membrane permeability also prevents potassium loss. Potassium-sparing diuretics exert a mild diuretic effect because only a small amount of the

IN SIGHT 7-2 Pathology Insight: Congestive Heart Failure

Congestive heart failure, or pump failure, is the inability of the heart to pump sufficient blood to meet the body's demands. Back-pressure from stagnant blood slows down the venous blood return to the heart. When the right ventricle fails, congestion of organs and extremities results. The patient's legs become swollen, especially at the end of the day, and the liver becomes enlarged due to fluid retention. The enlarged liver presses on nerves, which causes pain and nausea. Pressure in the abdominal veins can lead to an accumulation of fluid in the abdominal cavity (ascites). Left ventricular failure leads to pulmonary congestion and edema as fluid builds up in the alveoli. This accumulation of fluids in the lungs causes shortness of breath (dyspnea). Because there is less blood flowing to the major organs, their ability to function is impaired. The brain receives less blood, and this means less oxygen (hypoxia). The patient experiences confusion, loss of concentration, and mental fatigue. This also leads to changes in mental status. The kidneys cannot function properly, and this results in less urine formation (oliguria). Renal failure leads to abnormal retention of water and sodium, which leads to generalized edema. Patients with progressive congestive heart failure face life-threatening fluid overload and total heart failure. To compensate for decreased cardiac output, the body has adaptive mechanisms to try to meet the body's needs. As the failing heart tries to maintain a normal output of blood, it enlarges the pumping chambers to hold a greater blood volume. This increases the amount of blood pumped with each chamber's contraction. The heart also begins to increase its muscle mass. This allows for more force with each contraction. Along with this, the sympathetic nervous system helps out by activating adaptive processes to increase the heart rate, redistribute peripheral blood flow, and retain urine. These adaptive measures achieve almost normal cardiac output, but only for a short period of time. They eventually harm the pump because they require an increase in myocardial oxygen consumption. As the mechanism continues, myocardial reserve is exhausted. This leads to heart failure.

glomerular filtrate ever reaches the distal convoluted tubule. Common agents in this category include amiloride (Midamor), spironolactone (Aldactone), eplerenone (Inspra), and triamterene (Dyrenium). Adverse effects can include **hyperkalemia**.

CARBONIC ANHYDRASE INHIBITORS

Carbonic anhydrase inhibitors are low potency diuretics used to treat mild acute closed-angle glaucoma and chronic open-angle glaucoma (see Chapter 10). These diuretics act on the proximal convoluted tubule, so urine output is not significantly impacted. Carbonic anhydrase is active in formation of aqueous humor in the eye. By inhibiting carbonic anhydrase, these drugs decrease production of aqueous humor, thus lowering intraocular pressure. The most common carbonic anhydrase inhibitor is acetazolamide (Diamox). Acetazolamide may be given orally to cataract patients after surgery because pressure may build up in the eye as a response to manipulation of tissues.

OSMOTIC DIURETICS

Osmotic diuretics are highly potent. The mechanism of action of osmotic diuretics is unlike that of any diuretics previously described. Osmotic diuretics actually increase blood pressure and volume by drawing fluid out of tissues and into the circulatory system rapidly (Fig. 7-2). Thus, osmotic diuretics are contraindicated in patients with hypertension and edema. Osmotic diuretics are *not* used for management of chronic conditions such as congestive

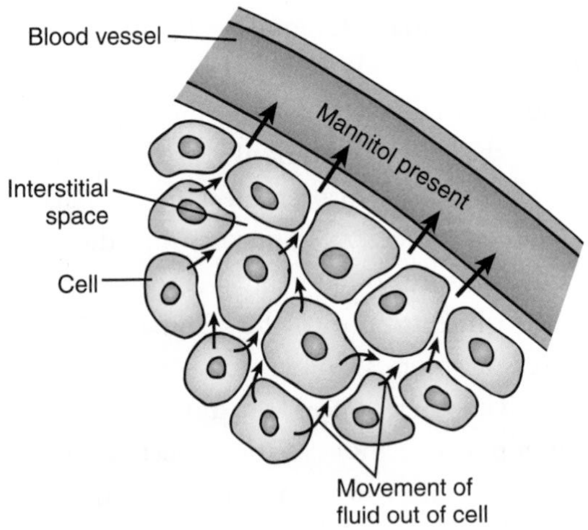

Figure 7-2 Mannitol causes a change in the osmolarity of blood, drawing interstitial and intracellular fluid into the bloodstream. This action eventually increases the amount of fluid excreted by the kidneys.

heart failure. Osmotic diuretics are used to prevent acute renal failure after cardiac surgery, to treat increased intracranial pressure, and to reduce intraocular pressure in open-globe procedures of the eye such as retinal detachment.

As the name implies, these drugs exert their effects through the process of osmosis. Remember, osmosis is the process of water moving through a semipermeable membrane from an area of lesser concentration of solute (e.g., sodium) to an area of greater concentration of solute. Water moves toward the diuretic agent present in the glomerulus, thus preventing the water from being reabsorbed. Water is then excreted with the diuretic agent in the urine. There is no significant change in sodium reabsorption, so electrolyte balance should remain relatively unaffected.

The most commonly used osmotic diuretic is mannitol (Osmitrol). Mannitol may be used to provide a rapid reduction in intraocular pressure in patients experiencing acute angle-closure glaucoma. It is administered intravenously, warmed, through a filter to prevent crystallization. Mannitol may also be given during some neurosurgical procedures to reduce intracranial pressure. In vascular procedures, particularly on the aorta, mannitol may be used to protect kidney function by increasing the volume of fluid entering the kidneys.

ADVANCED PRACTICES FOR THE SURGICAL FIRST ASSISTANT

CHAPTER 7—Diuretics

Key Terms

diuresis
hypokalemia

As discussed in the chapter, diuretics are administered for the management of several medical conditions: to decrease hypertension, to decrease edema (peripheral and pulmonary) in CHF, to decrease edema in renal or liver disorders, and to treat glaucoma. Diuretics achieve their treatment goals by bringing about a negative fluid balance, mobilizing excessive extracellular fluid, and reducing excess fluid volume. When the patient on diuretics is scheduled for surgery, preoperative evaluations are required. The surgical first assistant must understand the physiological effects on the body and any possible surgical complications that may arise from these medications. **Hypokalemia,** depletion of potassium in the blood serum, is often caused by the effects of diuretics on the kidneys. Thiazide and loop diuretics cause the highest rate of potassium loss. Diuretics increase the body's flow of urine **(diuresis)**. Although water and sodium are excreted from the body by the kidneys, other electrolytes such as potassium are also excreted. Potassium is one of the essential minerals needed by the body to maintain homeostasis. It helps regulate normal heart rhythm, blood pressure, and nerve connections. Potassium is also needed to convert blood sugar into glycogen for energy that can be stored in the muscles. Next to calcium and phosphorus, potassium is the most abundant mineral found in the body. Potassium cannot be produced by the body and must be replaced through diet or supplements. See Box A for a list of foods rich in potassium. Nearly 98% of the total potassium is found inside the cells, with the remaining 2% in the blood serum. Small fluctuations in the blood serum potassium may have adverse effects in the functions of the heart, nerves, and muscles. All patients on diuretic therapy are routinely tested preoperatively for blood serum potassium levels. Abnormal levels should be corrected prior to any elective surgical procedure.

POTASSIUM LEVELS

Potassium levels in the blood serum are identified through analysis of a blood sample. In most cases the test is part of a routine chemical analysis that also includes other minerals. A normal level of potassium is 3.5 to 5.0 mEq/L (milliequivalent per liter). A level of 3.0 mEq/L with symptoms or 2.5 mEq/L

BOX A Foods High in Potassium Content

- Apricots
- Bananas
- Beans
- Cantaloupe
- Chocolate
- Fish
- Honeydew
- Kiwi fruit
- Lima beans
- Meats
- Milk
- Oranges and juice
- Peaches
- Potatoes
- Poultry
- Prunes
- Pumpkin
- Raisins
- Spinach
- Sunflower seeds
- Sweet potatoes
- Tomatoes
- Vegetable juice
- Whole grains
- Winter squash
- Yogurt

with or without symptoms is considered severe hypokalemia and requires aggressive inpatient treatment. Patients with levels between 3.0 and 3.5 mEq/L are considered mildly hypokalemic and are usually treated on an outpatient basis with diet or oral supplements.

TREATMENT OF HYPOKALEMIA

Treatment of hypokalemia involves replacing the potassium with diet or a supplement to obtain and maintain a normal serum potassium level. Treatment by oral intake or a supplement is adequate for minor depletion of potassium and can be performed at home over a period of time. Because of the slow release of potassium into the system, oral replacement treatment is by far the best method for replacement without any serious side effects. Acute hypokalemia (level $>$ 2.5 mEq/L) is a serious life-threatening condition and needs to be replaced by intravenous administration of potassium, such as potassium chloride, as an inpatient. Cardiac monitoring is necessary because of possible arrhythmia caused by the fluctuations of potassium levels. Dosage required for correction is based on the accepted formula that 10 mEq/L of potassium chloride will increase the blood serum level by 0.1 mEq/L. Intravenous administration of 10 or 20 mEq/hour not exceeding 200 mEq/L is usually recommended for severe hypokalemia.

ALDOSTERONE

Although not technically a diuretic, aldosterone does affect kidney function. Aldosterone is a mineralocorticoid hormone produced by the adrenal cortex (see Chapter 8). It increases the reabsorption of sodium and water and the secretion of potassium in the kidneys. Aldosterone's action increases blood volume and thus blood pressure. Medications that interfere with aldosterone's action are used to treat hypertension. An example is spironolactone (Aldactone), which blocks the aldosterone receptor and so lowers blood pressure.

Advanced Practices Bibliography

Fulcher E, Fulcher R, Soto C: *Pharmacology principles and applications*, ed 2, 2009, Saunders/Elsevier.

Jensen SC, Peppers MP: *Pharmacology and drug administration for imaging technologists*, ed 2, St. Louis, 2006, Mosby/Elsevier.

Moscou K, Snipe K: *Pharmacology for pharmacy technicians*, St. Louis, 2009, Mosby/Elsevier.

Advanced Practices Internet Resources

AlgaeCal, Potassium Rich Foods - Foods High in Potassium: *www.algaecal.com/potassium-rich-foods.html*

Answers.com, Diuretics: *www.answers.com/topic/diuretics*

essortment, Health & Fitness: *www.essortment.com/health.html*

Advanced Practices: Learning the Language (Key Terms)

Using your textbook or a standard medical dictionary, look up and write the definitions of each term.

- diuresis
- hypokalemia

Advanced Practices: Review Questions

1. The term to describe a depletion of potassium in the blood serum is
   A. Hypovolemia
   B. Hypocalcemia
   C. Hypothermia
   D. Hypokalemia
2. Normal level of potassium in blood serum is ____________ mEq/L.
3. Describe the treatment for chronic and acute hypokalemia.
4. Which category of medication causes the highest rate of potassium depletion?
   A. Antibiotics
   B. Analgesics
   C. Diuretics
   D. Steroids
5. Name two food sources that are high in potassium.
6. How does aldosterone affect blood pressure?

KEY CONCEPTS

- Diuretics are agents administered to reduce the amount of fluid accumulating in patients with renal, hepatic, or cardiac dysfunction, as well as to relieve excessive intracranial or intraocular pressure. Excess fluid is removed through excretion of urine.
- Patients receiving long-term diuretic therapy have an increased risk of hypokalemia. If a surgical patient is hypokalemic, potential exists for cardiac dysrhythmias when under general anesthesia. To detect hypokalemia, blood chemistry analysis is performed preoperatively for all surgical patients taking diuretics. The sterile field should not be opened until the potassium levels are verified.
- Some surgical procedures require short-term intraoperative administration of diuretics. Diuretics are given intravenously in surgery during some ophthalmic, intracranial, and vascular procedures. An indwelling urinary catheter must be inserted on all surgical patients who may receive diuretics intraoperatively.
- The most common diuretics administered during surgery are mannitol (Osmitrol) and furosemide (Lasix).
- The hormone aldosterone also affects kidney function by increasing reabsorption of sodium and water.

Bibliography

Fulcher E, Fulcher R, Soto C: *Pharmacology principles and applications*, ed 2, 2009, Saunders/Elsevier.

Jensen SC, Peppers MP: *Pharmacology and drug administration for imaging technologists,* ed 2, St. Louis, 2006, Mosby/Elsevier.

Mosby's medical dictionary, ed 8, St. Louis, 2009, Mosby/Elsevier.

Moscou K, Snipe K: *Pharmacology for pharmacy technicians,* St. Louis, 2009, Mosby/Elsevier.

Shier DL, Butler JL, Lewis R: *Hole's human anatomy & physiology,* ed 12, New York, 2009, McGraw-Hill.

Internet Resources

MedlinePlus, Furosemide: www.nlm.nih.gov/medlineplus/druginfo/meds/a682858.html.

MayoClinic.com (search "Diuretics"): www.mayoclinic.com.

LEARNING THE LANGUAGE (KEY TERMS)

Using your textbook or a standard medical dictionary, look up and write the definitions of each term.

congestive heart failure (CHF)
creatinine
diuresis
diuretic
electrolyte
dysrhythmia
glaucoma
homeostasis
hyperkalemia
hypertension
hypokalemia
nephron

REVIEW QUESTIONS

1. How does the nephron work to eliminate waste products and excess water?
2. How do diuretics work?
3. Which structures of the nephron are affected by diuretics?
4. Why would a diuretic be prescribed for long-term use?
5. What is a common adverse effect of long-term diuretic therapy on a patient? How does that condition impact the administration of a general anesthetic?
6. What type of patient may come to surgery on long-term diuretic therapy?
7. Why are diuretics used intraoperatively?
8. Which diuretics are used intraoperatively?

CRITICAL THINKING

Scenario 1

Mrs. Hernandez is an 85-year-old female admitted to surgery for insertion of a hip prosthesis to treat a hip fracture. The surgical technologist assigned to transport the patient to the preoperative holding area performed a routine review of the patient's medical chart in the emergency department. The medical chart indicates that Mrs. Hernandez is being treated for chronic hypertension.

1. Knowing that she has a concurrent diagnosis of hypertension, which additional related items should be checked on her chart?
2. How might this situation affect the preparations going on in the surgery department?
3. What action or actions should the surgical technologist take prior to bringing the patient to preoperative holding?

Scenario 2

Mr. Van Nguyen is a 47-year-old male admitted to surgery for repair of a retinal detachment under general anesthesia.

1. Which diuretic may be administered intraoperatively?
2. The circulator should check the preference card for a standing order for what preoperative preparation of the patient specific to this situation?

CHAPTER 8 Hormones

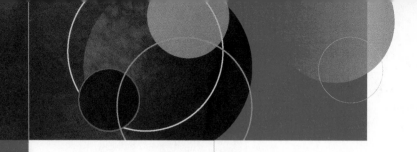

OBJECTIVES *After completing this chapter, you should be able to:*

1. Define terminology related to the endocrine system.
2. List endocrine glands and hormones secreted by each.
3. State the purpose for administration of each hormone.
4. Describe medical and surgical uses for hormones.
5. List hormones that may be administered from the sterile field.
6. List surgical procedures that may require administration of hormones from the sterile field.
7. Discuss safety issues regarding the use of epinephrine from the sterile field.

KEY TERMS

androgen
endometriosis
fibrocystic breast changes
palliatives

Hormones are chemicals released by endocrine glands into the bloodstream (Fig. 8-1). These diverse substances maintain homeostasis (relatively constant conditions in the body) by altering the activities of specific target cells. Functions regulated by hormones include reproduction, growth and development, and metabolism. Hormones have a wide range of actions and effects, and each hormone has a specific function at a specific location in the body. In addition to naturally occurring hormones, several synthetic hormones have been developed. Most hormones are administered as replacement therapy in the medical rather than the surgical setting. But some hormones are used in surgery and may be administered from the sterile back table during the course of a procedure.

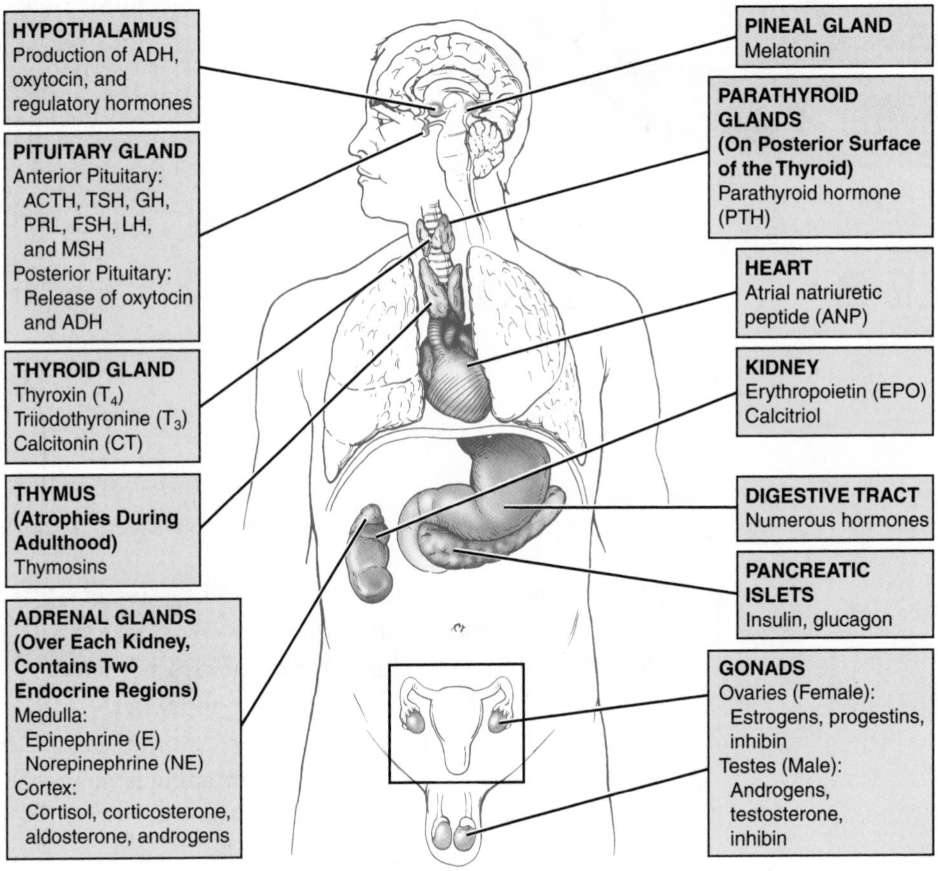

Figure 8-1 The endocrine system.

ENDOCRINE SYSTEM REVIEW

The endocrine system works with the nervous system to relay messages to maintain homeostasis. The endocrine system communicates by sending chemical messengers (hormones) to target cells located all over the body. Hormones are produced by endocrine glands and secreted into the extracellular space. They enter capillaries and are carried by the bloodstream to target cells. Hormones bind to receptor sites on cells and cause a change in cell physiology. Chemical messages take longer to work than those relayed by the nervous system, but effects generally last longer. Hormonal effects are many and varied, but actions on the body may be categorized into four main groups:

- Regulation of internal chemical balance and volume
- Response to environmental changes, including stress, trauma, and temperature changes
- Growth and development
- Reproduction

Hormones can be classified as steroid and nonsteroid. Steroid hormones are derived from cholesterol. In cellular mitochondria, enzymes convert cholesterol into pregnenolone, which is not a hormone, but the immediate precursor molecule to the synthesis of all steroid hormones. Steroid hormones are classified as glucocorticoids (primarily cortisol), mineralocorticoids (primarily aldosterone), estrogens, progestogens (progesterone), and **androgens** (male sex hormones; primarily testosterone). Nonsteroid hormones are synthesized from amino acids. The simplest hormones are amines, derived from a single amino acid. Amine hormones include epinephrine, norepinephrine, thyroxine, and triiodothyronine. Hormones made of short chains of amino acids are called peptide hormones. Antidiuretic hormone (ADH) and oxytocin are examples of peptide hormones. Protein hormones are longer, folded chains of amino acids. Examples of protein hormones are growth hormone (GH), parathyroid hormone (PTH), insulin, and glucagon (Box 8-1).

The vast majority of endocrine disorders are due either to hyposecretion or hypersecretion of hormones. Treatment for hyposecretion may include administration of hormones for supplement or for replacement. Hypersecretion may be treated medically with drugs to reduce secretion or surgically by gland removal, depending on indications.

Box 8-1 HORMONE CLASSIFICATIONS

Steroid	Nonsteroid
Aldosterone	Epinephrine
Cortisol	Norepinephrine
Estrogen	Thyroxine
Progesterone	Triiodothyronine
Testosterone	Antidiuretic hormone (ADH)
	Growth hormone (GH)
	Parathyroid hormone (PTH)
	Insulin
	Glucagon
	Oxytocin

ENDOCRINE GLANDS

PITUITARY GLAND

The pituitary gland, known as the "master gland," has a vital role in reproduction and growth, and it regulates the function of the renal system and thyroid gland. The pituitary gland is connected to the hypothalamus by a stalk called the infundibulum. It is divided into two lobes—the anterior or adenohypophysis and the posterior or neurohypophysis. The adenohypophysis communicates with the hypothalamus via factors released into the blood supply (Fig. 8-2). Hormones secreted by the adenohypophysis include GH (Insight 8-1), thyroid-stimulating hormone (TSH), adrenocorticotropic hormone (ACTH), prolactin (PRL), dopamine, and gonadotropic hormones, which include follicle-stimulating hormone (FSH) and luteinizing hormone (LH). The hypothalamus synthesizes oxytocin and vasopressin (also known as antidiuretic hormone, ADH) and transports those hormones to the neurohypophysis where they are released.

A pituitary hormone of particular importance to the surgical technologist is oxytocin. Oxytocin stimulates the uterine contractions necessary for normal labor and delivery. If a patient is unable to produce sufficient oxytocin naturally, it may be administered intravenously to induce labor. After delivery of the infant, the uterus must continue to contract in order to expel the placenta and to stop postpartum bleeding from the placental attachment site. After a cesarean section, oxytocin is administered intravenously by the anesthesia provider to supplement natural uterine contractions and slow postpartum bleeding. If uterine contractions are not firm enough, oxytocin may be injected directly into the uterine muscle. The scrubbed surgical technologist uses a syringe and a large-bore hypodermic needle (such as an 18-gauge) to draw up the desired dose of oxytocin from a properly-identified vial held by the circulator, changes needles, labels the syringe, and then passes the medication to the surgeon. Oxytocin is available as Oxytocin, Pitocin, and Syntocinon.

CAUTION

It is critical to avoid confusion of Pitocin with Pitressin. Pitocin is oxytocin, but Pitressin is vasopressin, which contains antidiuretic hormone (ADH) and oxytocin in a ratio of 20:1. Pitressin is used subcutaneously or intramuscularly to stabilize fluid balance in patients with diabetes insipidus. The surgical technologist must be alert to drug names that sound similar and carefully read the medication label. When in doubt, *always* clarify the order.

THYROID GLAND

The thyroid gland is a vascular structure consisting of two lobes joined by an isthmus. The largest of the endocrine glands, the thyroid is located below the larynx, on both sides of the trachea in the anterior neck. It sets the rate of body metabolism. In children, an underfunctioning thyroid (hypothyroidism) can stunt growth and delay mental development. Lack of thyroid hormones slows metabolism. An adult with hypothyroidism is sleepy, tires easily, is less mentally alert, has reduced endurance, and has a slow heart rate (bradycardia). Overfunctioning of the thyroid, or hyperthyroidism, causes restlessness, nervousness, sweating, and tachycardia (rapid heart rate). The most common cause of hyperthyroidism is Graves disease, an autoimmune disorder in which the body attacks the thyroid gland causing it to over-produce thyroxine.

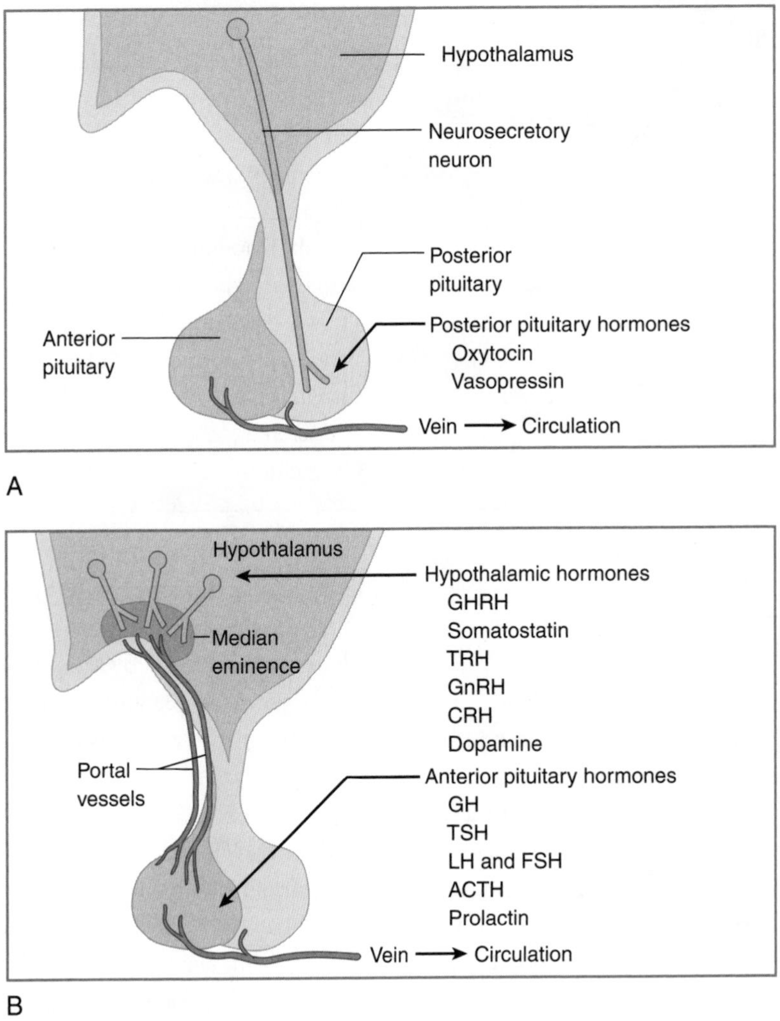

Figure 8-2 The pituitary gland is divided into two lobes—anterior (adenohypophysis) and posterior (neurohypophysis). **A,** The posterior lobe releases hormones that are produced by the hypothalamus (oxytocin and vasopressin). **B,** The anterior lobe releases hormones such as growth hormone and thyroid-stimulating hormone in response to signals from the hypothalamus. *(From Kester M, Karpa K, Quraishi S, et al:* Elsevier's integrated pharmacology, *St. Louis, 2007, Mosby.)*

The thyroid secretes three important hormones: thyroxine, triiodothyronine, and calcitonin. Thyroxine (T_4) and triiodothyronine (T_3) are regulated by TSH (thyrotropin), which is produced in the anterior lobe of the pituitary gland (adenohypophysis). These hormones are essential for normal growth and development; they also help regulate metabolism of carbohydrates, lipids, and proteins. Both T_3 and T_4 require iodine salts for production. Iodine salts are obtained from foods after absorption through the intestines. After absorption, iodine salts are transported by the bloodstream to the thyroid for use in hormone production. Calcitonin helps to control calcium and phosphate concentrations in the blood, and it is regulated by blood levels of these ions. Calcitonin can affect calcium and phosphate levels by inhibiting the rate of release from bone, increasing the rate of incorporation of these ions into bone, and increasing excretion of these ions by the kidneys.

Thyroid hormones are administered to treat hypothyroidism caused by disease or surgical removal of the thyroid gland. Naturally occurring thyroid hormone has been extracted from the thyroid gland of pigs (porcine) and is labeled as desiccated thyroid (Thyroid USP). Many types of synthetic thyroid hormone are available, including levothyroxine (Levothroid, Synthroid), liothyronine (T3, Triostat), liotrix (Thyrolar)—which is actually a combination of levothyroxine and liothyronine—and thyroglobulin (Proloid). Hypothyroidism is treated in

IN SIGHT 8-1 Biotechnology or Recombinant DNA Technology

Human growth hormone is used for long-term treatment of children with growth failure caused by hyposecretion of GH. Growth hormone obtained from domestic mammals such as cows and pigs does not work for humans. For many years the only source for growth hormone therapy was that extracted from the glands of human cadavers; however, this practice was terminated when several patients died from a rare neurological disease attributed to contaminated glands. So, another source had to be found. That source is biotechnology or recombinant DNA technology (see Chapter 1). This is defined as several techniques for cutting apart and splicing together different pieces of DNA. Segments of foreign DNA are transferred to another cell or organism, and the substances the DNA carries the code for are produced. Thus, these cells or organisms become factories for the production of the substances coded for by the inserted DNA.

For example, this process is carried out to make *Humulin* (human insulin). Although bovine and porcine insulin is similar to human insulin, the composition is slightly different. This difference can cause problems for a number of diabetic patients' immune systems, which produce antibodies against it. So researchers inserted the human insulin gene into a suitable vector (*Escherichia coli* bacterial cell) to produce an insulin that is chemically identical to what is produced in humans.

Another hormone that is produced using recombinant DNA technology is parathyroid hormone (PTH). This medication has a special side effect: when given in daily injections it promotes strong bones. Thus, it has also been approved as a treatment for osteoporosis.

the medical rather than surgical setting, so thyroid hormones are not administered from the sterile back table.

Antithyroid medications may be used to treat hyperthyroidism. Antithyroid medications are *not* hormones, but agents that interfere with the synthesis of thyroid hormones. A common antithyroid agent is methimazole (Tapazole), which may be used in the medical setting prior to surgery to reduce the size of a thyroid tumor or to inactivate thyroid tissue.

PARATHYROID GLANDS

The parathyroid glands are small, yellowish-brown ovals, approximately 6 mm in length, and frequently covered with adipose tissue. The glands are usually found embedded in the posterior surface of the thyroid gland. The number of parathyroid glands may vary from two to six, with 90% of the patients having four: two on each side of the thyroid gland. They produce PTH, or parathormone, which monitors circulating concentrations of calcium ions in the blood. Parathyroid hormone has four major functions: to stimulate osteoclasts, accelerating mineral turnover and the release of calcium from bone; to inhibit osteoblasts, reducing the rate of calcium deposition in bone; to enhance the reabsorption of calcium at the kidneys, reducing its loss via urine; and to stimulate the formation and secretion of calcitriol at the kidneys for the enhancement of calcium and phosphate absorption by the digestive tract. Inadequate amounts of PTH result in low calcium concentrations and hypoparathyroidism. This can cause a condition called tetany, characterized by prolonged muscle spasms involving the face and extremities. An example of a parathyroid hormone is teriparatide (Forteo), which is a synthetic version produced by biotechnology (recombinant DNA technology). Because hypoparathyroidism is treated medically, parathyroid hormones are not administered in surgery from the sterile back table.

If calcium concentrations become too high, hyperparathyroidism results. In this condition, bones can grow thin and brittle, skeletal muscles weaken, and the central nervous system is depressed. Surgical removal of parathyroid tissue may be indicated to treat hyperparathyroidism.

ADRENAL GLANDS

The adrenal glands are pyramid-shaped glands positioned on top of each kidney. The adrenals are highly vascular and consist of a central portion, the medulla, and an outer portion, the cortex (Fig. 8-3). The adrenal medulla produces, stores, and secretes the hormones epinephrine (adrenaline), norepinephrine (noradrenaline), and dopamine, collectively called catecholamines. The catecholamines are *sympathomimetic,* meaning they mimic effects of the sympathetic portion of the autonomic nervous system. Epinephrine and norepinephrine work with the sympathetic nervous system to prepare the body for the fight-or-flight response to stress. Effects of

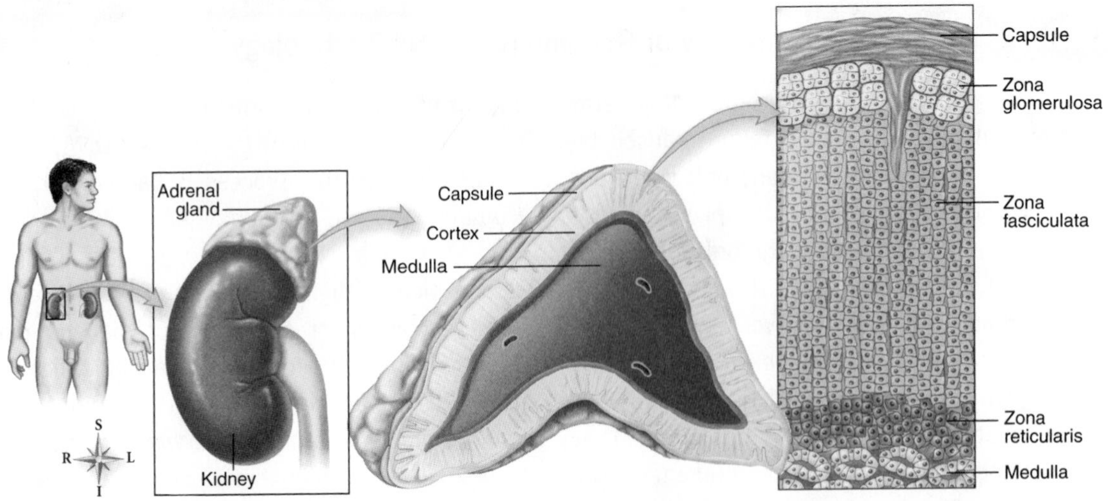

Figure 8-3 The adrenal gland consists of a central portion, the medulla, and an outer portion, the cortex. The medulla secretes epinephrine, norepinephrine, and dopamine. The adrenal cortex secretes glucocorticoid and mineralocorticoid hormones, collectively referred to as the steroid hormones. *(From Patton KT, Thibodeau GA:* Anatomy & physiology, *ed 7, St. Louis, 2010, Mosby/Elsevier.)*

these hormones include increased heart rate, increased force of cardiac muscle contraction, vasoconstriction, elevated blood pressure, increased respiratory rate, and decreased digestive system activity.

Epinephrine

Epinephrine is of particular interest to the surgical technologist because it is used frequently in surgery. Epinephrine is often used in combination with local anesthetics such as lidocaine to prolong anesthesia. When injected in dilute amounts (1:100,000 or 1:200,000), epinephrine causes local vasoconstriction; this means it reduces blood flow so it reduces the absorption rate of the anesthetic.

CAUTION

Epinephrine in local anesthetics is contraindicated for injection in areas of limited blood supply, such as fingers or toes. A local anesthetic agent containing epinephrine may have a red image on the label or red printing noting its concentration. The color red is used to provide a visual "alert," an additional safety measure, to help prevent inadvertent use of epinephrine when contraindicated.

MAKE IT SIMPLE

An easy phrase to remember when to avoid use of epinephrine in a local anesthetic is, "Don't use on fingers, toes, or tip of nose."

Concentrated epinephrine (1:1000) may be applied topically for hemostasis in limited areas. In middle ear procedures, for example, tiny pledgets of Gelfoam are typically dipped in epinephrine (1:1000) and applied to very small areas of capillary bleeding. In ear surgery, epinephrine 1:1000 is *only* used for topical application—*never* injection. If epinephrine 1:1000 is mistakenly injected, deadly tachycardia and hypertension may result (Insight 8-2).

The surgical technologist must exercise particular caution when identifying, labeling, and handling medications (see Chapter 4) for ear surgery, because two significantly different strengths of epinephrine are present on the sterile back table. As an example, in tympanoplasty, epinephrine 1:1000 is used for topical hemostasis in the middle ear while a local anesthetic with dilute epinephrine (1% lidocaine with epinephrine 1:100,000 or 1:200,000) is injected for hemostasis over a larger area. Both solutions are clear. To pass the correct medication at the correct time, the surgical technologist *must* know the route of administration for both strengths of epinephrine. The scrubbed surgical technologist must observe the delivery of these medications to the sterile field, and immediately label each drug—its identity *and* its strength—as it is accepted into the sterile field to avoid errors. In addition, topical strength epinephrine (1:1000) must *never* be kept in a syringe on the back table. Rather, a shallow container (such as a sterile Petri dish) should be used for topical epinephrine, to prevent the drug from being mistakenly drawn up into a syringe for injection.

INSIGHT 8-2 Epinephrine Error Tragedy

On December 15, 1995, 7-year-old Ben Kolb was admitted to Martin Memorial Hospital in Stuart, FL, for ear surgery. General anesthesia was administered, and after injection at the surgical site of what was thought to be lidocaine with epinephrine, Ben exhibited severe tachycardia and hypertension followed by cardiac arrest. Despite massive resuscitation efforts, he did not survive. After extensive independent investigation, it was determined that an unlabeled syringe thought to contain lidocaine with epinephrine actually contained only epinephrine (intended for topical use only).

In a tragic situation such as this, it is important to move beyond the tendency to simply blame individuals involved in the error. Full disclosure and candid discussion took place regarding what actually occurred and how changes could be implemented to prevent such errors in the future. It is vital that we work together to create an open and deliberate culture of safety in the operating room so that we can learn from medical mistakes and improve processes to protect our patients.

Steroids

Adrenal cortex hormones are classified in two major groups—glucocorticoids and mineralocorticoids—collectively known as steroids. The most important mineralocorticoid is aldosterone, which maintains homeostatic levels of sodium and potassium in the blood. Most significant to the surgical technologist are the glucocorticoids, which are used alone or in combination to reduce or inhibit the inflammatory response after surgical procedures such as shoulder arthroscopy or cataract extraction (see Chapter 10). Kenalog-40 and dexamethasone is an example of a combination of glucocorticoids that might be used intraoperatively in orthopedic surgery.

Glucocorticoids are used medically to help prevent rejection of donated organs (Insight 8-3), to reduce the inflammatory response in patients with arthritis, and with aldosterone as replacement therapy for Addison's disease (Insight 8-4). They are also used for the treatment of autoimmune disorders, to suppress hypersensitivity reactions, and to alleviate cerebral edema. Glucocorticoids administered for diseases such as arthritis are used as **palliatives**. Palliative drugs relieve symptoms, but they do not cure the condition or disease.

INSIGHT 8-3 Immunosuppressant Agents

Organ transplantation is the replacement of a diseased organ with a healthy donor organ. This procedure introduces foreign tissue into the recipient's system and will trigger the immune response, which can result in the destruction of the transplanted tissue. Thus, tissue must be matched between donor and recipient to avoid rejection. However, even with careful tissue matching, some incompatibilities will exist (except in cases of identical twins or autotransplantation). Glucocorticoids are used to prevent or alleviate the effects of the immune response when the response is detrimental. For transplant patients, the medication therapy will be lifelong or as long as the transplanted tissue is in place.

Glucocorticoids act by inhibiting synthesis of chemical mediators, such as histamines, and so reduce swelling, redness, warmth, and pain. They also suppress the infiltration of phagocytes to decrease lysosomal enzyme damage and suppress the proliferation of lymphocytes to reduce the immune component of inflammation.

When the immune system is suppressed with glucocorticoids, infectious organisms have the opportunity to multiply. Minor infections may become clinically significant after such therapy, so use in some patients, such as those with fungal or herpes infections, must be avoided. Glucocorticoids should be used cautiously in patients with diabetes mellitus, peptic ulcers, inflammatory bowel disorders, hypertension, congestive heart failure, or renal problems.

IN SIGHT 8-4 Pathology Insight: Addison's Disease

Addison's disease, also known as adrenocortical hypofunction, or adrenal insufficiency, occurs when the adrenal cortex does not secrete adequate amounts of steroid hormone. The disorder was first described by Thomas Addison in 1855, when the primary cause was tuberculosis. Today, however, autoimmune disease is the most common cause. Why? Because the body's circulating antibodies react specifically against adrenal tissue to destroy it. Tumors or hemorrhage of the adrenal glands can also cause the disorder, as can hypopituitarism—decreasing adrenocorticotropic hormone (ACTH) secretion—or abrupt withdrawal of long-term corticosteroid treatment. The disorder can occur at any age, even infancy, and is found in both males and females. Medical treatment involves replacement hormones such as prednisone or hydrocortisone and fludrocortisone. John F. Kennedy suffered from Addison's disease. He had almost no adrenal tissue; but by taking replacement hormones he was able to function in one of the world's most demanding jobs—the presidency of the United States (1960–1963).

Glucocorticoids may be administered orally, topically, intramuscularly, intraarticularly, intravenously, or by inhalation. These hormones may be long- or short-acting, depending on the agent used. Naturally occurring steroids include cortisone, hydrocortisone, aldosterone, and deoxycorticosterone. Many synthetic glucocorticoids have been produced. A partial list of synthetic steroid hormones includes synthetic cortisone (Cortistan, 32Cortone), synthetic hydrocortisone (Cortisol, Cortef, Solu-Cortef), prednisone (Deltasone), prednisolone (Delta-Cortef), methylprednisolone (Medrol, Depo-Medrol, Solu-Medrol), triamcinolone (Aristocort, Kenacort, Kenalog-40), fluticasone (Flonase, Flovent), dexamethasone (Decadron), and betamethasone (Celestone).

PANCREAS

The pancreas, which is posterior to the stomach and behind the parietal peritoneum, is divided into three anatomic areas: the head, which lies within the loop of the duodenum; the body; and the tail (Fig. 8-4). A unique feature of the pancreas is that it functions as an exocrine gland for digestion and as an endocrine gland for release of hormones. The exocrine pancreas is the primary source for the vital digestive enzymes amylase, lipase, and proteinase. A duct from the gland—the pancreatic duct—transports these digestive enzymes to the duodenum.

The endocrine portion of the pancreas is closely associated with blood vessels, which facilitate the transport of pancreatic hormones to the body. Pancreatic hormones are produced by clusters of cells called pancreatic islets or the islets of Langerhans. Pancreatic alpha (α) cells secrete glucagon and pancreatic beta (β) cells secrete insulin. Both of the pancreatic hormones, insulin and glucagon, regulate metabolism of glucose, a simple sugar used as an energy source. Glucagon is a protein; it stimulates the liver to break down glycogen into glucose, thus increasing blood sugar levels. Insulin, also a protein, stimulates the liver to form glycogen from glucose, thus lowering blood sugar levels.

Diabetes mellitus is the inability to effectively regulate glucose. There are two major types of diabetes; type 1 and type 2. Type 1 diabetes is caused by an autoimmune disorder in which the body attacks its own pancreatic β-cells. As a result, the body fails to produce insulin, so an outside source must be provided. Insulin was first obtained from animals, but human insulin (Humulin) is now produced via biotechnology. In type 2 diabetes, the body's tissues fail to respond to the action of insulin on target cells. Type 2 diabetes may be effectively managed with diet and exercise or administration of oral antidiabetic drugs, which include glyburide (Diabeta), pioglitazone (Actos), sitagliptin (Januvia), and metformin (Glucophage). Medications used to treat diabetes are not administered from the sterile back table.

OVARIES

The ovaries, located in the pelvic cavity, are paired glands that produce estrogen and progesterone. Estrogen and progesterone are critical to the development and maintenance of female sex characteristics, including the menstrual cycle, pregnancy, and lactation. These hormones are available in several forms—tablets, capsules, and oil (intramuscular use only)—and are administered to treat amenorrhea, dysmenorrhea, and the side effects of menopause. Estrogen and progesterone are used as oral contraceptives (birth control hormones) and may be used for hormone replacement therapy (HRT) after menopause or oophorectomy (Insight 8-5). Birth control hormones

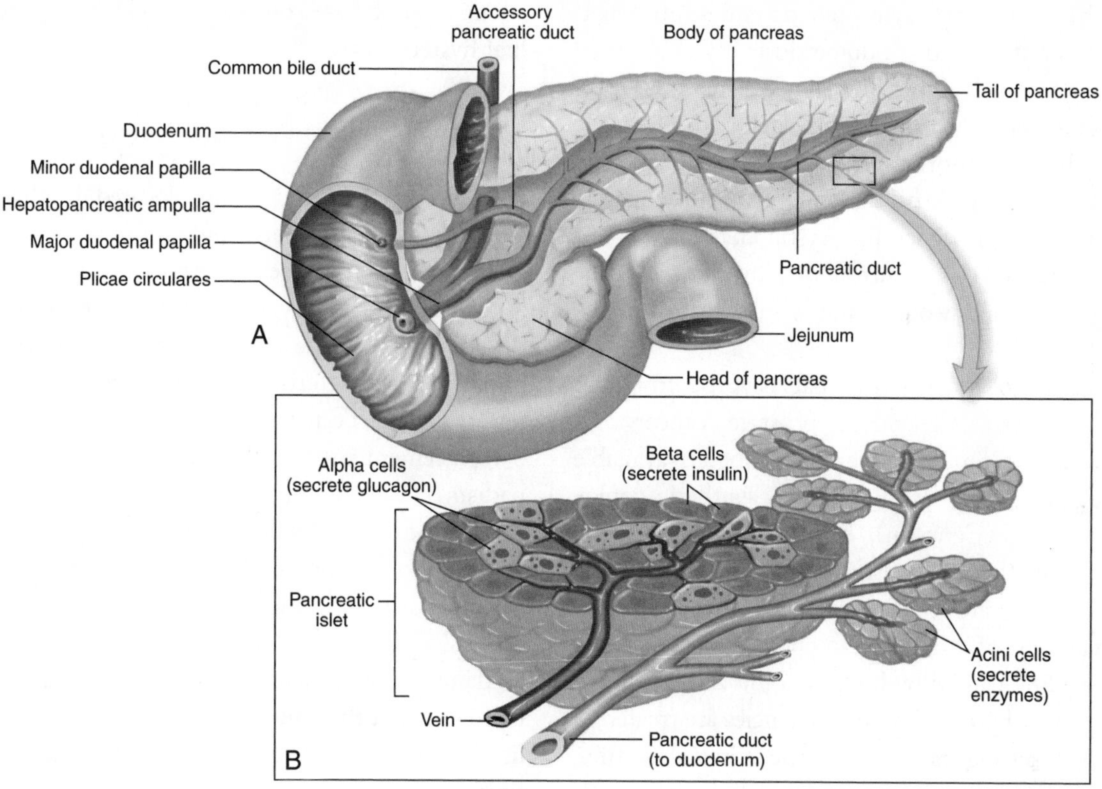

Figure 8-4 **A,** The pancreas is divided into three anatomic areas: the head, which lies within the loop of the duodenum; the body; and the tail. **B,** The exocrine cells of the pancreas secrete digestive enzymes into the pancreatic duct, which leads to the duodenum. The endocrine cells of the pancreas secrete hormones into the bloodstream. Pancreatic alpha (α) cells secrete glucagon and pancreatic beta (β) cells secrete insulin. *(From Patton KT, Thibodeau GA:* Anatomy & physiology, *ed 7, St. Louis, 2010, Mosby/Elsevier.)*

IN SIGHT 8-5 Pathology Insight: The Role of Estrogen in Osteoporosis

Osteoporosis is a disorder in which the skeletal system loses too much mineralized bone volume. Normal bones are remodeled throughout life. Until about age 30, bone formation exceeds bone resorption. Later, however, bone resorption outpaces formation; the result is a net bone loss of about 0.5% per year after age 30. After menopause, bone resorption is accelerated in women because estrogen production decreases. Bone tissue needs estrogen in order to absorb calcium. Estrogen also increases vitamin D metabolism—a process necessary for calcium absorption from the intestines. Without proper levels of estrogen in the body, the amount of calcium stored in bones is diminished and bones become more porous—that is, osteoporotic. The skeleton weakens, so it is less able to support body weight. Osteoporotic bone can be seen on routine spine radiographs. The shape of the bone is the same, but the image is less distinct; this suggests porous, or weaker, bone.

A more sensitive test is a bone-density scan known as dual x-ray absorptiometry, or DEXA. Many times, however, the first indication of osteoporosis is a fracture—in the femur at the hip, in the radius near the wrist, or as compression fractures of the vertebrae. Over time, osteoporotic symptoms include loss of height, stooped posture, and back pain. Estrogen replacement, also known as hormone replacement therapy (HRT), to treat osteoporosis is controversial. The Women's Health Initiative (WHI) demonstrated that HRT reduces the risk of hip fractures, but presents significant risk for stroke and blood clots especially in older women. As a result, HRT is not recommended for most post-menopausal women solely to improve bone density.

may also be used to treat symptomatic **endometriosis** if pregnancy is not desired. Endometriosis is an abnormal condition in which functional endometrial tissue is found situated outside of the uterus, such as in the pelvic cavity. Birth control hormones may also be used to treat symptoms of **fibrocystic breast changes**. Approximately 50% of women experience fibrocystic changes in their breasts—fluid-filled sacs surrounded by fibrous tissue that may become swollen and painful during the menstrual cycle.

Estrogens are also used for palliative treatment of advanced androgen-dependent prostate cancer and metastatic breast cancer. Common estrogens available are conjugated estrogens (Premarin), synthetic conjugated estrogens (Cenestin), and estradiol (Estrace). One type of synthetic progesterone (progestin) available is medroxyprogesterone (Provera). Provera may be used in the treatment of secondary amenorrhea or abnormal uterine bleeding caused by hormonal imbalances.

Estrogen and progesterone deficiencies are treated in the medical setting rather than the surgical setting, so they are not routinely administered from the sterile back table. A rare exception is a cream form of estrogen, which might be used on vaginal packing placed after vaginal hysterectomy.

TESTES

The testes are paired glands located in the scrotum. Endocrine cells are distributed throughout the testes and produce male sex hormones called **androgens**. Androgens, primarily testosterone, are critical for the development of male sex organs and maintenance of secondary sex characteristics. Androgens, especially testosterone (Depo-Testosterone, Delatest), are administered if replacement therapy is indicated, as seen in hypogonadism. Testosterone may also be used to treat some types of advanced breast cancer in females. The androgen danazol (Danocrine) may be used to treat diseases in females such as endometriosis. In addition, patients scheduled for an endometrial ablation may be placed on danazol therapy a few weeks prior to surgery to reduce the volume of the endometrial layer. Androgens are utilized in the medical setting rather than the surgical setting, so these hormones are not administered from the sterile back table.

ADVANCED PRACTICES FOR THE SURGICAL FIRST ASSISTANT

CHAPTER 8—Hormones

Key Terms

euthyroid
hypercalcemia
hypocalcemia

CLASSIFICATION OF HORMONES

Hormones are classified by the following characteristics: their target site (as TSH); whether they are steroid or nonsteroid in chemical composition; and if they are water soluble and can cross the cell's plasma membrane (hydrophilic) or not (hydrophobic). Hydrophilic hormones are derived from amino acids, peptides, and proteins. Hydrophobic hormones include steroids, which are derived from cholesterol. The more common classification is into steroid and nonsteroid categories. Steroid hormones include cortisol, aldosterone, estrogen, progesterone, and testosterone. Note that estrogen, progesterone, and testosterone are also sex hormones. Nonsteroid hormones include the remainder of those as described and listed in this chapter. Hormones that are not used completely are inactivated by enzymes in the blood or in intracellular spaces, and excreted primarily in the urine, with some found in bile. Most have short half-lives of approximately 10 to 20 minutes and so exert their effects rapidly. Some, however, have effects that last for several hours for prolonged stimulation of an organ.

TREATMENT OPTIONS

The thyroid and the parathyroid glands are among the most common glands of the endocrine system to be affected by a disorder and/or a disease. Treatment usually requires both drug therapy and surgery. The hormones secreted by these glands are essential for homeostasis; therefore any abnormal secretion must be corrected. The medical therapy is usually directed by an endocrinologist while surgical removal requires an endocrine surgeon (general or head and neck surgeon). The advanced practitioner acting as a surgical first assistant may only be exposed to the surgical aspect but should also have knowledge of the medical component. It is important to understand how each affects the other.

THYROID GLAND

As previously described in the chapter, the thyroid consists of two lobes connected by the isthmus and secretes hormones. Ideally, it is important for the surgical patient to be **euthyroid** prior to any procedure. If the patient is hyperthyroid (an over-functioning of the gland and thus overproduction of thyroid hormones), medical management with anti-thyroid agents or radioactive iodine ablation is indicated. If the patient is not managed a condition called thyroid storm, or hyperthyroid crisis, could occur. This is a failure of the body to tolerate increased thyroid hormones in response to a stressor (such as surgery). Thyroid storm is defined as an acute, life-threatening, thyroid hormone–induced hypermetabolic state, also referred to as thyrotoxicosis. Specifically, thyroid storm is a decompensated state of thyrotoxicosis that can cause death unless recognized early and treated aggressively. It is precipitated when the metabolic, thermoregulatory, and cardiovascular mechanisms that compensate for thyrotoxicosis fail. Symptoms include hyperpyrexia, cardiac arrhythmias, mental status changes, congestive heart failure, diaphoresis, agitation, and hemodynamic instability. If left untreated, thyroid storm can lead to congestive heart failure, cardiovascular collapse, coma, and death within 24 hours. In the past thyroid storm occurred intraoperatively and postoperatively from thyroid surgery, in patients with Graves disease and in some cases with toxic nodular goiter. It can also occur after administration of iodine-rich contrast media during radiologic studies. Presently, thyroid storm is rare due to prompt recognition, appropriate medical workup, and preoperative treatment (Table A). If the patient is hypothyroid (under-functioning of the gland), medical management with thyroid hormone replacement therapy is indicated before surgery. This condition, in its advanced stage known as myxedema, is characterized by hypothermia, CO_2 retention, and bradycardia. There may be emergency situations in which the patient must have surgery and is not euthyroid. When this occurs, the surgeon and anesthesia personnel will decide the best medications and treatment plan preoperatively and intraoperatively.

PARATHYROID GLANDS

Parathyroid glands are located in the neck, usually posterior to the thyroid gland. The glands may be found within the thyroid gland, in adipose tissue under the thyroid gland, or in the mediastinum. Incidentally, it is possible for the patient to have anywhere from 2 to 12 parathyroid glands. As stated in the chapter, they secrete PTH, which is responsible for regulating calcium levels in the body. Over-functioning of the parathyroid glands causes the secretion of too much PTH. Hyperparathyroidism is the most common disorder causing the patient's blood calcium level to be elevated. Hypoparathyroidism is responsible for low levels of calcium. Both conditions may be treated with medication therapy (Table B); however, most cases of hyperparathyroidism are treated surgically.

Table A Medical Treatment of Thyroid Disease

Medicine	Treatment of	Action	Therapeutic Dosage	Side Effects
methimazole (Tapazole)	Hyperthyroidism	Inhibits thyroid hormone synthesis	Initially 15-60 mg/day in three doses PO; maintenance 5-15 mg q8h	Rash, urticaria, headache, GI tract symptoms
propylthiouracil (PTU)	Hyperthyroidism	Inhibits conversion of T_3 and T_4 hormones	Initially 300-400 mg/day; Maintenance 100-150 mg/d, PO	Rash, hair loss, GI symptoms, loss of taste, drowsiness, decreased white blood cells, decreased platelets
Synthetic Thyroid Replacement Medications				
Medicine	**Treatment of**	**Action**	**Therapeutic Dosage**	**Side Effects**
levothyroxine sodium (Levothroid)	Hypothyroidism	Increases metabolic rate, replaces thyroid hormones (T_4)	1.7 mcg/kg/day PO	Nausea, vomiting, diarrhea, cramps, tremors, nervousness, insomnia, headache, weight loss
liothyronine (Synthroid)	Hypothyroidism	Replaces thyroid hormones (T_3)	5.25 mcg/day PO	Nausea, vomiting, diarrhea, cramps, tremors, nervousness, insomnia, headache, weight loss

PO, Per os.

Table B Medical Treatment of Parathyroid Disease

Medicine	Condition	Action	Therapeutic Dosage	Side Effects
calcitriol (Rocaltrol)	Hypoparathyroidism, hypocalcemia	Enhancement of calcium deposits in bones	0.25–0.50 mcg/day PO	Weakness, headache, nausea, vomiting, dry mouth, constipation
calcium	Hypoparathyroidism	Replaces calcium	500 mg bid, PO after meals.	
teriparatide (Forteo)	Osteoporosis, for those at high risk for fractures	Increases the number and action of osteoblasts	20 mcg/day SC	Dizziness, headache, depression, hypertension, vomiting, diarrhea

BLOOD SERUM CALCIUM LEVELS

Calcium is the most abundant and important mineral in the body. It is responsible for building and repairing bones and teeth as well as helping nerve function. It is necessary for muscle contraction, blood clotting, and proper function of the heart. Maintaining a normal level of calcium is essential for homeostasis and it must be replaced continuously by diet or supplemental agents. Ninety-nine percent of calcium is stored in the bones with the remaining 1% found in the blood. The normal lab value of calcium is 9.0 to 10.5 mg/dL (milligrams per deciliter) but may vary somewhat from lab to lab. A patient with a lab value lower than the normal is considered to have **hypocalcemia** while patients with values higher than normal have **hypercalcemia**. Hypocalcemia may be caused by radical surgery in the central neck including total thyroidectomy and radical neck dissection. Patients undergoing any central neck procedure will need to have calcium levels tested immediately postoperatively. A drop in the serum calcium level to less than 7.0 mg/dL may be treated with calcium gluconate administrated intravenously. The usual initial IV dose for hypocalcemia: 7 to 14 mEq calcium (15-30 mL calcium gluconate) IV in 50 to 100 mL normal saline or D5W over 15 to 30 minutes; may follow with infusion of 0.3% to 0.8% solution (30-40 mL calcium gluconate in 500-1000 mL IV solution) administered over 3 to 12 hours. Faster infusions may result in cardiac dysfunction or cardiac arrest. Hypercalcemia may be caused by over-functioning of one or more parathyroid glands. This is usually treated with surgical intervention as described later.

HYPERPARATHYROIDISM

Hyperparathyroidism is described as an oversecretion of PTH causing high calcium levels (hypercalcemia) in patients. There are two basic types of hyperparathyroidism: primary and secondary. Primary hyperparathyroidism, the most common disorder, is often caused by at least one diseased gland (usually adenoma) that over-stimulates the secretion of PTH. Surgical removal of the affected gland is usually required. The most common procedure today is minimal invasive excision of the affected gland with rapid PTH study. The gland is localized with the use of a sestamibi scan performed preoperatively in the nuclear medicine department. At the beginning of the procedure a blood sample is drawn and processed to identify the amount of serum PTH. A small incision is made over the location of the affected gland and the gland is surgically removed. The half-life of PTH is about 10 minutes: therefore, after this time, a second blood sample is drawn and processed in the same manner as the first. If the results reveal that the serum PTH level has dropped by at least 50%, it is accepted that only one gland was affected and the surgical procedure is concluded. Postoperative calcium levels are closely monitored for 24 hours.

Secondary hyperparathyroidism is a result of renal failure, which stimulates the parathyroid glands to secrete more PTH. This condition, when treated with hypocalcemic or vitamin D analogue medicine, produces limited results. Surgical management is still the most effective treatment. The surgical procedure requires that all but one half of the parathyroid glands is removed. With only one half of the gland functioning, the PTH level is reduced dramatically. Some surgeons will choose to transplant the remaining half gland in the sternocleidomastoid muscle for easy access if more gland needs to be removed at a later date.

HYPOPARATHYROIDISM

Hypoparathyroidism is a condition in which the parathyroid glands do not secrete an adequate amount of PTH, rendering the patient hypocalcemic. This condition is caused by inadvertent excision of all parathyroid tissue during a total thyroidectomy, and is referred to as true hypoparathyroidism found in 3% to 5% of total thyroidectomy. Postoperative calcium levels are monitored after total thyroidectomy to determine any functioning parathyroid tissue. If levels are low, replacement parathyroid hormone is prescribed. Another type of hypoparathyroidism, termed pseudohypoparathyroidism, is a rare, inherited familiar disorder. Females are twice as likely to inherit the condition as males. Both disorders are treated with a hypercalcemic medicine to regulate the calcium levels. There is no surgical procedure to correct this disorder.

Advanced Practices Bibliography

Fulcher E, Fulcher R, Soto C: *Pharmacology principles and applications*, ed 2, 2009, Saunders/Elsevier.

Moscou K, Snipe K: *Pharmacology for pharmacy technicians,* St. Louis, 2009, Mosby/Elsevier.

Advanced Practices Internet Resources

Answers.com, What kinds of molecules are hormones?: *www.answers.com/topic/what-kinds-of-molecules-are-hormones*

Cleveland Clinic, Center for Continuing Education, Disease Management Project (select Endocrinology): *www.clevelandclinicmeded.com/medicalpubs/diseasemanagement/*

Hypercalcemia: *www.clevelandclinicmeded.com/medicalpubs/diseasemanagement/endocrinology/hypercalcemia/*

Drugs.com, calcitonin nasal: www.drugs.com/mtm/calcitonin-nasal.html

endocrineweb:

http://www.rxlist.com/rocaltrol-drug.htm

http://www.rxlist.com/forteo-drug.htm

Introduction to Endocrinology & Endocrine Surgery: *www.endocrineweb.com/whatisendo.html*

Parathyroid Function: *www.endocrineweb.com/function.html*

emedicine, Thyroid Storm: *www.emedicine.com/ped/byname/thyroid-storm.htm*

Forteo: *www.forteo.com/Pages/index.aspx*

http://www.medicinenet.com/liothyronine_sodium/article.htm

HealthCentral.com, Drug Library, Proloid: http://www.rxlist.com/levothroid-drug.htm *www.healthcentral.com/peoplespharmacy/408/drugs/brand/62_overview/Proloid.html*

Labtestonline.org: *www.labtestonline.org/understanding/analytes/calcium/multiprint.html*

MedicineNet.com, Calcitonin Nasal Spray: *www.medicinenet.com/calcitonin_nasal_spray/article.htm*

New York Thyroid Center, Surgical Procedures, Thyroid Surgery: *http://cpmcnet.columbia.edu/dept/thyroid/parasurgHP.html*

PathologyOutlines.com, LLC, Parathyroid Gland, Copyright 2001–2003: *www.pathologyoutlines.com/parathyroidpf.html*

Vancouver General Hospital Pharmaceutical Sciences, calcium gluconate: *www.vhpharmsci.com/pdtm/monographs/calciumgluconate.htm*

WebMD,

Health Conditions: *http://my.webmd.com/hw/health-guide-atoz/stm159483.asp*

Hyperthyroidism: *www.webmd.com/search/search_results/default.aspx?sourceType=undefined&query=hyperthyroidis http://www.drugs.com/pro/methimazole.html*

http://www.drugs.com/pro/propylthiouracil.html

Advanced Practices: Learning the Language (Key Terms)

Using your textbook or a standard medical dictionary, look up and write the definitions of each term.

- euthyroid
- hypercalcemia
- hypocalcemia

Advanced Practices: Review Questions

1. What two endocrine glands are most commonly affected by a disorder or disease?
2. At the time of any thyroid surgery, it is best for the patient to be in the state of ____________.
   A. Hyperthyroid
   B. Hypothyroid
   C. Euthyroid
   D. Thyrotoxicosis
3. List three symptoms of thyroid storm.
4. Which is the most common disorder of the endocrine system that may cause a patient's blood calcium to be elevated?
   A. Hyperthyroidism
   B. Hyperparathyroidism
   C. Hypothyroidism
   D. Hypoparathyroidism
5. Describe the common causes of primary and secondary hyperparathyroidism.
6. What is the most common cause of hypoparathyroidism?
7. What happens to hormones that are not used completely in the body?

KEY CONCEPTS

- The endocrine system works with the nervous system to relay chemical messages called hormones.
- Hormones maintain homeostasis by altering activities of specific target cells.
- Hormones' activities include: regulation of internal chemical balance and volume, response to environmental changes, growth and development, and reproduction.
- Most endocrine disorders are due to hyposecretion or hypersecretion of hormones and are treated with medications administered from the medical setting.
- Some hormones are synthesized by biotechnology, also called recombinant DNA technology.
- Hormones most commonly administered in surgery are oxytocin, epinephrine, and the glucocorticoids.
- Additional caution must be used when handling concentrated epinephrine at the sterile back table to avoid inadvertent injection.

Bibliography

Fulcher E, Fulcher R, Soto C: *Pharmacology principles and applications*, ed 2, 2009, Saunders/Elsevier.

Kester M, Karpa K, Quraishi S, et al: *Elsevier's integrated pharmacology*, St. Louis, 2007, Mosby.

Moscou K, Snipe K: *Pharmacology for pharmacy technicians*, St. Louis, 2009, Mosby/Elsevier.

Stoelting R, Miller R: *Basics of anesthesia*, ed 5, Philadelphia, 2007, Churchill Livingstone/Elsevier.

Internet Resources

CNN.com: *Medical groups release new safety recommendations, questionnaires: Effort aimed at reducing hospital errors.* http://archives.cnn.com/2000/HEALTH/05/19/hospital.errors/index.html. Accessed May 7, 2010.

The Orlando Sentinel, Health-Care Industry: *Heal Thyself.* www.krupnicklaw.com/site/press/healing.htm. Accessed May 7, 2010.

Time.com: *Doctor's Deadly Mistakes.* www.time.com/time/magazine/article/0,9171,992809,00.html. Accessed May 7, 2010.

LEARNING THE LANGUAGE (KEY TERMS)

Using your textbook or a standard medical dictionary, look up and write the definition of each term.

androgen
endometriosis
fibrocystic breast changes
palliatives

REVIEW QUESTIONS

1. What is the general purpose of the endocrine system?
2. Why are the following hormones administered?
  a) Thyroid hormones
  b) Cortisone
  c) Testosterone
  d) Insulin
  e) Estrogen
  f) Oxytocin
3. Why would a male receive a female hormone? Why would a female receive a male hormone?
4. What is the purpose of Pitocin? What is the purpose of Pitressin?
5. Which surgical procedures may involve the administration of hormones from the sterile back table?
  a) Which hormones may be administered?
  b) How will each of those hormones be administered?
  c) What is the purpose of each of those hormones?
6. What is the purpose for administration of epinephrine 1:100,000? Which route is used? What is the purpose for administration of epinephrine 1:1000? Which route is used?
7. What safety measures must be employed when using epinephrine from the sterile back table?

CRITICAL THINKING

1. Can you think of other medications that are given for palliative purposes?
2. What are the strengths of epinephrine normally encountered in the surgical setting?

Scenario

Joseph Goldstein is a 55-year-old man scheduled for a total thyroidectomy. His diagnosis is carcinoma of the thyroid gland. Answer the following questions as they relate to Mr. Goldstein's procedure.

1. What other endocrine glands would be involved in this procedure?
2. Where are these other glands located?
3. How will the removal of the thyroid and these other glands affect the patient postoperatively?
4. What can be done to correct any imbalances caused by removing the thyroid glands?

CHAPTER 9

Medications that Affect Coagulation

OBJECTIVES *After completing this chapter, you should be able to:*

1. Define terms related to blood coagulation and medications that affect coagulation.
2. Describe the physiology of blood clot formation.
3. List agents that affect coagulation by category.
4. Identify the category of various agents that affect coagulation.
5. State the purpose of each category of medications that affect coagulation.
6. Describe the action of medications that affect coagulation.
7. List uses, routes of administration, side effects, and contraindications for agents that affect coagulation.
8. Describe the impact of preoperative oral anticoagulant therapy on the surgical patient.
9. List examples of surgical procedures in which agents that affect coagulation may be administered.
10. Compare and contrast administration route, onset of action, antagonist, and purpose of parenteral and oral anticoagulants.
11. List the administration route for each medication that affects coagulation.
12. Discuss aspects of heparin dosing from the sterile back table.

KEY TERMS

anticoagulants
coagulants
hemostatics
thrombolytics

Blood naturally contains both **coagulants**, which promote clotting, and **anticoagulants**, which inhibit clotting. Normally, anticoagulants are dominant; they keep blood in liquid form. But when damage occurs to blood vessels, the body's coagulation mechanism begins clot formation to prevent excessive blood loss. At times, it becomes necessary to enhance or assist natural coagulation. During surgical intervention, the blood

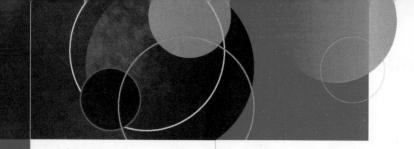

supply to an area may be disrupted, causing blood loss. Intraoperatively, damaged blood vessels are controlled with the use of thermal hemostasis (electrosurgical unit) or mechanical hemostasis (such as ligatures or hemostatic clips). The natural coagulation process usually works effectively on damaged capillaries, arterioles, and venules. But this process may be assisted. Topical **hemostatics** are coagulants used on areas of capillary bleeding as an adjunct to natural hemostasis. And when natural coagulation factors are absent or insufficient, systemic coagulants are used to restore or enhance the coagulation process. Although systemic coagulants are usually administered in the medical setting, they may be given immediately preoperatively or intraoperatively.

Conversely, blood coagulation may also be undesirable. Systemic *anti*coagulants are used to prevent or delay the onset of the coagulation sequence during surgical procedures performed on blood vessels, for example. Heparin is one such systemic anticoagulant. It is routinely administered intravenously by the anesthesia provider and topically from the sterile back table during peripheral and cardiovascular surgical procedures to prevent adverse clotting. Most other systemic anticoagulants are administered in the medical setting to prevent conditions such as deep vein thrombosis (DVT) or pulmonary embolism (PE). Patients on long-term anticoagulation require special consideration when under-going an invasive surgical procedure, because of their delayed coagulation time.

When a blood clot, or thrombus, forms within an intact blood vessel, a mechanism in the blood acts to dissolve the clot naturally. If the natural anticoagulation process is inadequate, **thrombolytics** may be administered to speed clot breakdown. Thrombolytics are agents used to help speed the breakdown of existing blood clots as seen in conditions such as DVT, PE, coronary artery thrombosis, and myocardial infarction.

PHYSIOLOGY OF CLOT FORMATION

The body's coagulation mechanism prevents blood loss due to trauma or damage to small blood vessels. (Trauma to large blood vessels, however, requires surgical intervention—thermal or mechanical hemostasis—to control blood loss.) Damage to a small blood vessel causes spasm, which causes a platelet plug to form, which leads to coagulation. In fact, blood clot formation

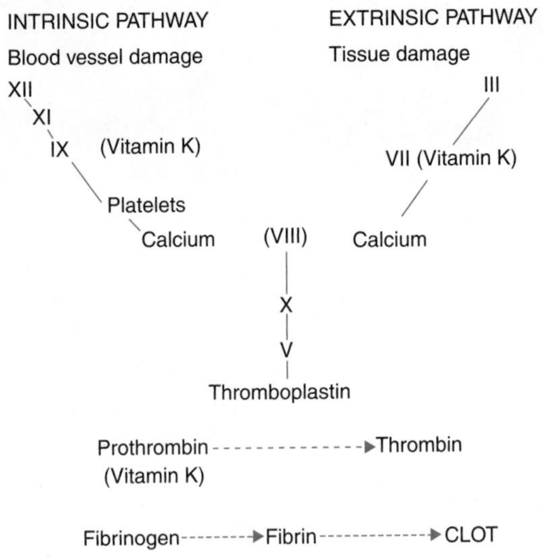

Figure 9-1 Blood coagulation pathways.

is a cascade of events occurring in three basic stages (Fig. 9-1):

Stage 1: Thromboplastin (also known as prothrombin activator) is formed.

Stage 2: Thromboplastin converts prothrombin (known as factor II) into thrombin.

Stage 3: Thrombin converts fibrinogen (known as factor I) to fibrin.

Fibrin is a mesh of protein threads—a net that traps blood cells to form a clot (Fig. 9-2).

Stage 1 involves two different mechanisms for the formation of thromboplastin—the extrinsic pathway

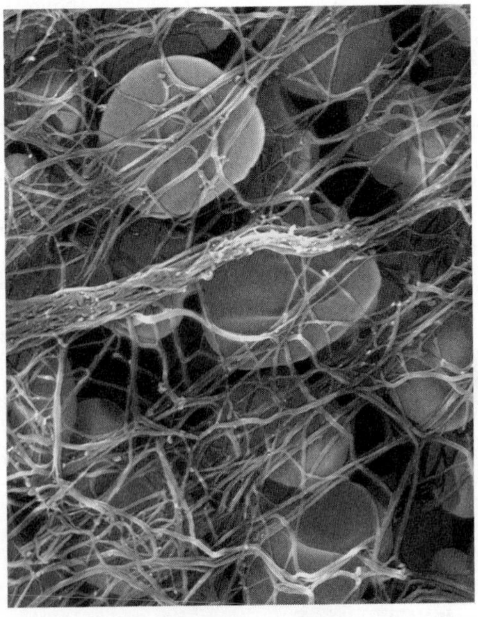

Figure 9-2 Image of fibrin net trapping red blood cells. *(Copyright Dennis Kunkel Microscopy, Inc.)*

and the intrinsic pathway. The *extrinsic* pathway is initiated by factors outside the blood. It is triggered by a clotting factor released from damaged tissue, that is, tissue thromboplastin, or factor III. The extrinsic pathway can produce a clot in seconds. Tissue thromboplastin (factor III) combines with antihemophilic factor (AHF) VIII and calcium to activate the Stuart-Prower factor X. When activated, factor X reacts with proaccelerin (factor V) and calcium to form thromboplastin.

The *intrinsic* pathway is initiated by substances contained in the blood. This pathway is more complex and takes several minutes. When a blood vessel is damaged, the Hageman factor (factor XII) is activated. Factor XII then activates plasma thromboplastin antecedent (PTA; factor XI), which activates plasma thromboplastin component (PTC; factor IX). Then, as in the extrinsic pathway, activated factor IX combines with antihemophilic factor and calcium to activate factor X and factor X reacts with proaccelerin (factor V) and calcium to form thromboplastin.

The clotting cascade requires calcium at all stages—that is, calcium enables many of the steps. Vitamin K also plays a vital role in coagulation. It is required, for example, to synthesize prothrombin (factor II), proconvertin (factor VII), PTC (factor IX), and the Stuart-Prower factor (X). See Table 9-1 for a summary of blood coagulation factors.

Occasionally, clotting may take place within an unbroken blood vessel; this abnormal clotting is called thrombosis. If it forms in an artery, such a clot (thrombus) may cut off blood supply to an area. If a thrombus forms in a vein, it may inhibit return of blood to systemic circulation. Or a venous clot may break off and become an embolus—traveling to the heart, brain, or lungs—causing severe complications, even death. Blood clots may dissolve naturally; this is because blood normally contains a clot-dissolving enzyme, fibrinolysin. But if the body's natural declotting mechanism is inadequate, medical or surgical intervention may be required. For example, arterial embolectomy may be necessary when blood clots form in the femoral, popliteal, or tibial artery. If a blood clot forms in a vein, medical treatment may be sufficient. With bed rest and administration of a thrombolytic agent, such a clot may dissolve.

Table 9-1 BLOOD COAGULATION FACTORS

Factor	Name	Function
I	Fibrinogen	Converted to fibrin
II	Prothrombin	Converted to thrombin
III	Tissue thromboplastin	Triggers extrinsic pathway
IV	Calcium	Essential in all three stages of clotting
V	Proaccelerin	Accelerates conversion of prothrombin to thrombin
VI		Factor VI is no longer believed to be involved in blood coagulation.
VII	Proconvertin	Essential for extrinsic pathway
VIII	Antihemophilic factor	Accelerates activation of factor X
IX	Plasma thromboplastin component (Christmas factor)	Essential for intrinsic pathway; accelerates activation of factor X
X	Stuart-Prower factor	Essential for intrinsic and extrinsic pathways
XI	Plasma thromboplastin antecedent	Essential for intrinsic pathway; accelerates activation of factor IX
XII	Hageman factor	Essential for intrinsic pathway
XIII	Fibrin-stabilizing factor	Strengthens fibrin clot

COAGULANTS

Coagulants are drugs that promote, accelerate, or make possible blood coagulation. There are two major categories of coagulants: hemostatics and systemic coagulants. Hemostatics are topical agents used almost exclusively in the surgical setting. Systemic coagulants are generally used in the medical setting.

HEMOSTATICS

Hemostatics are agents that enhance or accelerate blood clotting at a surgical site. These agents serve as adjuncts to natural coagulation, which controls minor capillary bleeding. Thus, traditional hemostatics are not effective against arterial or major venous bleeding. Recently however, hemostatic agents such as QuikClot have been developed to treat severe traumatic bleeding on the battlefield. These agents are not intended for use in the routine surgical setting.

Hemostatics used in surgery are applied topically in the form of films, powders, sponges, or solutions. Several different types of hemostatic agents are available (Box 9-1), and each is supplied in sterile packaging for delivery to the sterile field.

Absorbable Gelatin

Absorbable gelatin hemostatics are animal in origin, made from purified porcine skin gelatin USP. Applied topically, with pressure, to bleeding sites, these agents are thought to be mechanical, rather than chemical, in their mode of action. Gelatin hemostatics are absorbed completely in four to six weeks, depending on such factors as the amount used and the surgical site. Gelatin hemostatics may be used dry or moistened with saline; however, they should not be used in the presence of infection and they should never be placed intravascularly. Examples of gelatin hemostatics include Gelfilm as well as Gelfoam powder and sponges (Fig. 9-3) and Surgifoam. Dry Gelfilm has the consistency of stiff cellophane; moistened, it becomes pliable. As a pliable film, it can be cut into desired shapes and sizes. It is approved for use in neurosurgery, thoracic, and ocular surgery. Gelfoam powder can be made into a paste by mixing with saline. The powder form promotes granulation tissue, so it may be used on areas of skin ulceration. Gelfoam sponges are also available. They come in several sizes (Table 9-2) for various applications, and may be cut into desired shapes. Gelfoam is commonly used in orthopedic, general, and neurosurgical procedures. Gelfoam is also used in otologic surgery such as tympanoplasty. It is cut into tiny pieces called pledgets, which

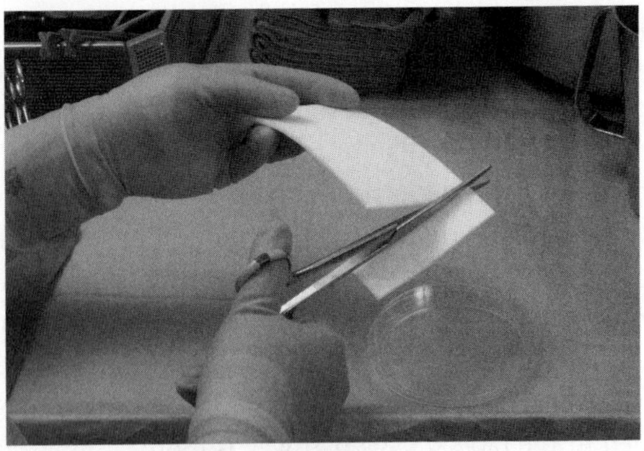

Figure 9-3 Absorbable gelatin hemostatic agents may be cut into desired shapes and sizes.

Box 9-1 TOPICAL HEMOSTATICS BY CATEGORY

Absorbable Gelatin
- Gelfilm
- Gelfoam powder
- Gelfoam sponge
- Surgifoam

Microfibrillar Collagen Hemostat
- Avitene
- Instat MCH

Oxidized Cellulose
- Oxycel
- Surgicel
- Surgicel Nu-Knit

Absorbable Collagen Sponge
- Collastat
- Helistat
- Hemopad
- Instat
- Superstat

Thrombin (see Table 9-4)

Miscellaneous Agents
- Bone wax
- Chemical hemostatics
  - Tannic acid
  - Silver nitrate
  - Monsel solution

Table 9-2 GELFOAM SPONGE SIZES

Manufacturer's Code	Actual Size
12-7	2 cm × 6 cm (12 cm^2)
50	8 cm × 6.25 cm (50 cm^2)
100	8 cm × 12 cm (100 cm^2)
200	8 cm × 25 cm (200 cm^2)

may be used to pack the area around a tympanic graft or to apply a very small amount of epinephrine (topically) on bleeding surfaces inside the middle ear (see Chapter 8).

Gelfoam is also available in a kit, combined with human thrombin, sterile saline, and a 10-mL syringe marketed as Gelfoam Plus. A Gelfoam sponge contained in the kit is moistened with a thrombin solution containing 125 units/mL and applied to a bleeding surface.

Absorbable gelatin is also available in "flowable" form, which conforms to uneven bleeding surfaces and enables clot formation. Flowable gelatins include Floseal and Surgiflo. Floseal Hemostatic Matrix is a combination of gelatin granules and topical human thrombin, contained in a kit that includes items needed for preparation and application. Surgiflo Hemostatic Matrix is supplied in a kit containing the agent and other items necessary to prepare it for use and application. It can be mixed with sterile saline or a thrombin solution at the time of preparation.

CAUTION

Consult package inserts for detailed information and directions for the appropriate preparation and use of flowable gelatins. The scrubbed surgical technologist must become familiar with each new hemostatic product developed so that it can be properly prepared for use.

Absorbable Collagen Sponge

Absorbable collagen sponges are made from purified bovine collagen. The sponge is cut to desired shape and applied with pressure to a bleeding site. When applied to bleeding surfaces, the sponge promotes platelet aggregation. Collagen may reduce the bonding strength of methyl methacrylate (bone cement), so it should not be applied to bone prior to placement of a prosthesis requiring cement fixation. Examples of absorbable collagen sponges are Collastat, Helistat, Hemopad, and Instat.

Microfibrillar Collagen Hemostat

Avitene MCH is a dry, fibrous preparation of purified bovine corium collagen (Fig. 9-4). Direct application to bleeding surfaces attracts platelets to the substance, thus triggering further platelet aggregation leading to formation of a fibrin clot. Avitene should be applied with dry instruments only, as it will adhere to wet surfaces. Wetting also decreases its hemostatic efficiency. In addition, contact with nonbleeding surfaces must be avoided as adhesions may result. Excess Avitene should be removed by irrigation within a few minutes. Avitene is available in powder form (called "flour") in amounts of 0.5 g, 1 g, and 5 g. Avitene is also available in sheets of various sizes and is packaged in delivery devices for endoscopic (Endo-Avitene) and specialty applications.

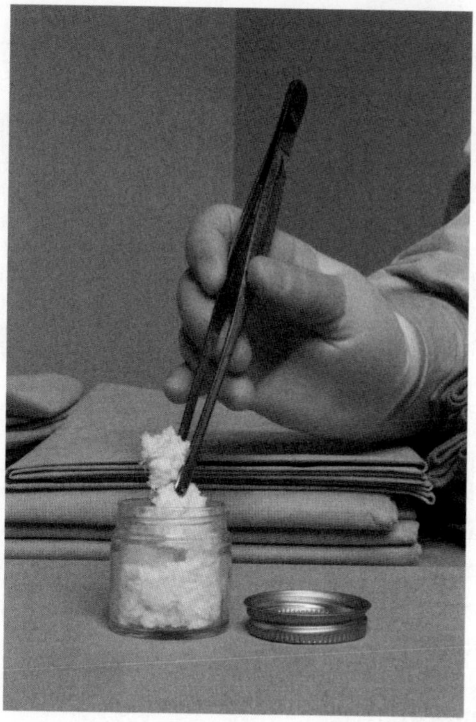

Figure 9-4 Avitene MCH is a microfibrillar collagen hemostatic agent.

Instat MCH is derived from bovine deep flexor tendon, a source of pure collagen. The microfibrillar form allows the surgeon to grasp only the amount needed with a forceps. Onset of action is 2 to 4 minutes. Instat MCH is absorbable, but removal is recommended. It is available in 0.5- and 1-g containers.

Oxidized Cellulose

The hemostatic action of oxidized cellulose is not yet clearly understood. When applied to bleeding surfaces, oxidized cellulose swells, becoming a gelatinous mass that serves as a nucleus for clotting. Oxidized regenerated cellulose (OCR) is the newer version, manufactured by dissolving cellulose and extruding it as a continuous fiber. OCR is absorbable, but removal is recommended after hemostasis is achieved. It is available in knitted gauze strips or fiber form and is best applied when dry. The fiber form can be grasped with dry tissue forceps in the specific amount needed. The gauze form may be cut to desired shape and size. OCR is commonly used in neurosurgery and otorhinolaryngology. Examples of oxidized regenerated cellulose include Surgicel gauze, Surgicel Nu-Knit (a knitted fabric), and Surgicel Fibrillar all available in

Table 9-3 SURGICEL, SURGICEL NU-KNIT, AND SURGICEL FIBRILLAR SIZES

Surgicel	Surgicel Nu-Knit	Surgicel Fibrillar
0.5 × 2 inches	1 × 1 inches	1 × 2 inches
2 × 3 inches	1 × 3.5 inches	2 × 4 inches
2 × 14 inches	3 × 4 inches	4 × 4 inches
4 × 8 inches	6 × 9 inches	

multiple sizes (Table 9-3). Surgicel absorbable hemostat is also bactericidal and effective against a wide range of gram-positive and gram-negative microorganisms. OCR has a low pH and should not be used with any agent containing bovine or human thrombin.

Thrombin

Thrombin is a topical liquid hemostatic agent of bovine origin (Thrombin-JMI, Thrombinar, Thrombostat). Some patients may develop antibodies against bovine thrombin, which resulted in an FDA "Black Box" warning. It may come prepared in a spray bottle kit or in a powder form that must be reconstituted with sterile water or saline (Fig. 9-5). Thrombin should be used immediately after preparation, or it should be refrigerated and used immediately after reconstituting. Thrombin works by catalyzing the conversion of fibrinogen to fibrin, thus increasing the speed of the natural clotting mechanism. Thrombin may be applied topically in solution or as a powder or in combination with a gelatin sponge. Thrombi-Gel is a combination of bovine thrombin and calcium chloride freeze-dried into a gelatin sponge, also available in nonwoven gauze form (Thrombi-Pad).

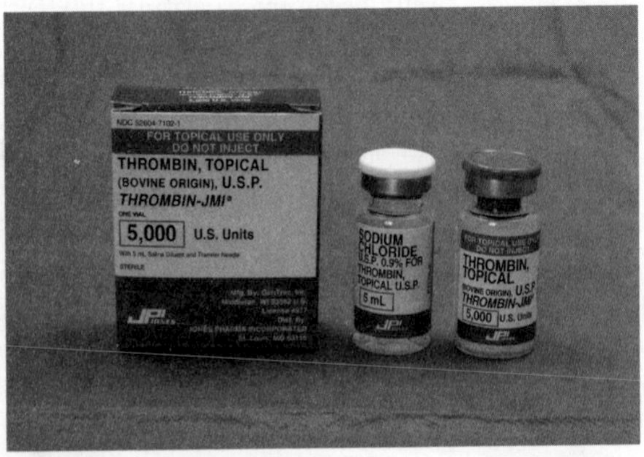

Figure 9-5 Thrombin must be reconstituted with sterile water or saline.

CAUTION

Thrombin must *never* be introduced into large blood vessels because significant intravascular clotting and death may result. In addition, to avoid inadvertent injection, thrombin should *never* be kept on the sterile back table in a syringe.

Thrombin is measured in units rather than milligrams and comes in strengths from 1000 to 20,000 units for different applications. The speed of thrombin's clotting action depends on the concentration used—typically 100 units/mL (1000 units of thrombin with 10 mL of diluent). Concentrations as high as 2000 units per milliliter may be used if needed. Areas of profuse bleeding, as in liver trauma, may require the highest concentration of thrombin.

Thrombin has also been derived from humans and is available as thrombin, topical human (Evithrom) from human plasma and the first recombinant form, topical recombinant thrombin (Recothrom). Topical human thrombin (Evithrom) comes in a frozen solution that must be thawed prior to topical administration. It is available in vials of 2 mL, 5 mL, or 20 mL containing 800 to 1200 units/mL of human thrombin and is approved for use in combination with gelatin sponges. Recothrom is supplied in 5000-unit and 20,000-unit vials of powder, which must be reconstituted with sterile saline to make a solution of 1000 units of thrombin per milliliter. It is approved for use with gelatin sponges. It is contraindicated for use in patients with known hypersensitivity to hamster proteins or snake proteins.

Thrombin is also combined with microfibrillar collagen in a surgical hemostatic agent called Vitagel. This product is combined with the patient's own plasma (fibrinogen and platelets), which is withdrawn at the beginning of the procedure.

In addition, thrombin is used in combination with other agents to form fibrin sealants. Fibrin sealant (Tisseel) contains human thrombin, human fibrinogen, and a synthetic fibrinolysis inhibitor. It is available in a freeze-dried kit that requires reconstituting prior to use and also in a frozen prefilled syringe that requires thawing prior to administration. Both forms are supplied in 2-mL, 4-mL, and 10-mL volume sizes. Fibrin sealant (Evicel) is supplied in a kit of 2 syringes containing human fibrinogen (BAC2) and human thrombin in frozen solutions. These agents must be thawed prior to use. A spray applicator is included in the kit and it is available in 2 mL, 4 mL, and 10 mL volumes with syringes containing equal volumes of fibrinogen and thrombin. See Table 9-4 for a list of hemostatics containing thrombin.

Table 9-4 HEMOSTATIC AGENTS CONTAINING TOPICAL THROMBIN

Generic Name	Brand Name
thrombin, topical (bovine)	Thrombin-JMI, Thrombinar, Thrombostat
thrombin (bovine) gelatin sponge	Thrombi-Gel
thrombin (bovine) nonwoven gauze	Thrombi-Pad
thrombin, topical (human)	Evithrom
thrombin, topical (recombinant)	Recothrom
thrombin and microfibrillar collagen	Vitagel
fibrin sealant	Tisseel
fibrin sealant	Evicel
thrombin, topical (human) and gelatin granules	Floseal

Tissue sealants are agents related to fibrin sealants, but are used for different purposes (Insight 9-1).

Miscellaneous Agents used as Hemostatics

Bone Wax

Bone wax is a topical hemostatic agent made from beeswax. It comes packaged for sterile delivery in a foil-type wrapper inside a peel-back package (Fig. 9-6). Bone wax

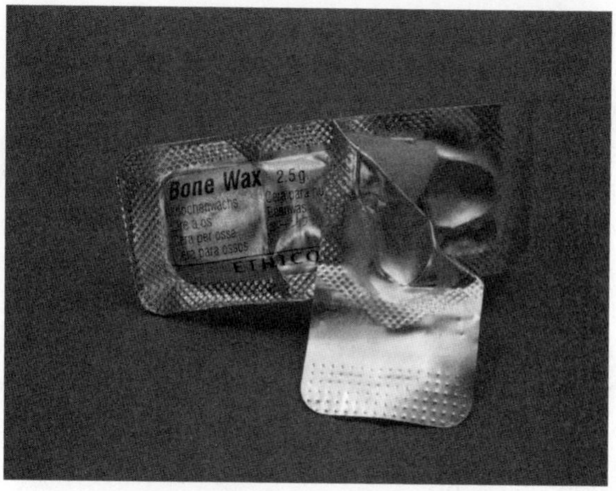

Figure 9-6 Bone wax comes packaged for sterile delivery in a foil-type wrapper inside a peel-back package.

is used primarily in orthopedics and neurosurgery to control bleeding on bone surfaces. It acts as a mechanical barrier rather than as a matrix for clotting. Bone wax is a pliable, opaque, waxy substance that is sparingly applied directly onto bone. It may harden when kept outside of the foil package for extended periods of time. There have been reports of complications including chronic inflammation and granuloma formation attributed to the use of bone wax.

Chemical Hemostatics

Some hemostatic agents, such as tannic acid and silver nitrate, chemically cauterize bleeding surfaces. Tannic acid is a powder made from an astringent plant. Applied topically to mucous membranes, it helps stop capillary bleeding. Tannic acid may be used after tonsillectomy

IN SIGHT 9-1 Tissue Sealants

Tissue sealants are sometimes confused with the hemostatic purpose of fibrin sealants. Tissue sealants are most often used to seal the small perforations left after suturing a tissue layer, such as a blood vessel or the dura. Tissue sealants can be from a natural source or a synthetic source. BioGlue is a natural protein-binding agent made from purified bovine serum albumin (BSA) and glutaraldehyde. It is supplied in a dual-chambered syringe with a special applicator tip in volumes of 2 mL, 5 mL, and 10 mL. It may be used in cardiovascular surgery.

Synthetic tissue sealants include CoSeal and DuraSeal, hydrogels made from polyethylene glycol. CoSeal may be used in vascular surgery. It swells up to 4 times its volume in 24 hours and is available in dual-syringe kits in volumes of 2 mL, 4 mL, and 8 mL. DuraSeal is used as an adjunct to closure of the dura. It is also supplied in a dual-syringe system. It is unique in that it is colored blue for easy identification during application.

Dermabond is a synthetic agent, cyanoacrylate, used to close small skin incisions, such as those used for laparoscopic cholecystectomy.

It is easy to get so many different sealants mixed up, so the surgical technologist must stay current with the introduction of new products in surgery, their purposes, uses, and unique preparation directions.

in combination with other agents such as 1% Neo-Synephrine (phenylephrine, a vasoconstrictor). Another example is mixing tannic acid with a combination of agents (which include glycerin, propylene glycol, Zephiran [benzalkonium] chloride, ephedrine sulfate, and phenylephrine solution) to form Simiele solution. A tonsil sponge is saturated with the tannic acid and Neo-Synephrine mixture or the Simiele solution and applied to the tonsillar fossa to control minor bleeding.

Silver nitrate is another cauterizing agent, especially when mixed with potassium nitrate. This combination is molded onto applicator sticks (which come in 6- and 12-inch lengths) and is used to cauterize wounds. It can also remove granulation tissue or warts. Silver nitrate sticks also come in 18-inch lengths for use with a sigmoidoscope. The applicator tips are moistened with water and applied to the desired area for treatment. Silver nitrate has a caustic effect on mucous membranes and should not be used around eyes. It may also discolor the treatment site with repeated application.

Another chemical hemostatic agent is Monsel solution, a deep brown solution of ferrous sulfate, sulfuric acid, and nitric acid diluted with water or available as a paste. Monsel solution may be applied to the bleeding surface remaining after a cervical cone biopsy.

CAUTION

Monsel solution may be easily confused with another brown-colored solution on the back table for cervical cone biopsy, Lugol solution (see Chapter 6). Lugol solution is a mild iodine solution used to stain the cervix to reveal the area of dysplasia for biopsy. If Monsel solution is applied to the cervix instead of Lugol solution, the biopsy area may be damaged by the cauterization effects of the acids. The scrub and circulator must verify both solutions during delivery to the back table, the containers must be labeled immediately, and the name of the agent called out as it is handed to the surgeon to avoid this dangerous medication error.

SYSTEMIC COAGULANTS

Systemic coagulants are agents that replenish deficiencies in the natural clotting mechanism. If needed, systemic coagulants are usually administered preoperatively. Occasionally, the anesthesia provider may administer a systemic coagulant intraoperatively. Systemic coagulants may be used to replace calcium, vitamin K, or some of the coagulation factors in the blood. Such deficiencies in coagulation substances may be due to heredity, as in hemophilia, or they may be acquired, as a vitamin K deficiency.

Box 9-2 SYSTEMIC COAGULANTS

Calcium Salt
Calcium chloride

Vitamin K
Konakion
Mephyton
AquaMephyton

Blood Coagulation Factors

Antihemophilic factor (VIII)
Hemofil-M
Koate-HT
Monociate

Factor IX complex
Profilnine SD Heat-treated
Proplex T

Systemic coagulants may be administered intravenously, intramuscularly, orally, or subcutaneously, depending on the medication used. See Box 9-2 for a summary of systemic coagulants.

Calcium Salts

Calcium, which is the body's most common mineral, is critical for numerous body functions, including blood coagulation. If calcium levels fall during surgery, natural coagulation becomes less efficient, so calcium salts may be administered intravenously to assist the mechanism. During transfusions, for example, anesthesia providers must monitor blood calcium levels very closely because the processing of donated blood tends to strip it of calcium. Typically, an injection of a 10% solution of calcium chloride ($CaCl_2$) is used to restore calcium levels intraoperatively. Calcium may also be given preoperatively. In the medical setting, calcium may be given by mouth (in tablet form) or injected intramuscularly.

CAUTION

Calcium salts are not given to patients with a history of malignant hyperthermia (MH). Why? Because one aspect of MH is increased calcium release from muscle cells (see Chapter 16).

Vitamin K

Vitamin K is a fat-soluble vitamin; it promotes blood clotting by increasing synthesis of coagulation factors. Recall that vitamin K is necessary to synthesize prothrombin (factor II), proconvertin (factor VII), PTC (factor IX), and the Stuart-Prower factor (X). In the surgical patient, a deficiency in vitamin K can lead to excessive bleeding. Decreased vitamin K levels are seen in patients on oral anticoagulants, such as coumarin derivatives. Some antibacterial therapies also cause vitamin K deficiency. If needed, vitamin K may be administered orally or by subcutaneous injection preoperatively, but it takes up to 24 hours to produce an acceptable effect. When surgery is needed urgently, vitamin K may be given intravenously, but there is an increased risk of anaphylaxis and it takes approximately 6 hours to produce an acceptable effect. When emergency surgery is necessary and cannot be delayed for vitamin K, fresh frozen plasma may be administered 10 to 15 mL/kg for immediate hemostasis (4-6 units in a 70-kg adult).

Vitamin K is also used in the medical setting to counteract anticoagulant-induced prothrombin deficiency. It does not directly counteract oral anticoagulants, but stimulates prothrombin formation by the liver. Vitamin K will not counteract the action of heparin. Administration of vitamin K intravenously has resulted in severe anaphylactic reactions; therefore, it is given intravenously only when other routes are not feasible and when the risks have been recognized and considered. Vitamin K is available as phytonadione (Mephyton) for oral administration or as vitamin K (AquaMEPHYTON) for injection.

Blood Coagulation Factors

Deficiency of any clotting factor interferes with effective coagulation. Two blood factors administered intravenously in the medical setting are antihemophilic factor (AHF), known as factor VIII, and factor IX complex. Factor VIII, a plasma protein essential for conversion of prothrombin to thrombin, is prepared from human blood plasma. This factor is absent in patients with hemophilia A and must be administered intravenously as needed prior to an operative procedure. Antihemophilic factor is available as Hemofil-M, Koate-HS, and Monociate. Factor IX complex is a concentrate of dried plasma fractions—mainly coagulation factors II, VII, IX, and X. Factor IX complex may be administered preoperatively as needed in patients with hemophilia B. It is also used in the medical setting to reverse coumarin-induced hemorrhage. Factor IX complex is available as Profilnine SD and Proplex T.

ANTICOAGULANTS

Anticoagulants are drugs that prevent or interfere with blood coagulation. Anticoagulants are administered in the medical setting to prevent venous thrombosis, pulmonary embolism, acute coronary occlusions after myocardial infarction (MI), and strokes caused by an embolus or cerebral blood clot. Anticoagulants do not dissolve existing clots; rather, they help to prevent new clots from forming. A surgical patient with a history of arterial stasis, or who must be immobilized for a prolonged period of time after surgery, may be placed on prophylactic anticoagulant therapy. Anticoagulants are used in surgery to help prevent clot formation as a response to trauma or manipulation of blood vessels. Patients receiving anticoagulants are carefully monitored for signs of hemorrhage, a common side effect. Minor hemorrhage may be evident as bruising, nosebleed (epistaxis), blood in urine (hematuria), or bloody stools (melena).

PARENTERAL ANTICOAGULANTS

Parenteral anticoagulants are drugs administered intravenously, subcutaneously, or topically that interfere with blood clotting. Heparin sodium is the most commonly used parenteral anticoagulant and it is used in both medical and surgical settings. It is a highly negatively-charged sugar molecule derived from porcine intestinal mucosa. Heparin acts by binding to antithrombin III (AT III, a protein), which greatly increases AT III's ability to inhibit the action of coagulation factors thrombin, Xa, and IXa. Binding with AT III enables heparin to work at several points in the clotting cascade by inhibiting factor X, interfering with the conversion of prothrombin to thrombin, and by inactivating thrombin, thus preventing conversion of fibrinogen to fibrin. Heparin also interferes with platelet aggregation. Heparin binds nonspecifically to plasma proteins, which may account for the variation of effects among patients. It is metabolized in the liver by heparinase. Heparin is considered safe for administration in pregnant patients because heparin does not cross the placenta to reach the fetus.

Heparin is measured in units rather than milligrams and is available in doses of 10 to 10,000 units/mL for injection (see Caution) and it is available in parenteral form only. Heparin injection is available in 1-mL single-dose vials containing 1000, 5000, or 10,000 units/mL (Table 9-5). Hep-Lock catheter flush heparin is supplied in 10 units/mL and 100 units/mL. Onset of action is rapid, usually within 5 minutes, with duration of 2 to 4 hours. Adverse reactions include increased risk of hemorrhage and thrombocytopenia (decrease in platelets), so heparin is contraindicated in patients with existing severe

Table 9-5 HEPARIN STRENGTHS

Strength	Volume
SINGLE-USE VIALS	
Heparin Injection	
1000 units/mL	1 mL
5000 units/mL	1 mL
10,000 units/mL	1 mL
HEP-LOCK FLUSH	
10 units/mL	1 mL
100 units/mL	1 mL

thrombocytopenia. Coagulation studies (Insight 9-2) are used to monitor heparin's therapeutic action.

If a high risk of PE or DVT exists, heparin may be administered preoperatively by subcutaneous injection at least 1 hour prior to a surgical procedure. Interestingly, orthopedic procedures are known to be associated with a higher risk of DVT and PE than other categories of major surgical procedures.

Heparin is the primary anticoagulant used intraoperatively, most commonly in peripheral and cardiovascular procedures. For example, it is administered intravenously by the anesthesia provider 3 minutes prior to placement of an arterial occluding clamp. Three minutes is usually sufficient to allow systemic distribution of heparin, helping to prevent the formation of blood clots caused by arterial stasis and vessel manipulation. It may be of historical interest to note that some older types of vascular graft materials had to be preclotted prior to insertion to minimize blood loss. Preclotting a graft required saturation with blood, which had to be withdrawn *prior* to systemic heparinization to be effective.

According to the FDA, "Serious injuries and deaths have been associated with the use of heparin, a blood-thinning drug that contained active pharmaceutical ingredient (API) from China. The adverse events have included allergic or hypersensitivity-type reactions, with symptoms such as low blood pressure, angioedema, shortness of breath, nausea, vomiting, diarrhea, and abdominal pain. In February 2008, Baxter Healthcare Corporation recalled multi-dose and single-dose vials of heparin sodium for injection, as well as HEP-LOCK heparin flush products. After launching a far-ranging investigation, FDA scientists identified a previously unknown contaminant in the heparin." This resulted in a change to the United States Pharmacopeia (USP) monograph for heparin, effective October 1, 2009. This action now requires that all manufactured heparin undergo testing to detect impurities. It also reconciles the USP unit dose with the WHO International Standard (IS) unit dose, which will result in approximately a 10% reduction in the potency of the heparin marketed in the United States. This change may impact the surgical use of heparin in vascular procedures because it is administered as a bolus intravenous dose and an immediate anticoagulant effect is necessary. Dosage adjustments may be made to accommodate the change.

CAUTION

Careful attention must be paid to identifying the correct strength of heparin administered, because 1 mL of heparin can contain 10 units, 100 units, 1000 units, 5000 units, or 10,000 units. Remember that the dose of drug administered is the strength *times* the volume. It is possible to administer the same volume of heparin, yet give a dose 1000 times more than ordered. The circulator and scrub must always read aloud and verify the number of *units* of heparin placed in solution for irrigation, as well as the volume. The container must be carefully labeled and the scrub must repeat the solution strength to the surgeon when passing it.

INSIGHT 9-2 Blood Coagulation Studies

Two laboratory tests are routinely used to assess blood coagulation. Prothrombin time (PT, pro-time) is an evaluation of the extrinsic and common coagulation system. PT is used to monitor anticoagulant therapy by vitamin K antagonists such as warfarin. PT screens for adequate amounts of factors I, II, VII, and X. Partial thromboplastin time (PTT) and activated partial thromboplastin time (APTT) evaluate the intrinsic and common coagulation pathways. PTT is used to monitor heparin therapy. PTT screens for deficiencies of all coagulation factors except VII and XIII. Previously, results of PT varied by the method used and so were reported with the appropriate reference range. The reporting of PT results has been standardized with the use of the International Normalized Ratio (INR). The INR is the PT ratio obtained using the World Health Organization's (WHO) reference preparation as the source of thromboplastin.

Heparin is also frequently used from the sterile back table during peripheral and cardiovascular procedures. A dilute solution, such as 5000 units of heparin in 1000 mL of normal saline, is commonly used as a topical arterial irrigant.

Heparin may be used from the sterile back table in many types of vascular procedures. During a femoral embolectomy, heparin is administered directly into the affected artery (intra-arterial) through an arterial irrigating catheter to clear the artery of remaining clot or embolic debris. In cardiovascular procedures requiring extracorporeal circulation, heparin is administered through the cardiopulmonary bypass pump to prevent coagulation of blood in the pump tubing. Heparin, in various strengths, is also used during placement of a venous access port or catheter. This is considered an intravenous administration of heparin because ports and catheters distribute medication directly into a vein. Again, proper identification—and careful labeling—of different strengths of heparin on the back table is mandatory (Fig. 9-7). For instance, a port or catheter may be flushed prior to insertion with a mild heparin solution, such as 10 units/mL; then when it is in position, it may be flushed with a solution of 100 units/mL. The scrubbed surgical technologist is responsible for passing the correct heparin solution at the correct time. It is imperative that the scrubbed surgical technologist call out the strength of heparin when passing it to the surgeon.

The antidote for heparin is protamine sulfate, a parenteral anticoagulant that binds with and inactivates heparin. Protamine is a highly positively charged protein, isolated from salmon. Recall that heparin is a highly negatively charged molecule. By binding to heparin, protamine interferes with heparin's ability to bind to AT III and exert its effects to inhibit clotting. Protamine may be used to treat a heparin overdose, or to reverse heparin-induced anticoagulation. Protamine is administered by slow intravenous injection. In surgery, protamine may be administered by the anesthesia provider prior to wound closure if anticoagulation is still evident. If it is necessary to reverse heparin after cardiopulmonary bypass, 1 mg of protamine may be administered for every 100 units of heparin that was given. It is important to note that protamine must be refrigerated, so it is obtained just prior to administration.

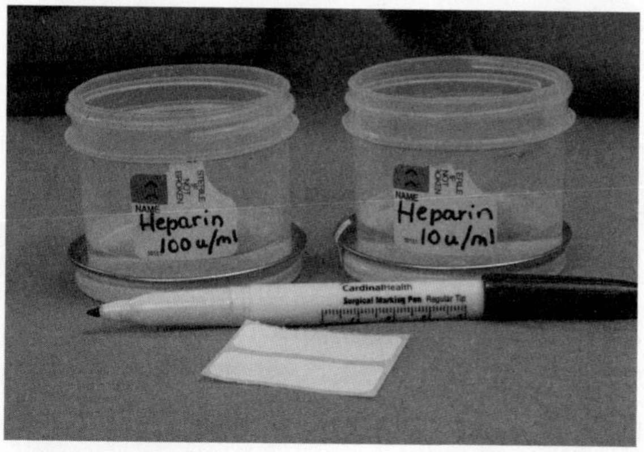

Figure 9-7 Heparin solutions on the sterile back table must be labeled.

Low-molecular-weight Heparins

Unfractionated heparin was the first line of treatment for many years, but it has been replaced in many situations by low-molecular-weight heparins (LMWHs). These smaller molecules are used for the same purposes as regular heparin, such as preventing or treating DVT and PE. Like traditional heparin, LMWHs bind to AT III and increase its activity but LMWHs have a lower affinity for plasma protein binding, so there is less variability among patients. LMWHs can be used outside the hospital setting because patients and their caregivers can be taught to administer the drug subcutaneously. Unlike unfractionated heparin, some LMWHs cannot be reversed reliably with protamine. LMWHs include dalteparin (Fragmin), tinzaparin (Innohep), and enoxaparin (Lovenox).

Enoxaparin is a LMWH used to prevent postoperative DVT following hip or knee replacement. Derived from porcine intestinal mucosa, enoxaparin is administered by subcutaneous injection. A preparation of the drug can be sent home with the patient, avoiding prolonged hospitalization for anticoagulant therapy. Enoxaparin is contraindicated in patients with active major bleeding or those with hypersensitivity to heparin or pork products. It should not be given in combination with other anticoagulants, including aspirin. Side effects include local irritation, pain at the injection site, fever, and nausea. Rare adverse effects include hemorrhagic complications and thrombocytopenia. When necessary, enoxaparin may be *partially* reversed by protamine (1 mg protamine slowly IV for 1 mg of enoxaparin).

CAUTION

Low-molecular-weight heparin and factor Xa inhibitor contain an FDA "Black Box" warning regarding epidural or spinal hematomas. "Epidural or spinal hematomas may occur in patients who are anticoagulated with low-molecular-weight heparins (LMWH), heparinoids, or fondaparinux sodium (Arixtra) and are receiving neuraxial anesthesia or undergoing spinal puncture. These hematomas may result in long-term or permanent paralysis."

Factor Xa Inhibitor

Fondaparinux (Arixtra) is a factor Xa inhibitor used for postoperative and long-term prophylaxis of DVT and PE in orthopedic fracture, total joint, and abdominal surgery patients. It is a synthetic chemical, identical in structure to the part of the heparin molecule that binds with AT III. Fondaparinux selectively affects only factor Xa, without directly affecting thrombin. It is administered subcutaneously *only*, no earlier than 6 to 8 hours after surgery once daily in a dose of 2.5 mg/day for 5 to 9 days. There is no reversal agent for fondaparinux.

ORAL ANTICOAGULANTS

Oral anticoagulants are used for long-term medical management of thromboembolic disease such as deep vein thrombosis or pulmonary embolism. Oral anticoagulant therapy is also used to prevent blood clots associated with cerebrovascular thromboembolic disease. Warfarin sodium (Coumadin), a coumarin derivative, is a widely prescribed oral anticoagulant. Coumarin derivatives act by inhibiting vitamin K activity in the liver, thereby preventing formation of coagulation factors II, VII, IX, and X. Warfarin, which is highly bound to plasma proteins (see Chapter 1), is metabolized in the liver and excreted in the urine. The onset of action of warfarin is prolonged, usually 12 to 72 hours, and its duration is 5 to 7 days. The effectiveness of warfarin therapy is assessed by measuring prothrombin time (PT), which should be approximately twice normal. More food, drug, and herbal interactions are associated with warfarin than with any other drug, so all other medications must be closely monitored. Herbal supplements must be closely monitored as well. Some common side effects include hemorrhagic episodes such as epistaxis, hematuria, and bleeding gums. The antidote for excessive warfarin anticoagulation is vitamin K.

Oral anticoagulant therapy poses a particular problem when a patient requires surgical intervention. In select cases, warfarin may be temporarily discontinued about 1 week prior to an elective surgical procedure. However, patients on oral anticoagulants who require emergency surgery exhibit prolonged bleeding times. As discussed previously, fresh frozen plasma may be administered to infuse coagulation factors in emergency situations. Meticulous hemostasis is also necessary to minimize blood loss in patients on oral anticoagulant therapy.

Aspirin (acetylsalicylic acid or ASA) is also considered an oral anticoagulant; it prevents clot formation by inhibiting platelet aggregation. Aspirin may be given after myocardial infarction or recurrent transient ischemic attacks (TIAs) to reduce risk of further incidence. The administration of just 300 mg of aspirin can double normal bleeding time for up to 7 days. Thus, if possible, patients on aspirin therapy should discontinue use at least one week prior to elective surgery.

THROMBOLYTICS

Thrombolytics (Table 9-6) are agents given intravenously in the medical setting to help dissolve blood clots. These drugs activate plasminogen to form plasmin, which digests fibrin. And when fibrin breaks down, the clot dissolves. Thrombolytics are used to treat acute myocardial infarction when coronary artery thrombosis is present. Anticoagulant therapy may be used in conjunction with thrombolytic agents, because clot formation is an ongoing process. The major side effect of thrombolytics is significant hemorrhage, so patients are closely monitored. Mild side effects include skin rash, itching, nausea, and headache. Examples of first-generation thrombolytics include streptokinase (Streptase), a protein synthesized by β-hemolytic streptococci, and urokinase (Abbokinase, Kinlytic), derived from human neonatal kidney cells grown in culture. Streptokinase is no longer available in the United Sates and urokinase was reintroduced in the United States in 2002.

Two second-generation thrombolytics are alteplase (Activase) and tenecteplase (TNKase). Both are thrombolytic agents produced by recombinant DNA technology. They are a biosynthetic form of a naturally occurring enzyme, human tissue-type plasminogen activator (t-PA). These agents are administered intravenously in the medical setting to reduce patient mortality in acute

Table 9-6 THROMBOLYTICS

Generic Name	Trade Name
streptokinase	Streptase
urokinase	Abbokinase, Kinlytic
alteplase	Activase
tenecteplase	TNKase

myocardial infarction. Tenecteplase is administered in a bolus and alteplase is given in a 90-minute infusion. In specific cases, alteplase may also play a role in the treatment of strokes, pulmonary emboli, and peripheral vascular occlusions. Because t-PA is a human enzyme, fewer allergic and hypersensitivity reactions occur with alteplase and tenecteplase than with first-generation thrombolytic agents. Another advantage of t-PA is its ability to act specifically—targeting clots rather than exerting systemic effects.

ADVANCED PRACTICES FOR THE SURGICAL FIRST ASSISTANT

CHAPTER 9—Medications that Affect Coagulation

Key Terms

aggregation
antiplatelet medicines
anticoagulation therapy
DVT
INR
prothrombin time
thrombocytopenia

ANTICOAGULATION THERAPY

A common medication protocol that affects the vascular system is **anticoagulation therapy.** It is crucial that the surgical first assistant be familiar with medications and how this therapy is used in the preoperative, intraoperative, and postoperative settings. In anticoagulation therapy the blood clotting action is diminished or eliminated. It can be implemented as short-term or long-term therapy. A higher degree of anticoagulation carries a higher risk of bleeding. These patients must be thoroughly educated on the effects of anticoagulation medications, and they are closely monitored while the therapy is in progress. There are various medications used for anticoagulation depending upon the conditions being treated and the length of time the treatment is required (Table A).

SHORT-TERM THERAPY

Short-term anticoagulation therapy is utilized intraoperatively on vascular procedures and for the postoperative prevention of **deep vein thrombosis** (DVT) or pulmonary embolism (PE) in the surgical patient. The most common medication used for short term therapy is heparin sodium. It is the medicine of choice for intraoperative anticoagulation because of its relatively short half-life (one hour). For example, in cardiac surgery using cardiopulmonary bypass, the usual dosage with heparin sodium administered intravenously is not less than 150 and up to 400 u/kg (units per kilogram of patient weight). This will obtain total anticoagulation of the patient's blood. The surgeon should be notified after one hour has lapsed since the last dosage. Additional doses may be required to maintain anticoagulation for the remainder of the procedure. Protamine sulfate is administered to reverse the effects of heparin sodium. Protamine sulfate should be administered very slowly to prevent hypotension. As stated, heparin sodium is used as the first line of treatment for DVT and PE. In addition, it is utilized for acute intravascular thrombosis. Therapy is started with an initial intravenous dose of 5000 units followed by a continuous heparin drip throughout the acute phase. For complete anticoagulation an intravenous drip of heparin sodium is administered at a rate of 20,000 to 40,000 units per day.

CAUTION

Heparin sodium comes in many strengths from 100 to 5,000 u/mL. Always check the strength before mixing or allowing administration of this medication.

Table A Anticoagulant and Antiplatelet Medications

Drug	Route	Indications	Dosage	Side Effects
ANTICOAGULANTS				
heparin sodium	SC, IV bolus, IV drip	Treat thromboembolism, DVT, PE, prevent blood clotting	80-100 u/kg IV bolus, 20,000-40,000 qd IV drip	Bleeding, itching, burning
enoxaparin sodium (Lovenox)	SC, IV	Prophylactic treatment and acute treatment of DVT and MI	30-40 mg SC qd or bid postop*	Anemia, diarrhea, nausea, thrombocytopenia
warfarin sodium (Coumadin)	PO	Long-term prophylaxis for thromboembolism	2.5-10 mg/day x 4 days then individualized dependent on the prothrombin time	Rash, fever, nausea, abdominal cramps, anorexia, diarrhea
ANTIPLATELETS				
aspirin	PO	Prophylaxis for MI, stroke, TIA	81-650 mg/day	Bleeding, bruising, GI symptoms
clopidogrel (Plavix)	PO	Prophylaxis for MI, stroke, TIA, and thromboembolism	75 mg/day	Heartburn, dizziness, aching muscles, GI discomfort, headache
dipyridamole (Persantine)	PO	Prophylaxis for thromboembolism	75-100 mg/day	Abdominal distress
	PO	Reduce damage from MI, prevent recurrence, prevent complications during heart bypass surgery	75-100 mg/day	Headache, dizziness, itching

**Note: One dose of enoxaparin sodium can also be given 12 hours preoperatively when used prophylactically.*
DVT, Deep vein thrombosis; GI, gastrointestinal; MI, myocardial infarction; PE, pulmonary embolism; TIA, transient ischemic attack.

LONG-TERM THERAPY

Long-term anticoagulation therapy is usually necessary for patients with vascular disease and/or vascular implants such as stents or heart valves. It carries the high risk of bleeding, which can be a major or life-threatening complication. The risk of thrombus or embolus formation must outweigh the risk of bleeding. Warfarin sodium (Coumadin) is the most common medication for long-term anticoagulation to treat any thromboembolic condition such as DVT and PE. It is also used to prevent thrombus formation for patients with atrial fibrillation. Warfarin is an oral anticoagulant that suppresses the amount of vitamin K produced in the liver. When the amount of vitamin K is reduced, clotting factors II, VII, IX, and X are suppressed. Warfarin's medication levels peak a few days after its administration, and it remains in the body for 2 to 5 days after it has been discontinued.

Warfarin sodium prolongs the clotting time that is assessed by the **prothrombin time** (PT) laboratory test and must be closely monitored. Laboratory values of PT may be different between specific labs depending upon the type of reagent used. In order to control this variability, the international normalized ratio (INR) laboratory test was introduced. This has been widely accepted as the test of choice to monitor and adjust the effects of warfarin sodium in order to maintain the appropriate level of anticoagulant in the patient. The effects of warfarin sodium can be different among the patient population, making dosage difficult to control, especially at the beginning of the therapy. Initial and maintenance dosages of warfarin sodium are individualized according to the INR results. The INR is mathematically calculated from a PT (clotting time). Therapeutic ranges of anticoagulants are controversial within the medical community. It is commonly accepted that an INR range of 2.0 to 3.0 is sufficient to maintain a level of anticoagulation that is beneficial for the treatment of most thromboembolus conditions. Patients should be monitored for bruising, bloody stools, bleeding gums, and hematuria.

Enoxaparin sodium (Lovenox), a sterile aqueous solution, is a LMWH. It comes in prefilled syringes and multiple-dose vials for subcutaneous and intravenous use. Unlike heparin, the medication may be administered by patients at home using a prefilled syringe (with physician prescribed dosage) and injecting it (subcutaneously) into the fatty tissues of the abdomen. Enoxaparin sodium is indicated in the prophylactic treatment of DVT in abdominal surgery, hip and knee replacement, and for treatment of DVT with or without PE. **Thrombocytopenia**, or low platelet count, can occur with enoxaparin sodium use. Therefore, blood tests for platelet monitoring are performed.

Other oral medications that affect the clotting factor of blood are **antiplatelet medicines**. These drugs suppress **aggregation** (clumping) of platelets. The most common is aspirin, which is often discounted by health care workers as a drug therapy. Aspirin (commonly abbreviated as ASA) is used mainly for prophylactic coverage to prevent the formation of a thrombus in arteries. Patients at risk for MI, stroke, or TIA will benefit from aspirin therapy. Tablets come in strengths of 81 mg, 162 mg, 325 mg, or 500 mg and are taken orally. Aspirin reaches its maximum effect on platelets within 30 minutes after administration. Due to its long acting effects, patients requiring surgery of any kind should discontinue the use of aspirin at least 7 days prior to their procedures. Adverse effects include heartburn, gastrointestinal symptoms, and nausea.

Other antiplatelet medications include clopidogrel (Plavix) and dipyridamole (Persantine). These medicines may be prescribed individually or be used in combination with an anticoagulation medication. Indications for use as a stand-alone therapy are usually in patients with high risk for or history of a thromboembolic event. These include prevention of MI, stroke, and TIA. These medications have relatively long half-lives and should be discontinued several days in advance of any surgical procedures.

Clopidogrel (Plavix) is prescribed to prevent formation of thrombus in arteries. Like aspirin, clopidogrel is used as a prophylactic therapy for patients with history or high risk for arterial thromboembolic event, MI, stroke, or TIA. Recommended dosage is 75 mg/day orally. Its peak effect may take up to 4 days to be reached. Common side effects may include gastrointestinal discomfort, headache, dizziness, aching muscles, and heartburn. Excessive bruising may also occur while taking this medication.

Dipyridamole (Persantine) is used to prevent thrombus in patients who have had heart valve surgery. As stated, it may also be used in combination with other medications (such as aspirin) to reduce the damage from a MI, to prevent a recurrence, and to prevent complications during heart bypass surgery. Usual dosage is 75 to 100 mg orally four times a day. Common side effects may include abdominal distress, dizziness, headache, and itching.

CAUTION

When epidural/spinal anesthesia or spinal puncture is done, patients anticoagulated or scheduled to be anticoagulated with low-molecular-weight heparins or heparinoids are at risk of developing an epidural or spinal hematoma. This can result in long-term or permanent paralysis. The risk increases with the use of an indwelling epidural catheter and by traumatic or repeated epidural/spinal punctures.

{Note} *Antiplatelet medicines have no benefit for use in venous thrombus conditions.*

Advanced Practices Bibliography

Fulcher E, Fulcher R, Soto C: *Pharmacology principles and applications*, ed 2, 2009, Saunders/Elsevier.

Mosby's medical dictionary, ed 8, St. Louis, 2009, Mosby/Elsevier.

Moscou K, Snipe K: *Pharmacology for pharmacy technicians*, St. Louis, 2009, Mosby/Elsevier.

Advanced Practices Internet Resources

Bayer HealthCare: *Bayer Aspirin FAQs.* http://www.wonderdrug.com/faq.htm.

Diener HC, Cunha L, Forbes C, et al: European Stroke Prevention Study 2. Dipyridamole and acetylsalicylic acid in the secondary prevention of stroke, *J Neurol Sci* 143(1):1–13, 1996. http://linkinghub.elsevier.com/retrieve/pii/S0022510X96003085. Accessed July 21, 2010.

Drugs.com: *Dipyridamole.* www.drugs.com/pro/dipyridamole.html.

HealthSquare.com: *Persantine.* www.healthsquare.com/newrx/per1331.htm.

MedlinePlus: *Drugs, Herbs and Supplements.* www.nlm.nih.gov/medlineplus/druginfo/medmaster/a682830.html-20k.

RxList: *Heparin.* www.rxlist.com/heparin-drug.htm.

RxList: *Lovenox.* www.rxlist.com/lovenox-drug.htm.

RxList: *Persantine (dipyridamole USP).* www.rxlist.com/persantine-drug.htm.

sanofi-aventis: *Frequently Asked Questions About LOVENOX.* www.lovenox.com/consumer/prescribed-lovenox/faq.aspx#q8.

sanofi-aventis: *Lovenox.* www.lovenox.com/consumer/default.aspx.

sanofi-aventis: *Lovenox Prescribing Information.* http://products.sanofi-aventis.us/lovenox/lovenox.html#Boxed%20Warning.

http://stroke.emedtv.com/plavix/plavix-dosage.html.

http://www.rxlist.com/plavix-drug.htm.

Advanced Practices: Learning the Language (Key Terms)

Using your textbook or a standard medical dictionary, look up and write the definitions of each term.

- aggregation
- antiplatelet medicines
- anticoagulation therapy
- DVT
- INR
- prothrombin time
- thrombocytopenia

Advanced Practices: Review Questions

1. Why is it necessary for patients on anticoagulation therapy to be closely monitored?
2. What type of procedures may require short-term anticoagulation therapy?
3. What condition is treated with short-term anticoagulation therapy postoperatively?
4. The most common medication used for short-term anticoagulation is __________ and its normal dosage is __________ u/kg of patient weight.
5. One indication for long-term anticoagulation therapy is ____________________.
6. How does warfarin produce its anticoagulation effect?
7. List three oral anticoagulant medications and an indication for each.

KEY CONCEPTS

- Blood naturally contains both coagulants and anticoagulants, but anticoagulants are normally dominant because they keep blood in its flowing, liquid form.
- Blood coagulation is a process that minimizes blood loss when small blood vessels are disrupted. The formation of a blood clot is the result of a three-stage cascade of events.
- Clot formation may be initiated via two different pathways—extrinsic or intrinsic.
- Thrombosis is the formation of a blood clot within an unbroken blood vessel. If natural coagulation or anticoagulation is inadequate, medical or surgical intervention may be necessary.
- Drugs that affect blood coagulation fall into two main categories: coagulants and anticoagulants.
- Coagulants assist the body's natural clotting mechanism. Coagulants applied topically during surgery to control minor bleeding and capillary oozing are called hemostatics.
- Anticoagulants work to prevent undesired clotting, slow the normal clotting mechanism, or help break up existing clots.
- Anticoagulants fall into three basic categories: parenteral anticoagulants, oral anticoagulants, and thrombolytics.
- Heparin is the most common parenteral anticoagulant used in surgery, usually during peripheral and cardiovascular procedures.
- Thrombolytics are administered intravenously to break up existing blood clots.

Bibliography

Fulcher E, Fulcher R, Soto C: *Pharmacology principles and applications,* ed 2, 2009, Saunders/Elsevier.

Kester M, Karpa K, Quraishi S, et al: *Elsevier's integrated pharmacology,* St. Louis, 2007, Mosby.

Moscou K, Snipe K: *Pharmacology for pharmacy technicians,* St. Louis, 2009, Mosby/Elsevier.

Stoelting R, Miller R: *Basics of anesthesia,* ed 5, Philadelphia, 2007, Churchill Livingstone/Elsevier.

Internet Resources

Activase (Alteplase): www.activase.com/home/index.jsp.

ARIXTRA (fondaparinux sodium): www.arixtra.com/.

Baxter BioSurgery: *COSEAL (Surgical Sealant).* www.baxterbiosurgery.com/us/products/coseal/.

Baxter BioSurgery: *FLOSEAL Hemostatic Matrix.* www.baxterbiosurgery.com/us/products/floseal/.

Baxter BioSurgery: *TISSEEL (Fibrin Sealant)*. www.advancingbiosurgery.com/us/products/tisseel/index.html.

Covidien: *DuraSeal Dural Sealant System*. www.durasealinfo.com/DuraSealCranial/.

CryoLife: *BioGlue Surgical Adhesive*. www.cryolife.com/products/bioglue-surgical-adhesive.

Davol: *SURGICAL SPECIALTIES: Hemostasis, Avitene Flour*. www.davol.com/davol/content/avitene_flour.aspx.

Ethicon 360: *Surgicel*. www.ethicon360.com/products/surgicel-family-absorbable-hemostats.

Ethicon 360: *Surgiflo hemostatic matrix*. www.ethicon360.com/products/surgiflo-hemostatic-matrix.

Ethicon 360: *Surgifoam*. www.ethicon360.com/products/surgifoam-absorable-hemostat.

EVICEL Fibrin Sealant (Human): www.ethicon360.com/products/evicel-fibrin-sealant-human.

EVITHROM Thrombin, Topical (Human): www.ethicon360.com/products/evithrom-thrombin-topical-human.

Hospira: *Heparin Sodium Injection*, March, 2008. www.hospira.com/Files/heparin_sodium_injection.pdf.

INSTAT MCH Microfibrillar Collagen Hemostat: www.ethicon360.com/products/instat-mch-microfibrillar-collagen-hemostat.

Levy BS: Topical hemostasis agents: some tried and true, others too new, *J Fam Pract* 20(9), 2008. Available at: www.jfponline.com/pages.asp?aid=6652.

Orthovita: *Vitagel Surgical Hemostat*. www.orthovita.com/vitagel/.

Pfizer for Professionals: *Gelfoam Sterile Sponge*. http://media.pfizer.com/files/products/uspi_gelfoam_sponge.pdf.

RECOTHROM Thrombin, Topical (Recombinant): www.recothrom.com/.

sanofi-aventis: *Lovenox product monograph*. www.sanofi-aventis.ca/products/en/lovenox.pdf.

Thrombin-JMI: www.thrombin-jmi.com/.

TNKase: *TNKase prescribing information*. www.tnkase.com/full_pi.jsp.

U.S. Food and Drug Administration: *FDA Public Health Alert: Change in Heparin USP Monograph*. www.fda.gov/Drugs/DrugSafety/PostmarketDrugSafetyInformationforPatientsandProviders/ucm184502.htm update as of 4/7/2010 available at: www.fda.gov/Drugs/DrugSafety/PostmarketDrugSafetyInformationforPatientsandProviders/ucm207506.htm.

ZMedica: *QuikClot Adsorbent Hemostatic Agent for Healthcare Providers*. www.z-medica.com/military/Home.aspx. Accessed July 21, 2010.

LEARNING THE LANGUAGE (KEY TERMS)

Using your textbook or a standard medical dictionary, look up and write the definition of each term.

anticoagulants
coagulants
hemostatics
thrombolytics

REVIEW QUESTIONS

1. Why are hemostatics used? Can you name some?
2. What are systemic coagulants used for? Can you name some?
3. Name three surgical procedures that usually require heparin ready on the back table. In what strengths?
4. How does oral anticoagulant therapy affect the patient about to undergo a surgical procedure?
5. Why are thrombolytics administered?

CRITICAL THINKING

Scenario 1

You are scrubbed for a repair of an abdominal aortic aneurysm. The preference card indicates that Dr. Fromm wants 5000 units of heparin in 500 mL of saline for topical irrigation. The circulator can only find carpules containing 10,000 units/mL of heparin.

1. What is one solution to this problem?
2. What is another solution to this problem?

Scenario 2

Mr. Davis is a 67-year-old man admitted to surgery for an immediate laparoscopic cholecystectomy for acute cholecystitis. Review of his medical chart reveals that he is on coumadin (Warfarin).

1. What complications do you expect to see during this procedure?
2. What additional supplies should you bring in the room in preparation for these complications?
3. What actions may be taken during surgery to treat these complications?

CHAPTER 10 Ophthalmic Agents

OBJECTIVES *After completing this chapter, you should be able to:*

1. Describe the basic anatomy of the eye.
2. Define terminology related to ophthalmic medications.
3. State the purpose of each category of ophthalmic medications.
4. List examples of ophthalmic medications in each category.
5. Identify category of ophthalmic agents.
6. Describe how ophthalmic agents are used in surgery.
7. Identify categories of medications used to treat glaucoma.

KEY TERMS

constric t
cycloplegics
dilate
glaucoma
IOP
miotics
mydriatics

Ophthalmic surgical procedures often require the use of several categories of medications (Box 10-1) from the sterile back table. Initially, the scrubbed surgical technologist must properly identify and label all medications received into the sterile field. In addition, the surgical technologist must understand the purpose of each drug in order to pass it to the surgeon at the appropriate time. This is especially important during procedures where the operative microscope is used. The surgeon must focus attention and vision through the microscope lens and should not have to continually refocus away from the operative field. In this chapter we'll discuss definitions, purposes, routes, and agents in each ophthalmic drug category used in surgery. A review of basic anatomy is included for reference.

ANATOMY REVIEW

The eye (Fig. 10-1) is a complex sense organ that receives visual stimuli and transmits signals via the optic nerve (cranial nerve II) to the brain for interpretation. Accessory structures include eyebrows, eyelids, eyelashes, and the lacrimal system. The lacrimal system produces, distributes, and removes tears, which keep eye surfaces moist and clean. A thin, transparent mucous membrane called the conjunctiva lines the inside of the eyelids and the anterior surface of the eyeball (globe). Only about 17% of the globe is visible; the remainder is protected within the bony orbit where it is supported on a cushion of fat and fascia. The globe consists of three layers of tissue: fibrous, vascular, and nervous. The fibrous outer

Box 10-1 CATEGORIES OF AGENTS USED IN OPHTHALMIC SURGERY

Enzymes	Ophthalmic antibiotics
Irrigation solutions and lubricants	Anesthetics
Viscoelastic agents (OVD)	Anti-glaucoma agents
Miotics	Anti-inflammatory agents
Mydriatics and cycloplegics	Dyes

coat of the eye is composed of a dense, white connective tissue, called sclera. Sclera gives the globe its shape, provides protection, and can be seen through the conjunctiva as the "white" of the eye. The anterior covering of the eye is made of clear, nonvascular fibrous tissue called the cornea. The cornea does not contain blood vessels to provide its nourishment; rather, it is nourished by being bathed in a solution called aqueous humor and from oxygen in the air. It serves as the "window" of the eye. The area where the cornea and sclera meet is called the limbus. Deep to the limbus is a venous sinus called the canal of Schlemm.

The vascular layer of the eye is called choroid. The anterior, and thickest, portion of choroid is the ciliary body. The ciliary body secretes aqueous humor from structures called ciliary processes. Ciliary muscle arises in the ciliary body and attaches to the lens, altering its shape to accommodate near or distant vision. The iris is attached to the ciliary process and is positioned between the cornea and lens. The pigmented iris consists of radial and circular muscle fibers whose function is to change the size of its opening, called the pupil. The pupil regulates the amount of light entering the eye by **constricting** (making an opening smaller) or **dilating** (making an opening larger). The nervous layer of the eye, called the retina, is present only posteriorly and covers the choroid. Images focused onto the retina trigger sensory receptors characterized as rods and cones. Signals are then transmitted via the optic nerve to the occipital lobe of the brain for recognition.

The lens is positioned just behind the iris and serves to focus images onto the retina. The lens consists of protein fibers arranged in onion-like layers. The lens, which is normally transparent, is covered by a clear fibrous capsule and held in place by suspensory ligaments called zonula.

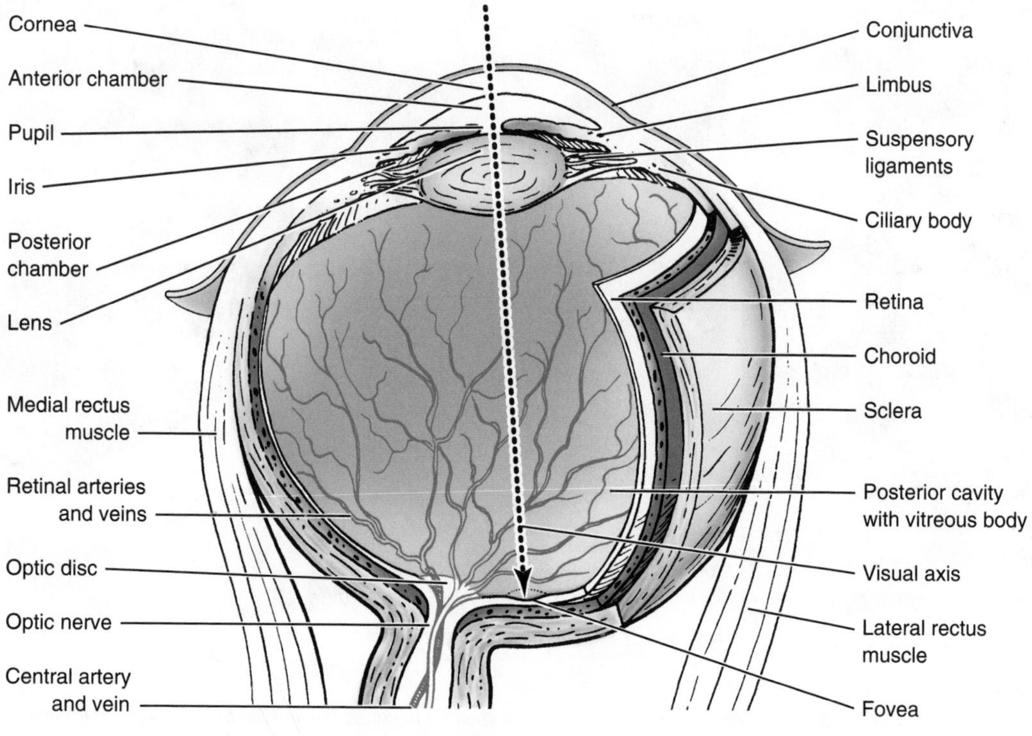

Figure 10-1 Anatomy of the eye.

MAKE IT SIMPLE

The parts of the ocular lens may be compared to a pitted fruit, such as a peach. The nucleus of the lens is like the pit of the fruit, the cortex of the lens is like the flesh of the fruit, and the lens capsule is like the skin of the fruit.

The interior portion of the globe contains two cavities, anterior and posterior, separated by the lens. The anterior cavity is further separated into anterior and posterior chambers. The anterior chamber is posterior to the cornea and anterior to the iris. The posterior chamber is behind the iris and anterior to the lens. The entire anterior cavity is filled with aqueous humor (fluid) secreted by the ciliary processes. Aqueous humor flows forward in the anterior cavity and drains through the trabecular meshwork into the canal of Schlemm. If a blockage occurs in the trabecular meshwork, intraocular pressure **(IOP)** builds, causing **glaucoma**. Glaucoma is the term used to describe a group of ocular conditions characterized by increased IOP. The posterior cavity, which is between the lens and retina, is filled with a thick substance called vitreous humor. Vitreous humor gives the globe its shape, keeps the retina in position, and contributes to IOP. Unlike aqueous humor, vitreous humor is not replaced.

The eye contains a barrier similar to the blood-brain barrier. The blood-eye barrier prevents effective absorption of most systemically administered medications. For this reason, the most common administration route for ophthalmic medications is topical application; as drops, suspensions, ointments, and on medicated disks or pledgets inserted onto the eye. A few agents may be given orally or parenterally. Ophthalmic agents administered topically enter systemic circulation through the conjunctival vessels and the nasolacrimal system. About 80% of eye drops enter the nasolacrimal system, then drain from nose to mouth and enter the stomach where absorption takes place. Figure 10-2 illustrates the proper steps for administration of topical ophthalmic solutions. After administration of the medications, compression of the lacrimal sac prevents rapid drainage of medication into the lacrimal system where it is carried away from the eye.

{NOTE} *It is important to follow aseptic technique when applying ophthalmic medications. The tip of the medication applicator should not touch the patient's tissue or the bottle is considered to be contaminated and must be discarded immediately after use. Also, such*

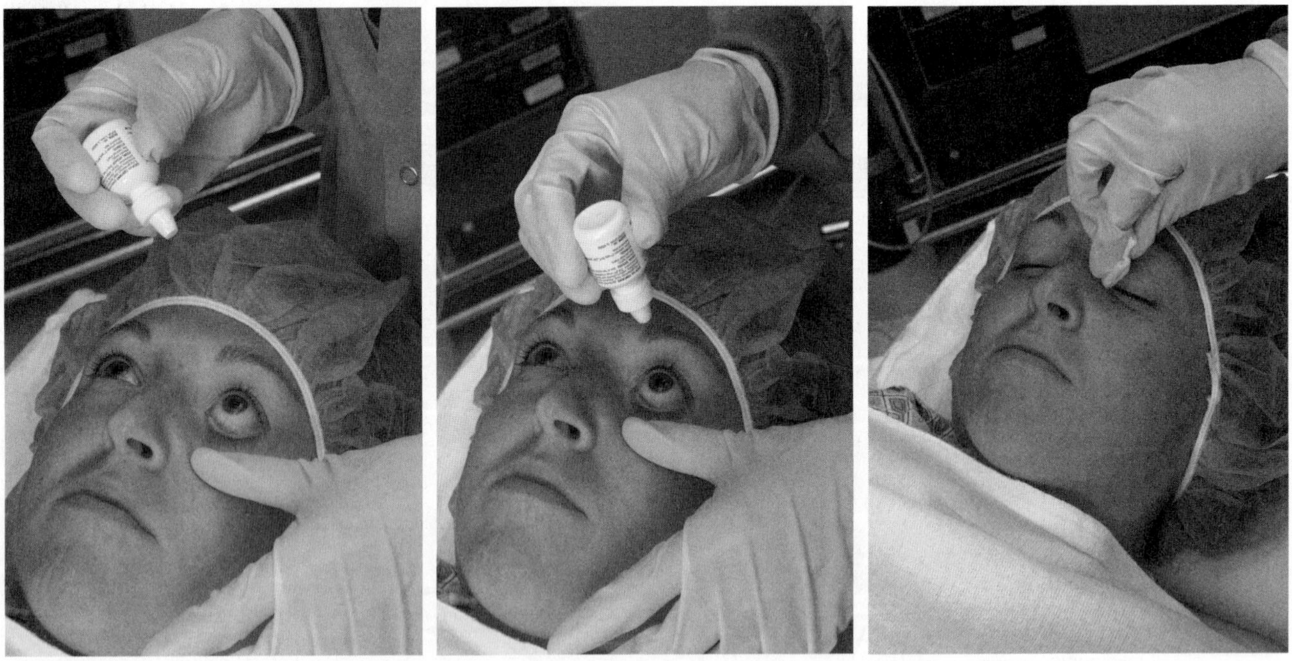

A B C

Figure 10-2 **Administration of eye drops. A,** Step 1: Gentle retraction of the lower lid to expose conjunctival sac. **B,** Step 2: Place drops or ointment onto the lower cul-de-sac. **C,** Step 3: Hold light finger pressure over lacrimal sac for approximately 1 minute; then, with eye closed, remove excess medication from the inner corner of the eyelid with a cotton ball.

contact could result in a corneal abrasion. When using ointments for the first time, the first quarter inch should be squeezed from the container and discarded.

Topical administration may limit a drug's effectiveness due to dilution by lacrimal fluid. Sustained-release delivery systems, such as pilocarpine ophthalmic (Ocusert), a wafer-thin disk used to produce miosis and decrease IOP, have been developed to overcome lacrimal medication dilution. The disk is placed into the lower conjunctival sac, where it delivers the appropriate amount of medication every hour for 7 days. The patient must remove and replace the wafer as directed. Other innovative medication delivery systems are being continually introduced. DuraSite is a drug delivery vehicle that binds drug molecules in matrix that enables release of the medication in a gel-like drop. Added to the antibiotic azithromycin, DuraSite extends the length of time the antibiotic is in contact with the ocular surface.

Another method for instilling ophthalmic medications preoperatively is with the use of pledgets. Medication-soaked pledgets are placed in the conjunctival cul-de-sac after the eye has been anesthetized with local anesthetic drops. An example of this method is instilling mydriatic or cycloplegic medication preoperatively. Antibiotic and local anesthetic medications can also be added to the pledget mixture (placing all medications into a sterile medicine cup), then inserting the pledget with sterile tissue forceps.

Intraoperatively, medications may also be administered directly into the anterior chamber of the eye, referred to as intracameral administration.

CATEGORIES OF OPHTHALMIC AGENTS

ENZYMES

Enzymes are proteins that act as catalysts; that is, they speed up chemical reactions. Hyaluronidase is a protein enzyme extracted from highly purified bovine (cattle) or ovine (sheep) testicular enzyme. This enzyme makes tissue more permeable to medications. Mixed with injectable local anesthetic agents, hyaluronidase increases the rate and extent of anesthetic diffusion through tissue for nerve block. For example, hyaluronidase may be added to 4 mL of 2% lidocaine or to 4 mL of 0.5% bupivacaine for peribulbar block. Hyaluronidase is available as bovine hyaluronidase (Amphadase) or ovine hyaluronidase (Vitrase). Vitrase is packaged sterile in vials and must be reconstituted with sodium chloride injection, then used immediately after preparation. Edema is the most frequently reported side effect of hyaluronidase.

{NOTE} *As of January 2001, hyaluronidase marketed as Wydase was no longer being produced by Wyeth-Ayerst Co. Wydase was the most common form of hyaluronidase used in ophthalmic procedures. It has been replaced by bovine hyaluronidase (Amphadase) or ovine hyaluronidase (Vitrase).*

Historically, alpha-chymotrypsin (Alpha-Chymar, Zolyse) was an enzyme injected during intracapsular cataract extraction (ICCE) to break down the suspensory ligaments (zonula) holding the lens in place. Alpha-chymotrypsin is a proteolytic enzyme; specifically, it dissolves the protein structure of fibrous connective tissue in the zonula. Current techniques of cataract extraction—phacoemulsification and extracapsular cataract extraction (ECCE)—leave the zonula intact, so the use of proteolytic enzymes for this purpose is infrequent today.

IRRIGATING SOLUTIONS AND LUBRICANTS

Irrigating solutions are used during ophthalmic procedures to cleanse the operative site and keep the cornea moist. The most common ophthalmic irrigating solution is balanced salt solution (BSS). BSS is a sterile, physiologically balanced irrigant. It is packaged in sterile containers of 15 mL and 30 mL for topical use from the sterile field; it also comes in bottles of 250 mL and 500 mL for infusion using administration tubing sets. During most ophthalmic procedures (and any other procedures that involve blood in the eye area) the scrubbed surgical technologist will periodically irrigate the cornea with BSS. Other ophthalmic irrigating solutions (A-K Rinse, Blinx, Irigate, HypoTears, Tearisol) are available for over-the-counter purchase.

Lubricants are agents in ointment form that are used to moisten and protect the eye. Ophthalmic lubricants may be used when a general anesthetic is administered for any surgical procedure. Under general anesthesia, eyelids are relaxed and the corneal reflex is absent. To prevent corneal drying or damage and maintain integrity of the epithelial surface, a non-ionic ointment/lubricant such as lanolin alcohol (Lacri-Lube) or polyvinyl alcohol (Liquifilm) is applied to each eye and the eyelids are taped closed. On emergence from anesthesia, patients may exhibit blurred vision; although this blurring is due to the ointment, they should be prevented from rubbing their eyes. Be alert to any patient allergic reactions to preservatives found in these medications.

CAUTION

It is possible to injure the cornea, even through closed eyelids. Always take precautions to avoid injury of the eye area.

VISCOELASTIC AGENTS

Viscoelastic agents are thick, jelly-like substances injected into the eye during certain ophthalmic procedures. These agents are often injected into the anterior chamber during cataract extraction (phacoemulsification) to keep the chamber expanded, to prevent injury to surrounding tissue, and to protect the cornea. Viscoelastic agents may also be used as a vitreous substitute or tamponade (compression). Examples of viscoelastic agents include sodium hyaluronate (Healon, Healon 5, Amvisc-Plus, Vitrax, Provisc), 2% hydroxypropyl methylcellulose (Ocucoat), and a combination of sodium chondroitin sulfate 4% and sodium hyaluronate 3% (Viscoat). Viscoelastic agents are supplied, premeasured, in sterile syringes with blunt-tipped cannulas. Most should be kept refrigerated until use. Side effects include a transient rise in IOP, iritis, corneal edema, and corneal decompensation. Note that the term *ophthalmic viscosurgical device* (OVD) is being used for viscoelastic agents because they are no longer considered as the only medications used to maintain space and coat ocular tissues. Rather, they are an integral part of cataract surgery and are being used in combinations as newer techniques for ophthalmic surgery are being developed. For example, the Duovisc viscoelastic system combines two viscoelastic materials, Viscoat and Provisc, into a single system to be used during a cataract procedure. Another OVD available is 1.4% sodium hyaluronate (Neocrom Cohesive).

MIOTICS

Miotics are medications that constrict the pupil by stimulating the sphincter muscle of the iris. Because constriction of the pupil (miosis) reduces IOP, miotics are frequently used in short-term treatment of glaucoma. Miotics may be used intraoperatively when pupillary constriction is indicated, as in laser iridectomy. Occasionally miotics are used to maintain the position of an implanted lens after cataract extraction. Miotics may be administered by injection or topical application. Side effects include eye, eyebrow, or eyelid pain; blurred vision; abdominal cramps; and diarrhea.

Acetylcholine chloride is a miotic agent available in a solution of mannitol marketed as Miochol-E. It may be used for initial treatment of chronic open-angle glaucoma and acute glaucoma; this is because miosis facilitates drainage of aqueous humor. Miochol-E may be injected during surgery to decrease IOP and to cause miosis if needed. Miosis lasts about 10 minutes. Miochol-E should be reconstituted immediately before use. Carbachol (Isopto Carbachol) is used topically to reduce IOP in glaucoma, and by injection (Miostat) into the anterior chamber as needed intraoperatively. Pilocarpine hydrochloride (Pilocar, Isopto Carpine), in 1% and 4% ophthalmic solution, is another topical miotic. Pilocarpine is also available in the Ocusert disk and in gel form (Pilopine HS gel) for sustained release administration. Pilocarpine (as acetylcholine) acts directly on the smooth muscle of the iris to stimulate miosis. Pilocarpine increases flow of aqueous humor through the trabecular meshwork, thus it is most useful in treating open-angle glaucoma.

MYDRIATICS AND CYCLOPLEGICS

Both **mydriatics** and **cycloplegics** are paralytic agents used to dilate the pupil prior to ophthalmoscopy. Both kinds of agents cause *mydriasis*—dilation of the pupil—by paralyzing the sphincter muscle of the iris. Cycloplegics also paralyze the accommodation mechanism. (This means that patients may be unable to see near objects clearly.) After topical instillation of mydriatics or cycloplegics, the lacrimal sac should be compressed for 2 to 3 minutes to avoid rapid systemic absorption of the medication (see Fig. 10-2). Common mydriatic agents are atropine and phenylephrine. Atropine sulfate (Atropisol, Isopto Atropine), an anticholinergic agent and a belladonna alkaloid, is available for ophthalmic use in solutions of 0.25% and 2%, and in ointment of 0.5% and 1% for topical application. Atropine may be used to dilate the pupil for a few weeks after surgery if needed. Atropine's onset is approximately 30 minutes, while peak effect is seen in 30 to 40 minutes; duration is 7 to 10 days. Atropine is also a potent cycloplegic. Homatropine hydrobromide (Isopto Homatropine) is similar to atropine, but has a faster onset of approximately 10 to 30 minutes, and a shorter duration of up to 3 days. Phenylephrine (Neo-Synephrine, AK-Dilate) is available in solutions of 2.5% and 10% for topical ophthalmic use. Its onset is approximately

30 minutes, with effects lasting 2 to 3 hours. Cycloplegic agents include cyclopentolate HCL (Cyclogyl, AK-Pentolate, Pentolair) available in 0.5% to 2% solutions and tropicamide (Mydral, Mydriacyl, Opticyl) available in 0.5% and 1% solutions. Side effects include tachycardia, photophobia, dry mouth, edema, conjunctivitis, and dermatitis.

OPHTHALMIC ANTIBIOTICS

Antibiotics are frequently used in ophthalmology to treat external ocular infections and as prophylaxis against postoperative infections. Ophthalmic antibiotic preparations include aminoglycosides such as gentamicin, neomycin, and tobramycin. Interestingly, no nephrotoxicity or ototoxicity has been noted with ophthalmic use of aminoglycosides (see Chapter 5). Gentamicin (Garamycin, Genoptic) is available in 0.3% solution or ointment, tobramycin (Tobrex) in 0.3% solution or ointment, and neomycin in a solution of 2.5mg/mL or ointment 5mg/g. Tobramycin may be combined with the anti-inflammatory agent dexamethasone in TobraDex solution or ointment. Neomycin is also available as Neosporin and Mycitracin, combined with polymyxin and bacitracin (commonly referred to as *triple antibiotic*). Other common ophthalmic antibiotics include bacitracin ointment (A-K Tracin, Baciguent) in 500 units/g, erythromycin (Ilotycin) 0.5% ointment, and sulfacetamide (Bleph-10, Sulamyd) in 10% and 30% solution and 10% ointment. Newer ophthalmic antibiotics include moxifloxacin (Vigamox) 0.5% solution, gatifloxacin (Zymar) 0.3% solution, ciprofloxacin (Ciloxan) 0.3% solution and 0.3% ointment, and triamcinolone with ciprofloxacin in a controlled-release system (DuoCat) for subconjunctival injection.

ANESTHETICS

Anesthetics are medications that interfere with normal transmission of pain impulses to the brain. Most ophthalmic surgical procedures require the use of a topical or an injected anesthetic agent. Cocaine solution (1% and 4%) was the initial topical anesthetic agent used in ophthalmology; but it is used rarely now. Two common topical ophthalmic anesthetics are tetracaine hydrochloride (Pontocaine) and proparacaine hydrochloride (Alcaine, Ophthaine). Both medications are available in a 0.5% ophthalmic solution. Their onset is under 1 minute, and duration is 10 to 20 minutes. Tetracaine is also available in gel form (TetraVisc, TetraVisc FORTE) for sustained contact time and increased anesthetic effect. Many ophthalmic procedures are scheduled with an anesthesia provider present to administer sedation and monitor the patient. This is called MAC—monitored anesthesia care (see Chapter 14).

Ophthalmic procedures requiring an extensive area of anesthesia are performed under a regional, retrobulbar (see Chapter 14) or peribulbar block. This type of anesthesia, which provides both sensory and motor (movement) block, is done with a local anesthetic, such as lidocaine or bupivacaine. In retrobulbar block, the agents are injected near the optic nerve (Fig. 10-3). In peribulbar block, the injections are made in the soft tissue superior (above) and inferior (below) to the eyeball. Other agents may be added to the anesthetic, such as hyaluronidase (Vitrase). Hyaluronidase, as discussed previously, is an enzyme mixed with anesthetics to increase diffusion of the anesthetic through the tissue, and to improve the effectiveness of the block. This is contraindicated if a malignancy is present. Another agent added to an anesthetic is epinephrine. Epinephrine is a powerful vasoconstrictor; it is used to prevent rapid absorption of the anesthetic, thereby prolonging the block.

ANTIGLAUCOMA AGENTS

The word *glaucoma* is a general term that refers to a group of conditions characterized by increased IOP. There are two main causes for this condition: either aqueous humor is overproduced, or the drainage mechanism is blocked. Normal IOP is between 10 and 22 mm Hg and pressure greater than 25 mmHg is considered abnormal. This pressure damages the optic nerve and may cause blindness. Although glaucoma is easily treated in the medical setting, untreated it can lead to blindness.

{NOTE} *Most anti-glaucoma agents discussed in this section are administered in the medical setting rather than in the surgical setting.*

The most common form of glaucoma is chronic open-angle glaucoma. In open-angle glaucoma, the trabecular meshwork cannot drain aqueous fluid effectively. A far rarer form is narrow-angle glaucoma (also called angle-closure glaucoma), which may be acute or chronic and is found in only about 5% of all glaucoma patients. Angle-closure glaucoma is caused by an abnormally narrow junction between the cornea and iris, blocking the flow of aqueous humor into the trabecular meshwork. Surgical treatments for angle-closure glaucoma include iridectomy and trabeculectomy.

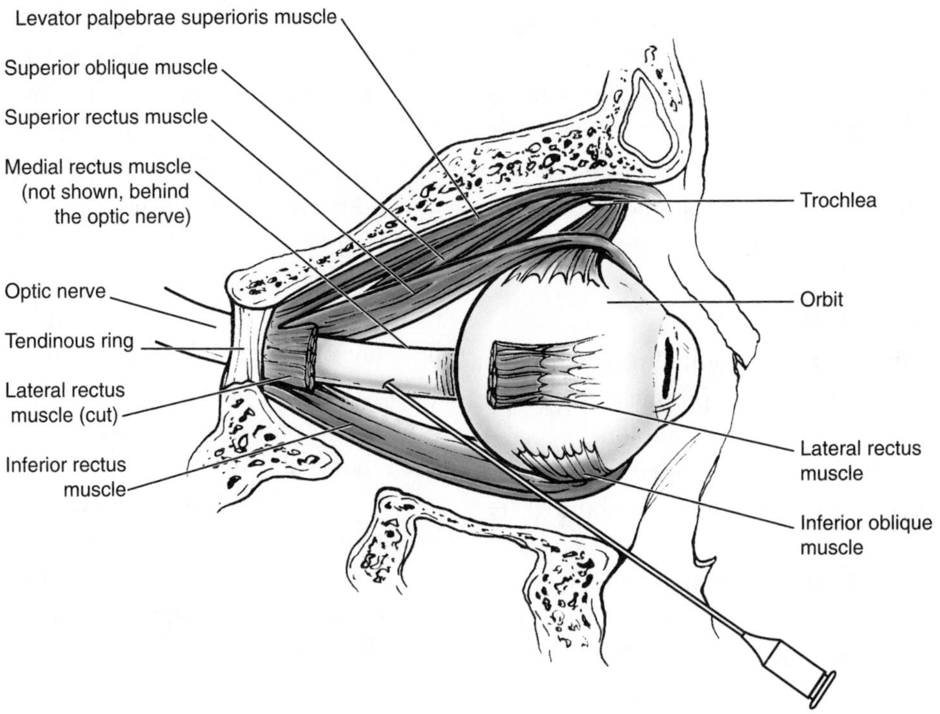

Figure 10-3 Retrobulbar block.

Because pupillary constriction (miosis) may open the trabecular meshwork and facilitate drainage of excess fluid, short-term treatment often involves the use of miotic agents (as discussed previously). However, long-term management of increased IOP may be accomplished with several different types of agents including prostaglandin analogues, miotics, β-adrenergic blockers, α-adrenergic agonists, and diuretics (see Chapter 7), particularly carbonic anhydrase inhibitors (Box 10-2).

Carbonic anhydrase is an enzyme present in the ciliary body; it catalyzes secretion of aqueous humor. A carbonic anhydrase inhibitor such as acetazolamide (Diamox) interferes with production of carbonic anhydrase; thus it reduces production of aqueous humor and decreases IOP. Acetazolamide, which reduces aqueous humor production by 50% to 60%, is administered orally to manage chronic open-angle glaucoma, or given intravenously to treat acute angle-closure glaucoma. With oral administration, ocular effects are seen in 1 to 2 hours, with a duration of 3 to 5 hours. Other carbonic anhydrase inhibitors include brinzolamide (Azopt) and dorzolamide (Trusopt). Side effects may include lethargy, anorexia, drowsiness, nausea, vomiting, and hypokalemia.

Osmotic diuretics may also be used for short-term treatment of glaucoma. By raising the osmotic pressure of blood, osmotic diuretics cause fluid to be drawn out of the eye, lowering IOP. Ocular effects of osmotic diuretics last about 4 hours. Osmotic diuretics may be used immediately before surgery to reduce IOP, or they may be given during procedures to treat retinal detachment to aid in scleral closure. Osmotic diuretics are also used in cases of acute angle-closure glaucoma to facilitate the response of the iris muscle to miotics. The most common osmotic diuretic used in ophthalmic surgery is mannitol (Osmitrol). Mannitol in a 5% to 20% solution is given intravenously in a dose of 0.25 to 2 g/kg of patient weight. For example, 500 mL of a 20% mannitol solution may be administered over a period of 30 to 60 minutes. When mannitol is administered preoperatively, an

Box 10-2 CATEGORIES OF MEDICATIONS USED TO TREAT GLAUCOMA

Carbonic anhydrase inhibitors	β-Adrenergic blockers
Osmotic diuretics	Cholinergics (miotics)
α-Adrenergic agonists	Prostaglandin analogues

indwelling urinary catheter is usually inserted into the patient's bladder to accommodate resulting diuresis (increased excretion of urine). Maximum effect is noted approximately an hour after administration. Other osmotic diuretics used in ophthalmology include glycerin 50% solution (Glyrol, Osmoglyn, Ophthalgan) and isosorbide 45% solution (Isordil, Isonate), both administered orally. Side effects from osmotics are commonly headache, nausea, vomiting, and diarrhea.

Another category of medications used to treat glaucoma is the α-adrenergic agonists (also called sympathomimetics), administered as eye drops. These agents are considered the third line of treatment for glaucoma, reducing production of aqueous humor and increasing outflow. Examples of these agents include apraclonidine (Iopidine), brimonidine (Alphagan), epinephrine, and dipivefrin (Propine), a prodrug that is converted to epinephrine in the eye.

A group of medications known as β-adrenergic blockers are also used to treat glaucoma. By blocking β-adrenergic receptor sites, these drugs reduce aqueous fluid production. Systemic side effects of β-adrenergic blockers include decreased heart rate and blood pressure. Timolol (Timoptic) is used to treat chronic open-angle glaucoma. Although its exact mechanism is not yet known, it has been reported to decrease production of aqueous humor and increase outflow. Timolol, in 0.25% or 0.5% ophthalmic solution, is administered in a dosage of one drop in the affected eye twice a day. One dose of timolol may reduce IOP for up to 24 hours. Unlike miotics, no accommodation problems are noted with use. Other β-adrenergic blockers include betaxolol (Betoptic) 0.5% solution, metipranolol (Optipranolol) 0.3% solution, and levobunolol (Betagan) 0.25% and 0.5% solution. Side effects include mild ocular irritation, eye pain, headache, decreased corneal sensitivity, transient dry eye syndrome, and blurring of central vision.

MAKE IT SIMPLE

The names of β-adrenergic blockers usually end in "-olol."

Currently, the first line of glaucoma treatment is a group of drugs known as prostaglandin analogues (PGA). These agents significantly reduce IOP by increasing uveoscleral outflow, a different route than the trabecular meshwork. PGAs may be used alone or in combination with other categories of agents such as carbonic anhydrase inhibitors or β-adrenergic blockers. Bimatoprost (Lumigan 0.03%), latanoprost (Xalatan 0.005%), and travoprost (Travatan 0.004%) are all prostaglandin analogues.

ANTI-INFLAMMATORY AGENTS

Two categories of anti-inflammatory agents are used in ophthalmology: steroids and nonsteroidal anti-inflammatory drugs (NSAIDs). Steroids are hormones (see Chapter 8) with a wide range of effects; they are used in ophthalmology to decrease ocular inflammatory response to trauma, to decrease corneal inflammation, to protect the eye from scarring, and postoperatively to decrease swelling. They are contraindicated in the presence of infection because steroids are not bactericidal and tend to hide the symptoms of infection. However, steroid preparations are also available in combination with antimicrobial agents. Examples are TobraDex, which combines the anti-inflammatory action of dexamethasone 0.1% with the antibiotic tobramycin 0.3%; PRED-G, which is prednisolone in combination with the antibiotic gentamicin; and Maxitrol ointment, which combines the antibiotics neomycin and polymyxin B with dexamethasone. Steroids may be administered via four routes: topical, systemic, periocular, or intravitreal. Common steroids used are betamethasone (Celestone suspension), dexamethasone (Maxidex suspension, Decadron ointment and solution), and prednisolone (Inflamase, Pred Forte suspension and solution).

Ocular NSAIDs are used to prevent or treat cystoid macular edema, iritis, and conjunctivitis. They are also used to reduce postoperative inflammation following cataract surgery. Ophthalmic solutions of ketorolac 0.5% (Acular), diclofenac 0.1% (Voltaren), nepafenac 0.1% (Nevanac), and bromfenac 0.09% (Xibrom) are available. NSAIDs may also be used to inhibit intraoperative miosis, particularly flurbiprofen 0.03% (Ocufen) and suprofen 0.1% (Profenal). Side effects include burning and stinging when administered.

DYES

Dyes, which are used to color or mark tissue, may also be used as diagnostic agents in ophthalmology. Ophthalmic dyes are instilled topically to diagnose abnormalities of the cornea and conjunctival epithelium or to locate foreign bodies. Dyes may also be used to observe the flow of aqueous humor or to demonstrate lacrimal system function. Examples of dyes used in ophthalmology are fluorescein sodium, rose bengal, and lissamine green. These dyes are available as individually wrapped sterile paper strips, which are moistened with a sterile solution and applied to the anterior surface of the eye. Fluorescein sodium (Fluor-I-Strip, Ful-Glo, AK-Fluor, Fluorescite) is a nontoxic, water-soluble dye that is applied to the cornea or conjunctiva to identify denuded areas of epithelium or foreign bodies. It diagnoses corneal abrasions by staining damaged or diseased corneal tissue bright green. A foreign body will be surrounded by a green ring. Fluorescein sodium should not be used with soft contact lenses, because they may absorb the dye. Rose bengal and lissamine green in 1% solutions stain devitalized cells better than fluorescein sodium. These dyes are primarily used for demarcation of devitalized conjunctival epithelium seen in "dry eye" syndrome (keratoconjunctivitis sicca, or KCS).

Indocyanine green (IC-Green) is a diagnostic dye used for ophthalmic angiography. It is given intravenously outside the surgical setting in order to visualize the choroidal vascular network. The dye leaks slowly from these choroidal capillaries, which allows vessels in the deeper tissues to be seen (because they are not masked by the dye). As these deeper layers are visualized, tumors and other problems that may not be detectable with regular angiography at this point can be located and treated. Indocyanine green is a fluorescent, sterile, water-soluble dye that comes in powder form and must be reconstituted with sterile water. Once prepared, it must be used within 10 hours. It contains sodium iodide, so caution must be used for patients with iodide allergies.

ADVANCED PRACTICES FOR THE SURGICAL FIRST ASSISTANT

CHAPTER 10—Ophthalmic Agents

Key Terms

extracapsular
intracapsular
phacoemulsification

CATARACT EXTRACTION

The surgical first assistant practicing in ophthalmology must combine the science of pathophysiology and anatomy of the eyes with a current knowledge of the pharmaceutical agents used in the treatment of eye disorders and surgical procedures. One of the most common eye disorders is cataracts. Cataracts are the leading cause of decreased vision in the United States, and globally the leading cause of blindness. About 5.5 million Americans have a cataract interfering with their vision with 400,000 new cases per year. By the age of 80, more than half of all Americans have cataracts. With surgical removal being the only treatment, cataract surgery represents the most common and successful of all surgical procedures today. More than 1 million cataracts are removed each year. A cataract is defined as an opacity or clouding of the crystalline lens of the eye. Although most cataracts are age related (senile cataract), they may be associated with other factors. These include trauma, metabolic diseases, congenital factors, prolonged corticosteroid usage, and exposure to radiation or ultraviolet (UV) light. Cataracts may develop in one or both eyes. Each cataract tends to "mature" or develop at a different rate. Therefore the patient's vision may be affected in one eye more than the other. Because of this differential, only one cataract is removed at a time. Cataract extraction is an intraocular procedure. Cataracts can be extracted by one of two methods: **intracapsular** or **extracapsular.** The most commonly performed surgical intervention for cataracts in the United States is extracapsular extraction with **phacoemulsification** and intraocular lens implant. It is not uncommon for the patient to be referred for surgery before the cataract has fully matured; that is, produces swelling and opacity of the entire lens. It is safer with less risk of complications and easier removal of the cataract before this stage.

Today's patient undergoing an ophthalmic procedure, such as cataract extraction, is most likely to have surgery performed on an ambulatory (same-day surgery) basis. This means the perioperative team must coordinate patient preparations in a very short period of time. The success of surgical intervention depends on the skills and knowledge of the team.

CAUTION

Medications that are intended for usage in the eyes are potent, and one medication error can result in permanent blindness. Therefore all medications and irrigating solutions should be confirmed and labeled immediately.

PREOPERATIVE MEDICATIONS

Preoperative medications are extremely important to the outcome of the procedure and to the patient's safety. Conventionally, preoperative preparation for cataract extraction involved the installation of multiple drops. These may include, but are not limited to, a mydriatic for maximum pupil dilation that is essential for lens extraction. A short acting mydriatic such as phenylephrine hydrochloride (Neo-Synephrine) 2.5% or 10% is preferred. This can be used alone or in combination with a cycloplegic. Tropicamide (Mydriacyl) 1% is a commonly used agent that causes cycloplegia (paralysis of accommodation, inhibits focusing) and it also has a mydriatic effect. Another mydriatic-cycloplegic is cyclopentolate (Cyclogyl) 1%. A non-steroidal anti-inflammatory agent such as ketorolac (Acular) 0.5%, flurbiprofen (Ocufen) 0.03%, nepafenac (Nevanac) ophthalmic, or prednisolone acetate (Omnipred) may be used to decrease the inflammatory process and to help maintain pupil dilation. A topical, broad spectrum anti-infective agent such as moxifloxacin (Vigamox) 0.5% or gatifloxacin (Zymar) 0.3% ophthalmic solution may be used to sterilize the eye to prevent the intraocular introduction of bacteria, and is prescribed for the patient postoperatively as well.

{NOTE} *Ophthalmic medications are sterile when opened. Take care to prevent contamination when handling the container.*

When prepping, povidone iodine ophthalmic solution (Betadine Ophthalmic) 5% is used. Usually one drop is inserted into the operative eye. The eye is closed and then the area around the site is prepped with regular povidone iodine prep solution.

ASSISTANT ADVICE

When administering topical mydriatics or cycloplegics for pupil dilation preoperatively, a patient with dark irises may need a larger dose because more pigment requires more of the medication to achieve the desired effect.

TOPICAL METHOD OF LOCAL ANESTHESIA

The topical method of local anesthesia for cataract extraction has increased in popularity. A combination of anesthetic eye drops such as tetracaine hydrochloride (Pontocaine) 0.5% is instilled into the eye and enhanced with infiltration anesthetic such as methylparaben-free (MPF) lidocaine (Xylocaine) 1% or 2%, which is placed into the anterior chamber through the incision. Lidocaine (MPF) 4% ophthalmic drops may also be used before and during the procedure. Another topical anesthetic agent used is proparacaine (Alcaine) 0.5%, which can be instilled into the operative eye one hour preoperatively, then every so many minutes (as 5-10) for a total of three doses (surgeon's preference).

{NOTE} *The patient may be given only topical local anesthesia to the eye and valium orally to calm nervousness. Therefore, it may not be necessary for the patient to be NPO (nil per os [nothing by mouth]) or have an intravenous (IV) solution started before the procedure.*

INTRAOPERATIVE MEDICATIONS

As discussed in the chapter, intraoperative medications may include balanced salt solution (BSS) used for intraocular irrigation and to moisten the cornea. A viscoelastic agent is injected into the anterior chamber to deepen and maintain the chamber, and widen the pupil to facilitate the use of the phacoemulsification. These agents, now known as ophthalmic viscosurgical devices (OVDs), include duovisc (Duovisc) or sodium hyaluronate (Healon GV). Following the placement of the intraocular lens implant, timolol (Timoptic, Betimol) 0.5% drops may be used to decrease IOP. A miotic such as acetylcholine chloride (Miochol-E) may be used immediately after delivery of the lens to achieve constriction of the iris. Note that moxifloxacin (Vigamox) or gatifloxacin (Zymar) and ketorolac (Acular) 0.5%, mentioned in Preoperative Medications, may be used again. An alternative to this is a subconjunctival injection of the corticosteroid and antibiotic. Some commonly injected corticosteroids (anti-inflammatory agents) may include betamethasone (Celestone) or dexamethasone (Decadron). Gentamicin sulfate (Garamycin) is a commonly used antibiotic for these injections. Some surgeons prefer to patch and shield the eye following the procedure.

When preparing irrigation solution used during phacoemulsification, a mixture of medications may be added to the BSS 500-mL bottle. These include epinephrine (1:1000) for control of bleeding and antibiotics such as vancomycin and/or gentamicin. Some surgeons are also adding ascorbic acid 1.76 mL to the BSS solution. It also aids in control of bleeding and helps decrease IOP.

ASSISTANT *ADVICE*

Irrigation of the eye is commonly performed during ophthalmic procedures to prevent drying of the cornea and to remove blood and debris from the operative site. This should be done from the inner canthus to the outer canthus of the eye to prevent the irrigation and debris from pooling. When irrigating the eye, IF POSSIBLE, turn the patient's head toward the affected side. This will help to prevent cross-contamination to the unaffected eye. Remember that the cornea is NEVER wiped with a radiopaque sponge because this would scratch its surface.

POSTOPERATIVE MEDICATIONS

The patient is usually released within a few hours postoperatively (unless there are any complications). Postoperative medications sent home with the patient will usually include the same topical anti-inflammatory agent (to reduce pain and swelling) and antibiotic agents used during the surgical procedure. The patient is instructed to avoid activities that could increase pressure in the eye and may also be sent home with a medication such as acetazolamide (Diamox) 500 mg, taken orally with food, to decrease IOP. Normally the patient is seen the next day for postoperative evaluation. See Box A for sample cataract order sheet.

Advanced Practices Bibliography

Fulcher E, Fulcher R, Soto C: *Pharmacology principles and applications*, ed 2, St. Louis, 2009, Saunders/Elsevier.

Moscou K, Snipe K: *Pharmacology for pharmacy technicians*, St. Louis, 2009, Mosby/Elsevier.

Rothrock J: *Alexander's care of the patient in surgery*, ed 13, St. Louis, 2007, Mosby/Elsevier.

Advanced Practices Internet Resources

Betimol.com: http://www.betimol.com.

Birch AA, Evans M, Redenbo E: Ultrasonic Localization of Retrobulbar Needles during Retrobulbar Block, *Reg Anesth Pain Med* 19(2):30, 1994. Available at http://journals.lww.com/rapm/Citation/1994/19021/Ultrasonic_Localization_of_Retrobulbar_Needles.30.aspx. Accessed July 22, 2010.

BOX A Sample Cataract Order Sheet

Preoperative Orders

1. Obtain operative consent for "Cataract extraction with intraocular lens implant" for the surgical eye. Left Right
2. NPO
3. Start IV of lactated Ringer's 1000 mL at keep vein open (KVO) rate
4. Preoperative eye drops: at least one hour before the procedure, but not more than 2 hours before, instill 1 drop of the following into the operative eye, then every 5 minutes 2 for a total of 3 doses:
   a) Proparacaine 0.5% (Alcaine)
   b) Tropicamide 0.5% (Mydriacyl)
   c) Phenylephrine 2.5% (Neo-Synephrine)
   d) Gatifloxacin 0.3% (Zymar)
5. Povidone iodine (Betadine Ophthalmic) 5% prep solution: 1 drop into operative eye after previous drops are administered, close eye, and prep area around the eye with povidone iodine solution (Betadine)

Intraoperative Orders

1. Prepare BSS 500 mL by adding epinephrine 1:1000 (1 mg/1 mL)
2. Proparacaine 0.5% 1 drop into operative eye after prep
3. For retrobulbar block draw up 4.5 mL of 1% lidocaine with epinephrine (1:100,000) and 0.5 mL of hyaluronidase (Wydase) in a 10-mL syring with a 25-gauge, 1½-inch, needle for use by surgeon
4. Have available for the surgical field for use by surgeon: sodium hyaluronate (Healon GV) for intraocular use . . . may instill immediately after the procedure
5. Antibiotic: instill 2 drops of gatifloxacin (Zymar) and timolol (Timoptic) immediately after the procedure

Postoperative Orders

1. To recovery room
2. Routine vital signs
3. Discontinue IV when taking PO fluids
4. Acetazolamide (Diamox) 250 mg PO with food
5. Remind patient not to rub or press on eye
6. Discharge to home with a driver when patient is alert and stable

Drugs.com: *Cyclogyl.* www.drugs.com/cons/cyclogyl-ophthalmic.html.

Drugs.com: *MIOCHOL-E (acetylcholine chloride intraocular solution).* www.drugs.com/pdr/miochol-e-system-pak.html.

Drugs.com: *Nevanac.* www.drugs.com/nevanac.html.

Drugs.com: *Ocufen Drops.* www.drugs.com/cdi/ocufen-drops.html.

Drugs.com: *Ofloxacin ophthalmic.* www.drugs.com/mtm/ofloxacin-ophthalmic.html.

Drugs.com: *Omnipred.* www.drugs.com/pro/omnipred.html.

Drugs.com: *Proparacaine Drops.* www.drugs.com/cdi/proparacaine-drops.html.

Drugs.com: *Timoptic Drops.* www.drugs.com/cdi/timoptic-drops.html.

Drugs.com: *Tobradex.* www.drugs.com/tobradex.html.

eMedicine from WebMD: *Cataract, Senile.* http://emedicine.medscape.com/article/1210914-overview.

The Free Dictionary: *Mature Cataract.* http://medical-dictionary.thefreedictionary.com/mature+cataract.

Medcompare.com: *Duovisc.* www.medcompare.com/details/33204/DuoVisc.html.

National Eye Institute: *Facts About Cataract.* www.nei.nih.gov/health/cataract/cataract_facts.asp.

Prevent Blindness America: *Facts & Myths about Cataracts.* www.preventblindness.org/resources/factsheets/Cataracts_MK08.PDF.

ReZoom: *Fact Sheet: Aging Vision and Cataracts.* www.rezoomiol.com/alt/files/CFSheet.pdf.
RxList: *Vigamox.* www.rxlist.com/vigamox-drug.htm.
RxList: *Zymar.* www.rxlist.com/zymar-drug.htm.

Advanced Practices: Learning the Language (Key Terms)

Using your textbook or a standard medical dictionary, look up and write the definitions of each item.

- extracapsular
- intracapsular
- phacoemulsification

Advanced Practices: Review Questions

1. Eye medications are considered
   A. Potent
   B. Weak
   C. Short acting
   D. Long acting
2. Multiple dosages of mydriatic drops may be needed to achieve pupil dilation on a patient with
   A. Blue eyes
   B. Brown eyes
   C. Glaucoma
   D. Diabetes
3. Which of the following agents would be used to achieve maximum pupil dilation?
   A. Neo-Synephrine
   B. Miostat
   C. Carbachol
   D. Timoptic
4. Betamethasone is what type of pharmacologic agent?
   A. Anti-inflammatory
   B. Antibiotic
   C. Diuretic
   D. Vasoconstrictor
5. A substance used to lubricate and support the shape of the eye during lens extraction, now known as an OVD is
   A. Healon
   B. Zymar
   C. Diamox
   D. Neo-Synephrine
6. The ophthalmic condition commonly treated with a miotic drug is
   A. Cataract
   B. Retinal detachment
   C. Pterygium
   D. Glaucoma

KEY CONCEPTS

- The eye is a complex sense organ comprised of many anatomic structures.
- The blood-eye barrier prevents effective absorption of most systemically administered medications, thus the most common method of administration for ophthalmic medications is topical.
- Enzymes are used to increase anesthetic diffusion through tissue for nerve blocks.
- Irrigating solutions cleanse the operative site and keep the cornea moist and lubricants are used to protect the cornea for patients undergoing general anesthesia for any category of surgical procedures.
- Viscoelastic agents are used to keep the anterior chamber expanded and to prevent injury to surrounding tissue.
- Miotics constrict the pupil and can be used for short-term treatment of glaucoma, and to maintain position of the lens after cataract surgery.
- Mydriatics and cycloplegics dilate the pupil by paralyzing the sphincter muscle of the iris.
- Ophthalmic formulations of antibiotics are used to prevent and treat ocular infections.
- Ophthalmic anesthesia is achieved with topical agents, and when a more extensive area is involved, a retrobulbar or peribulbar block can be administered.

- *Glaucoma* is a general term referring to a group of conditions characterized by increased intraocular pressure.
- There are several categories of medications that are used to treat glaucoma: carbonic anhydrase inhibitors, osmotic diuretics, α-adrenergic agonists, β-adrenergic blockers, cholinergics, and prostaglandin analogues.
- Steroids and NSAIDs are used as anti-inflammatory agents in ophthalmology.
- Steroid preparations are available in combination with antimicrobials.
- Dyes are used as diagnostic agents in ophthalmology.

Bibliography

Fulcher E, Fulcher R, Soto C: *Pharmacology principles and applications,* ed 2, St. Louis, 2009, Saunders/Elsevier.

Moscou K, Snipe K: *Pharmacology for pharmacy technicians,* St. Louis, 2009, Mosby/Elsevier.

Stoelting R, Miller R: *Basics of anesthesia,* ed 5, Philadelphia, 2007, Churchill Livingstone/Elsevier.

Internet Resources

Abbott Medical Optics: *Healon5 OVD Viscoelastic.* www.amo-inc.com/products/cataract/ovds/healon5-viscoelastic.

Alcon, Inc: *Cataract Surgery.* www.alcon.com/en/alcon-products/surgical.asp.

Alcon, Inc: *Eye Allergies.* www.alcon.com/en/alcon-products/pharmaceutical.asp.

ClinicalTrials.gov: *Nepafenac 0.1% Eye Drops, Suspension Compared to Ketorolac Trometamol 0.5% Eye Drops, Solution and Placebo.* http://clinicaltrials.gov/ct2/show/NCT00405730.

Daily Med, AMPHADASE (hyaluronidase) injection [Amphastar Pharmaceuticals, Inc.]: http://dailymed.nlm.nih.gov/dailymed/drugInfo.cfm?id=13960.

Glaucoma Research Foundation: *Glaucoma Medications.* www.glaucoma.org/treating/medication.php.

InSite Vision: *DuraSite Core Technology.* www.insitevision.com/durasite.

OCuSOFT, Inc: *TetraVisc FORTE, topical ophthalmic anesthesia.* www.ocusoft.com/media-newsroom/pr/introducing-tetravisc-forte.

Review of Ophthalmology: *Uveoscleral Outflow: A Better Way to Go?* www.revophth.com/index.asp?page=1_14600.htm.

WebMD: *Prostaglandin Analogs for Glaucoma.* www.webmd.com/eye-health/prostaglandin-analogs-for-glaucoma.

LEARNING THE LANGUAGE (KEY TERMS)

Using your textbook or a standard medical dictionary, look up and write the definitions of each item.

constrict
cycloplegic
dilate
glaucoma
IOP
miotic
mydriatic

REVIEW QUESTIONS

1. Why are enzymes used in ophthalmology?
2. What is the difference between a miotic and a mydriatic?
3. What types of ophthalmic medications are available in ointment form?
4. Which routes are used to administer ophthalmic medications?
5. How do various antiglaucoma agents work?
6. Can you name two ophthalmic anti-inflammatory agents?
7. Why are dyes used in ophthalmology?

CRITICAL THINKING

1. Obtain a list of ophthalmic medications used at your facility and answer the following questions.
   a) What local anesthetic medications are used?
   b) What viscoelastic agents are used?
   c) What miotics are used?
   d) What mydriatics and cycloplegics are used?
2. Do anesthesia personnel at your facility use ointments to help protect patients' eyes? If yes, what ointments are used?
3. List two ways in which aseptic technique is used to help prevent infections during ophthalmic surgery.

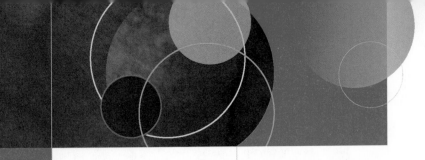

CHAPTER 11
Fluids and Irrigation Solutions

OBJECTIVES *Upon completion of this chapter you should be able to:*

1. Briefly describe the physiology of fluid loss in the surgical patient.
2. List fluid electrolytes and their functions crucial to homeostasis.
3. Define terms and abbreviations related to fluid replacement.
4. State objectives of parenteral fluid therapy in surgery.
5. List common intravenous solutions and their purposes in surgery.
6. List supplies needed to start an intravenous line.
7. List basic functions and types of blood.
8. State average adult circulating volume of blood, hemoglobin, and hematocrit values.
9. List the formed elements present in blood.
10. Define terms and abbreviations related to blood.
11. Briefly describe antigen-antibody interactions in blood types.
12. List and describe indications for blood replacement in the surgical patient.
13. List available options for blood replacement.
14. Describe components of whole blood used for replacement.
15. Define autologous and homologous blood donation.
16. Describe the process of intraoperative autotransfusion.
17. List and describe volume expander solutions used in surgery.
18. List and describe oxygen therapeutics used in clinical trials.
19. Describe the procedure for blood replacement in surgery using donor blood from the blood bank.
20. List and describe fluids used as irrigation solutions in surgery.
21. List and describe supplies and equipment used for irrigation.

KEY TERMS

agglutination
antibody
antigen
arrhythmia
autologous
autotransfusion
electrolyte
hematocrit
hemoglobin
hemolysis
homologous
hypercalcemia
hyperkalemia
hypernatremia
hypocalcemia
hypokalemia
hyponatremia
hypovolemia
intravenous
isotonic
metabolic acidosis

One of the primary goals of surgical patient care is to maintain the patient in as stable a physiologic state as possible. Because fluids are essential to survival, blood and fluid replacement are two of the most common means used in surgery to assist in maintaining homeostasis. Blood loss may be due to trauma or to the surgical procedure itself. The volume of blood lost must be carefully assessed and replaced if significant. The surgical patient's fluid and electrolyte balance must also be assessed and monitored. Most surgical patients will have preoperative fluid and food restrictions prior to surgery, so fluid replacement is usually indicated. This is accomplished by administering **intravenous** (IV) fluids and medications. Intravenous means administration of fluids or medications through a vein. They may be ordered for replacement of lost fluids, to maintain fluid and electrolyte balance, or to administer IV medications. *Replacement fluids* are often ordered to replenish losses due to hemorrhage (in surgery), vomiting and diarrhea (in the medical setting). *Maintenance fluids* sustain normal fluid and electrolyte balance. Additionally, fluids are used to irrigate body tissues during surgical procedures. These irrigation solutions must be physiologically acceptable to tissues while providing visualization, removing blood and debris, and adding medications to the surgical site. The surgical technologist will observe blood or fluid replacement and assist with irrigation procedures in the surgical suite daily.

FLUID AND ELECTROLYTE MANAGEMENT

PHYSIOLOGY REVIEW

In a healthy adult, approximately 60% of the total body weight is made up of fluids, **electrolytes,** and nonelectrolytes. Fluids are distributed into two distinct compartments: intracellular fluid (ICF) and extracellular fluid (ECF).

The major electrolytes break down into sodium (Na^+), chloride (Cl^-), potassium (K^+), calcium (Ca^{2+}), phosphate (HPO_4^{2-}), and magnesium (Mg^{2+}) ions. Other electrolytes are bicarbonate (HCO_3^-), sulfate (SO_4^{2-}), and carbonic acid (H_2CO_3). The nonelectrolytes present in normal body fluid are glucose, urea, and creatinine. Electrolytes have three main purposes in homeostasis: controlling the volume of body water by osmotic pressure, maintaining the acid-base balance, and serving as essential minerals. See Table 11-1 for a list of major electrolytes and functions. Altering of normal concentrations of these elements can result in serious, and possibly life-threatening, complications.

Chloride is the most abundant anion in extracellular fluid and helps regulate osmotic pressure between intracellular and extracellular spaces. Magnesium plays an important part in the sodium-potassium pump and also activates enzymes required to break down adenosine triphosphate (ATP). Phosphate is stored in teeth and bone and is released when needed. Phosphate is a necessary element in the formation of DNA and RNA, in synthesis of ATP, and in buffering of acid-base reactions.

Table 11-1 MAJOR ELECTROLYTES AND FUNCTIONS

Electrolyte	Chemical Symbol	Function
Sodium	Na^+	Osmotic pressure, nerve impulse transmission
Chloride	Cl^-	Osmotic pressure, aids digestion
Potassium	K^+	Osmotic pressure, acid–base balance, nerve impulse transmission
Calcium	Ca^{2+}	Bone growth and development, blood coagulation, enzyme activity, neuromuscular function
Magnesium	Mg^{2+}	Enzyme action in synthesis of ATP, muscle contraction, protein synthesis
Phosphate	$HPO_4{}^{2-}$, $H_2PO_4{}^-$	Acid–base balance
Bicarbonate	$HCO_3{}^-$	Acid–base balance
Sulfate	$SO_4{}^{2-}$	Acid–base balance
Carbonic acid	$H_2CO_3{}^-$	Acid–base balance

Two electrolytes with particular importance to surgery are calcium and potassium. Calcium is the most abundant mineral in the body and necessary for the formation and function of bones and teeth. Calcium is also involved in the blood-clotting process, neurotransmitter release, muscle contraction, and cardiac function. Too much calcium, **hypercalcemia**, or too little, **hypocalcemia**, can cause the heart to beat irregularly (cardiac **arrhythmias**), muscle spasms, and weak heartbeats. Normal calcium levels are 4.5 to 5.5 mEq/L. Potassium serves several critical functions in homeostasis. Potassium helps maintain fluid volume in cells, controls pH, and is vital in the transmission of nerve impulses. Either too much potassium, **hyperkalemia**, or too little, **hypokalemia**, causes serious metabolic problems. Because potassium is critical to neuromuscular function, cardiac arrhythmias are often seen in patients with potassium imbalances. Many elderly patients may be taking diuretics (see Chapter 7) and can easily become hypokalemic, so a potassium level must be determined on all surgical patients taking diuretics. Normal potassium levels are 3.5 to 5 mEq/L. A potassium or calcium imbalance is of special concern in surgical patients because of increased risk of cardiac arrhythmias or arrest when a general anesthetic is administered. Elective surgery may be postponed until potassium and calcium levels have been restored to a safe range.

{NOTE} *Potassium is an electrolyte that can be added at higher concentrations in premixed IV solutions, or added to the IV solution before infusion preoperatively.*

CAUTION

IV potassium can cause severe and potentially fatal cardiac rhythm disturbances. Thus, patients should be carefully monitored and when possible, oral potassium is preferable.

Sodium controls distribution of water in the body and maintains fluid and electrolyte balance. Sodium is the principle cation of extracellular fluid and vital to neuromuscular function. If there is too much sodium in the body, the condition is called **hypernatremia**. This condition frequently results from a relative water loss and the cells become dehydrated. If there is too little, it is called **hyponatremia**. This results from excessive water ingestion or retention, or inadequate sodium intake.

INTRAVENOUS FLUIDS

Appropriate fluid and electrolyte management are integral components of surgical patient care, both for maintaining homeostasis and also for positive surgical outcomes. Nearly every surgical patient will receive intravenous fluids. An IV drip is "started" on the patient for two purposes: to establish a direct access to the circulatory system for medication administration, and to administer parenteral fluids. IV fluids may be used at a slow rate (e.g., 30 mL/hr on an adult) to *keep the vein open* (KVO or TKO). Parenteral fluid therapy has three objectives: to maintain daily fluid requirements, to restore previous losses, and to replace current losses. To accomplish these objectives, several fluids are available and are used for specific purposes. The IV fluids most commonly used in the surgical setting are called *crystalloids*. These are solutions composed mainly of water with

Table 11-2 COMMON INTRAVENOUS FLUID COMPONENTS

Component	Abbreviation
Dextrose	D
Lactated Ringer	LR
Normal saline (0.9%)	NaCl, NS
Ringer lactate	RL
Saline	S
Sodium chloride	NaCl
Water	W

dissolved electrolytes, dextrose solutions, and multiple-electrolyte solutions. The names of IV solutions are abbreviated on their bags and containers. The abbreviation letters indicate the components of the solution and the numbers indicate the strength or concentration of the components in the solution. Numbers are often written as subscripts to the letters. For example, an IV solution of D5W indicates dextrose (D) is 5% of the concentration in water (W) (Table 11-2).

COMMON INTRAVENOUS FLUIDS ADMINISTERED IN SURGERY

Sodium chloride (NaCl) in a 0.9% solution (**isotonic**) is the agent of choice for fluid replacement or simple hydration and one of the most common IV fluid used in surgery. Sodium chloride is packaged in 1000-mL, 500-mL, 250-mL, and 100-mL bags for IV administration. It comes in a variety of concentrations (the amount of sodium chloride in solution) that include 5%, 3%, 0.9%, 0.45%, 0.33%, 0.225% (Fig. 11-2). Sodium chloride is used when chloride loss is greater than or equal to sodium loss, for treatment of **metabolic acidosis** (excess acid in body fluids) in the presence of fluid loss, and to replenish lost sodium. Sodium chloride is the IV fluid used when transfusing blood products, as it does not hemolyze (fill with fluid and rupture) blood cells.

TECH TIP

Normal saline (NS) and physiologic saline are common terms for 0.9% sodium chloride. The concentration of sodium chloride in normal saline is 0.9 g per 100 mL of solution. Another common IV saline concentration is 0.45% sodium chloride. Notice that 0.45% is one half the strength of 0.9% NaCl and it is sometimes written as 1/2 NS (for one-half normal saline). Other saline concentrations are 0.33% NaCl or 1/3 NS, and 0.225% NaCl or 1/4 NS.

MAKE IT SIMPLE

Normal saline is 0.9% sodium chloride.

Dextrose (D) is used in patients who require an easily metabolized source of calories: it is a natural sugar found in the body and provides energy for cellular activity. Dextrose is available in various concentrations in water and in normal saline. Dextrose in water is used to hydrate the surgical patient, spare body protein, and enhance liver function. Because the trauma and stress of surgery causes some water and sodium retention, intraoperative intravenous therapy often involves administration of limited amounts of dextrose 5% in water (D5W) (Fig. 11-1). Dextrose in water is also prepared in 2.5%, 10%, 20% 25%, 30%, 40%, 50%, 60%, and 70% solutions.

The percentage of solution determines the clinical use of dextrose. Lower concentrations (less than 10%) are utilized for: peripheral hydrations, providing calories, and assessing kidney function (if patients do not need electrolyte replacement). In higher concentrations, dextrose is used for reversing hypoglycemia, providing calories when less fluid is indicated, and with amino acids for total parenteral nutrition.

Dextrose is frequently used in saline solutions, for example 5% in normal saline (D5NS). It is packaged in bags of 1000 mL, 500 mL, 250 mL, and 150 mL. This fluid is used for temporary treatment of circulatory insufficiency and shock due to hypovolemia, in the absence of a plasma extender, and for early treatment with plasma for loss of fluid due to burns. Dextrose 10% in normal saline (D10NS) is supplied in 1000-mL and 500-mL bags and is used to replenish nutrients and electrolytes.

It should be noted that dextrose solutions given IV increase insulin and oral hypoglycemic requirements for the diabetic patient. Dextrose is not used in conjunction with transfusion of blood products because it causes **hemolysis** of blood cells.

Ionosol B (MB and T) and 5% dextrose injection are maintenance and replacement electrolyte solutions. They provide a source of water, electrolytes, and carbohydrates to cover hydration, insensible water loss, and urinary excretion. Ionosol comes packaged in 500-mL and 1000-mL plastic bags; Ionosol MB and T also come in a 250-mL size.

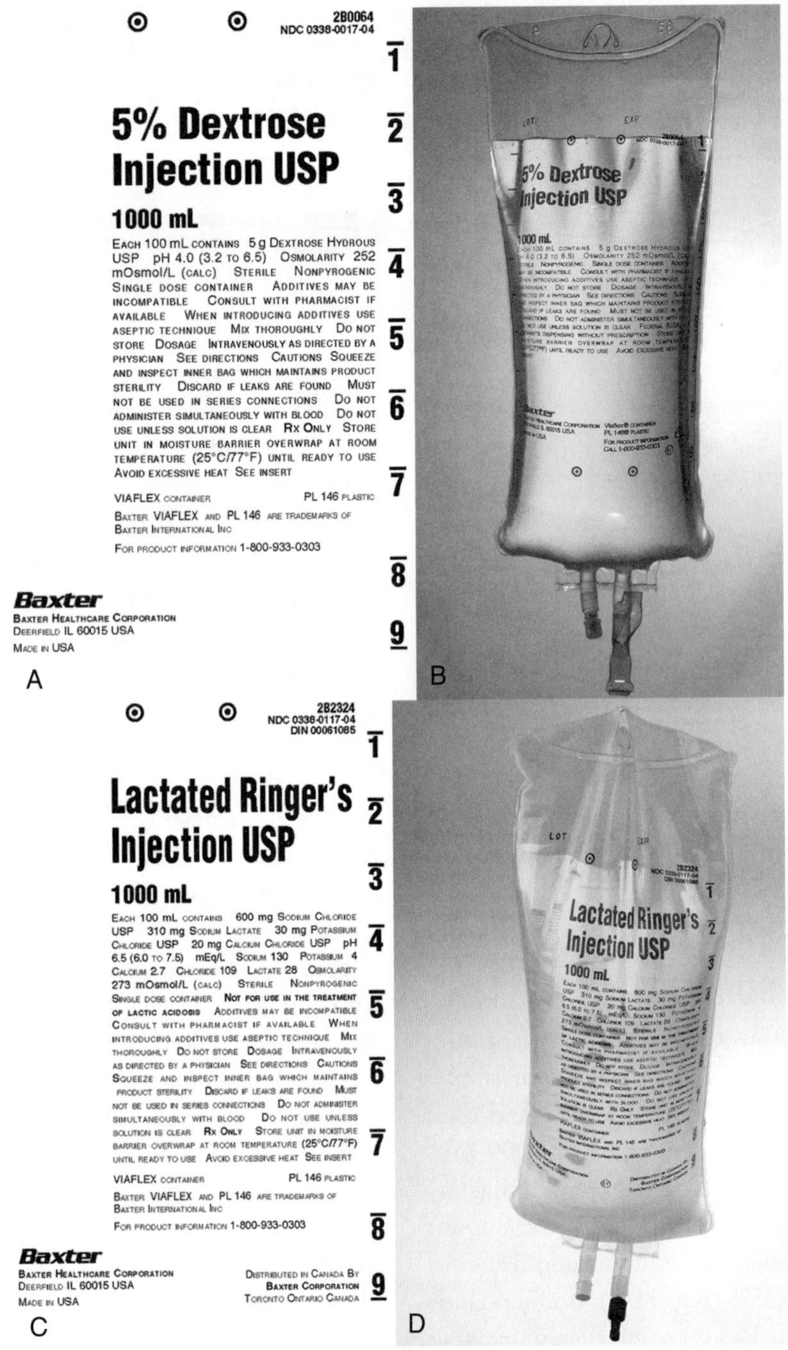

Figure 11-1 Five percent dextrose and lactated Ringer IV solutions, 1000 mL. *(Courtesy of Baxter Healthcare Corp. All rights reserved.)*

Lactated Ringer (LR), or Ringer lactate (RL), is a physiologic salt solution used to replenish the patient's electrolytes and for rehydration to stimulate renal activity. It is the other most common IV fluid used in surgery. Lactated Ringer solution, which is used to replace fluid lost from burns or severe diarrhea, closely resembles the composition of extracellular fluid. It should not be used in patients with the inability to metabolize lactate (found in the solution). Patients at high risk are those with liver disease, Addison disease (see Insight 8-2 later in this chapter), severe pH imbalances, shock, or cardiac failure. Hartmann solution is very similar to Lactated Ringer (except for its ionic concentration), and is often referred to as such (Fig. 11-1).

Plasma-Lyte and Isolyte E are electrolyte balanced solutions compatible with the pH of blood. They are used to treat the massive loss of water and electrolytes seen in

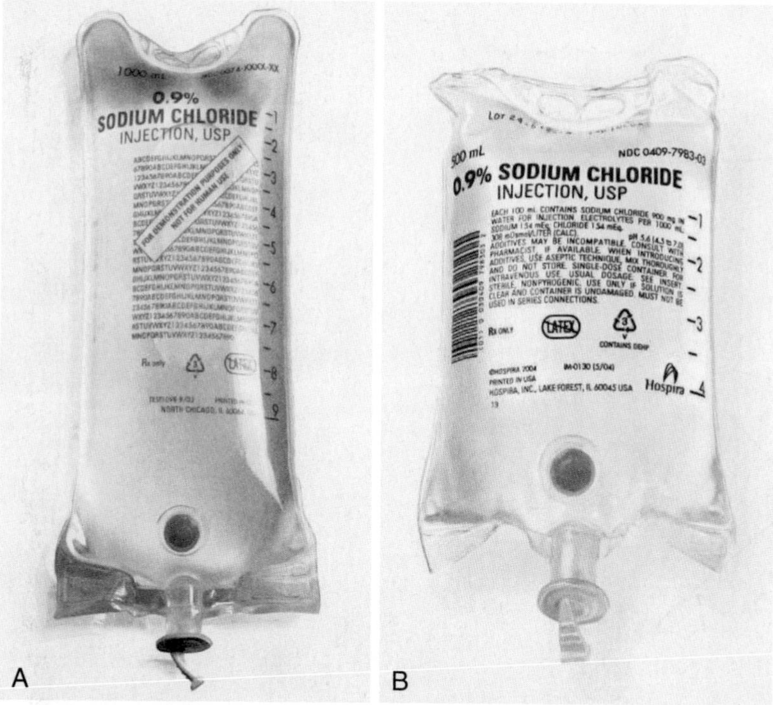

Figure 11-2 Normal saline (0.9% sodium chloride) 1000 mL and 500 mL. *(Courtesy of Hospira, Inc., Lake Forest, Ill. All rights reserved.)*

uncontrolled vomiting or diarrhea. The composition of these solutions is similar to the plasma portion of blood.

Intravenous Equipment and Supplies

An intravenous line is established in nearly all surgical patients prior to surgery. A flexible catheter, or Angiocath, (Fig. 11-3) is inserted via a needle into a vein, usually in the patient's hand or forearm. The needle is removed, leaving the catheter in the vein where it is taped securely in place. The *primary* IV tubing connects to the hub of the IV catheter and the other end is connected to a container of intravenous solution. This tubing contains a drip chamber, injection port, and roller clamp (Fig. 11-4). Fluids and most of the medications needed during surgery are administered through the intravenous line. A *secondary* IV tubing may be used with the primary tubing when giving medications via "piggyback." The secondary tubing is shorter and also contains a drip chamber and roller clamp. In this set-up, the secondary tubing is hung higher on the IV pole than the primary IV so that the secondary medication infuses first. Secondary lines are used with antibiotics. At times, the IV tubing may be placed in an electronic infusion pump system (Fig. 11-5).

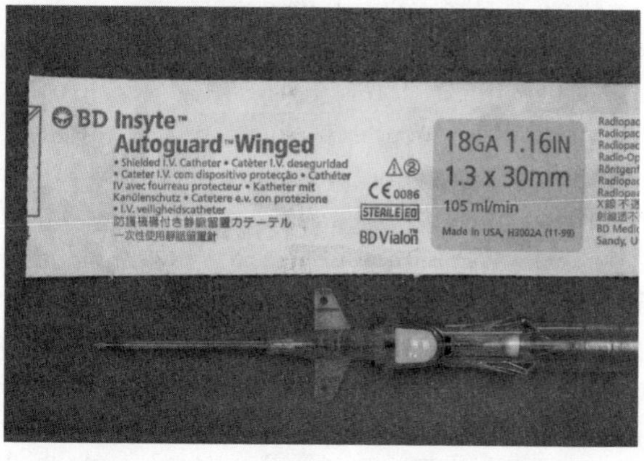

Figure 11-3 IV catheter.

TECH TIP

Make sure the IV tubing does not become kinked or compromised during patient positioning. Intravenous fluids must be able to run at the required rate. Even from the position of scrubbed surgical technologist, you can observe the drip chamber to see that the IV fluid is moving.

BLOOD REPLACEMENT

PHYSIOLOGY REVIEW

Blood performs several critical functions in maintaining homeostasis. It is used to transport oxygen, nutrients, wastes, hormones, and enzymes throughout the body.

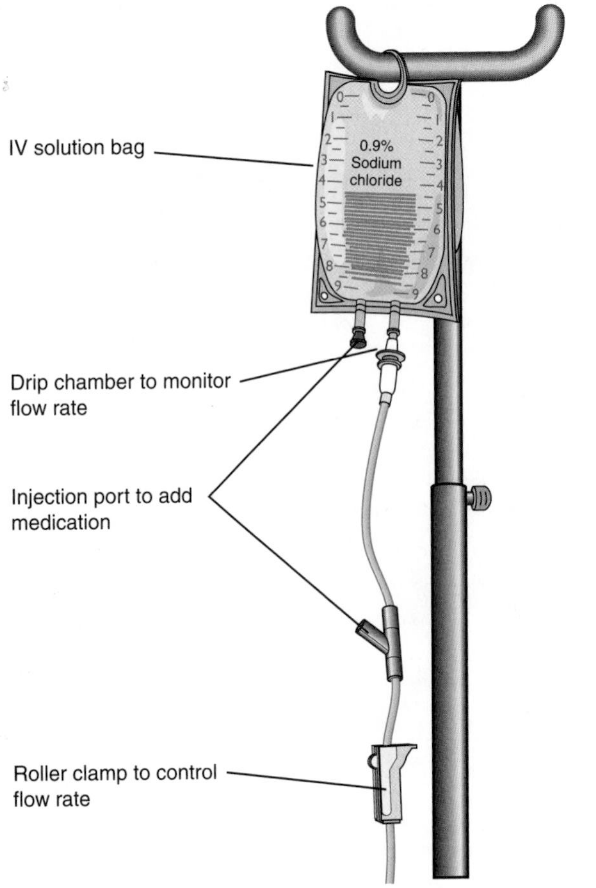

Figure 11-4 IV tubing.

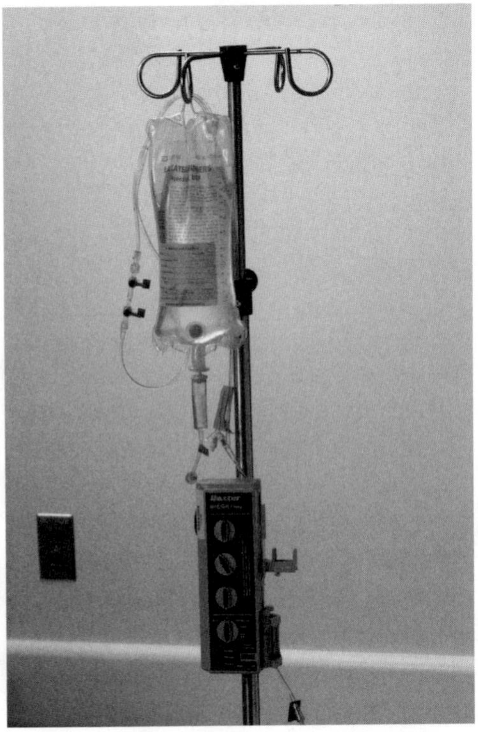

Figure 11-5 Electronic IV infusion pump and controller.

Blood also maintains the body's acid-base balance (pH), its temperature, and its water content. The immune response is carried through the circulatory system as well. Blood is so crucial to maintaining life processes that it has a self-protection mechanism—clotting—to prevent harmful loss.

In an average adult, the circulating blood volume is approximately 70 mL/kg of body mass. In order to keep the body functioning normally, this blood volume should be maintained. Some surgical patients are at high risk for substantial blood loss during surgery; these include patients needing cardiac and peripheral vascular procedures or those with trauma. The goal of blood replacement in scheduled surgical procedures is to maintain the circulating volume of blood as well as its oxygen-carrying capacity.

Blood consists of two main components: formed elements and plasma (fluid). The formed elements include erythrocytes (red blood cells or RBCs), leukocytes (white blood cells or WBCs), and platelets. Erythrocytes contain **hemoglobin**, a protein responsible for transport of oxygen and carbon dioxide between the lungs and the cells. Leukocytes provide protection against foreign microbes by phagocytosis and antibody production. Platelets mediate the clotting process.

Most surgical patients undergo laboratory tests to determine the amount of hemoglobin (Hgb) present in their blood. A normal hemoglobin level is 12 to 16 g/100 mL of blood in adult females and 14 to 18 g/100 mL in adult males. A low hemoglobin level indicates reduced oxygen-carrying capacity. Since oxygen levels must be optimum during general anesthesia, elective surgery may be canceled if the hemoglobin dips below normal levels. Another important measure of the oxygen-carrying capacity of the blood is **hematocrit.** Hematocrit is the volume of erythrocytes in a given volume of blood and is expressed as a percentage. Normal hematocrit levels range from 35% to 52%, varying by age and gender (Table 11-3).

In cases of known or anticipated blood loss, the patient's blood must be typed and cross-matched in order to administer compatible donor blood. The blood type is determined by proteins called **antigens** present on the surface of RBCs. Blood type is inherited, and there are many types and groupings based on the antigens present on the RBCs. The major groupings of concern in surgery are ABO and Rh. Patients may be type A, B, AB, or O. Type A blood contains the A antigen, type B has

Table 11-3 BLOOD VALUES

Parameter	Females	Males
Circulating blood volume	4-5 L (4.2-5.3 qt)	5-6 L (5.3-6.4 qt)
Hemoglobin	12-16 g/100 mL	14-18 g/100 mL
Hematocrit	35%-46%	40%-52%
Red blood cells	4.2-5.4 million/mm^3	4.7-6.1 million/mm^3
Platelets	150,000-4 million/mm^3	150,000-4 million/mm^3

the B antigen, type AB contains both, and type O blood has neither. Blood is also designated as Rh positive (Rh antigen present) or Rh negative (no Rh antigen present). Each person also has the corresponding **antibody** present in his or her plasma; that is, type A has anti-B, type B has anti-A, type O has both anti-A and anti-B, and type AB has neither (Fig. 11-6). If type A blood is administered to a type B patient, the recipient's antibodies will attack the donor RBCs, causing a potentially fatal transfusion reaction (Insight 11-1). A blood cross-match is performed to determine compatibility between the donor and the recipient. A sample of donor RBCs is mixed with the recipient's serum and the results are examined to determine compatibility. See Table 11-4 and Table 11-5 for more information on blood types.

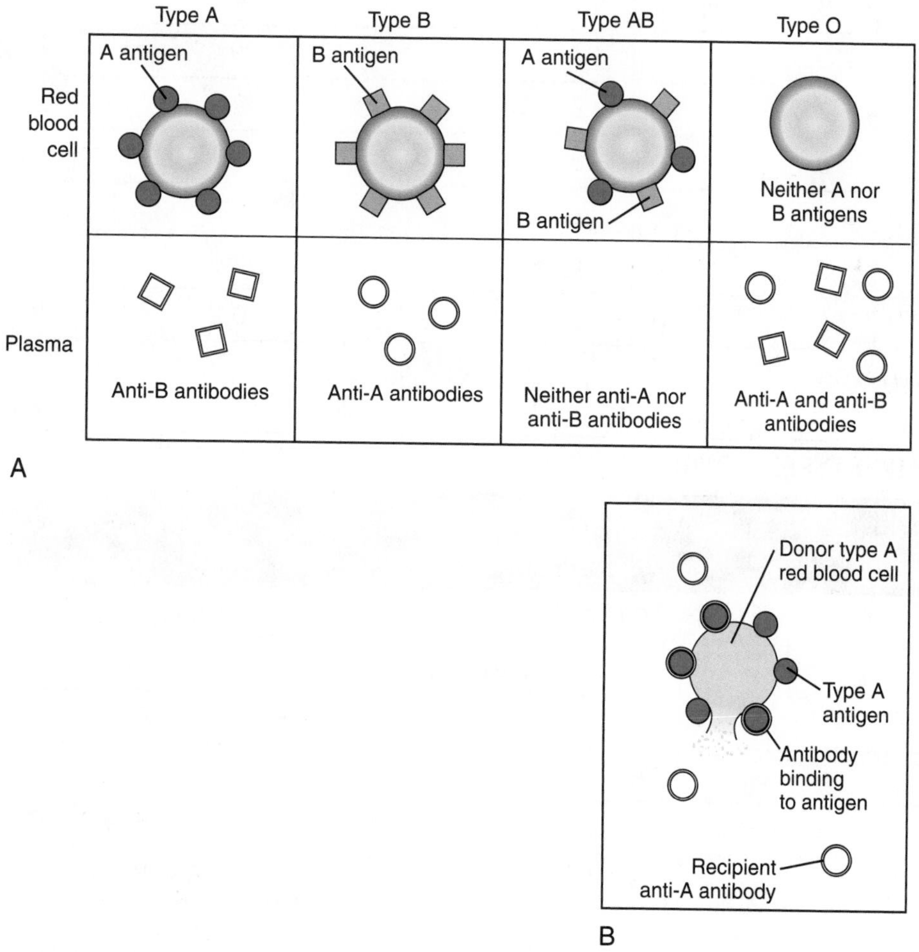

Figure 11-6 Antigen and antibody in blood types.

IN SIGHT 11-1 Hemolytic Transfusion Reaction

If blood is not properly typed and matched before being transfused, a serious and sometimes fatal reaction, called hemolytic transfusion reaction or hemolytic anemia, can occur. This can result from incompatible blood types or Rh factors and must be treated immediately. If the patient is under general anesthesia, the symptoms are a generalized diffuse blood loss and lowered blood oxygen saturation levels (because the red blood cells are not carrying sufficient oxygen). If any suspicious reactions occur during blood transfusion, the following steps should be taken:

1. Stop the transfusion.
2. Report immediately to the surgeon and the blood bank.
3. Send a sample of the patient's blood to the blood bank (to rule out a mismatch).
4. Return any unused portion of the blood unit and blood tubing to the blood bank.
5. Begin appropriate medication therapy, which usually includes steroid therapy as soon as possible.
6. Send urine samples to the lab in order to check for kidney function.

In some cases the patient may have to undergo renal dialysis in order to rid the system of mismatched blood.

Table 11-4 BLOOD TYPES–PERCENTAGE IN POPULATIONS

Blood Type	Caucasian (%)	African American (%)	Hispanic (%)	Asian (%)
O+	37	47	53	39
O−	8	4	4	1
A+	33	24	29	27
A−	7	2	2	0.5
B+	9	18	9	25
B−	2	1	1	0.4
AB+	3	4	2	7
AB−	1	0.3	0.2	0.1

Data from the American Red Cross.

Table 11-5 BLOOD TYPES–DONOR

Your Blood Type	Patients Who Can Receive Your Red Blood Cells	Patients Who Can Receive Your Plasma
O+	O+, A+, B+, AB+	O+, O−
O−	All blood types	O+, O−
A+	A+, AB+	A+, A−, O+, O−
A−	A+, A−, AB+, AB−	A+, A−, O+, O−
B+	B+, AB+	B+, B−, O+, O−
B−	B+, B−, AB+, AB−	B+, B−, O+, O−
AB+	AB+	All blood types
AB−	AB+, AB−	All blood types

Data from the American Red Cross.

RhoD immune globulin (RhoGam) is a medication used to treat possible blood compatibility reactions. It is an injectable blood product manufactured from human plasma that contains anti-D to suppress the immune response of an Rh-negative mother to an Rh-positive fetus. If the anti-Rh antibody is given right after delivery, it blocks the sensitization of the mother and prevents Rh disease from occurring in the woman's next Rh-positive pregnancy. This Rh disease could result in miscarriage in subsequent pregnancies if not treated. RhoD immune globulin is for intramuscular injection only and is routinely given to Rh-negative mothers who deliver Rh-positive babies.

For further explanation of the physiology of blood and labor and delivery, please refer to your anatomy and physiology textbook.

INDICATIONS FOR BLOOD REPLACEMENT

The first fully recorded blood transfusion occurred in France in 1667 when a 15-year-old male was given lamb's blood. Amazingly, the boy did not die, perhaps due to the small amount of blood he received. This method was popular for a time until transfusion reactions were recognized and reported. France banned transfusions in 1670 and soon other countries followed. Blood transfusions did not progress for 150 years. Dr. James Blundell performed many transfusions in the early 19th century (about half were successful), developed instruments for the process, and published his results. Since the discovery that all human blood is not alike in 1901 by Karl Landsteiner, many advances have been made in blood transfusion therapy. Today, blood transfusions are implemented with the knowledge that blood must be compatible in type and Rh factor. If unmatched blood is given, blood clumping or **agglutination** will occur.

The most common indication for blood replacement in surgery is **hypovolemia** (low circulating blood volume) seen most frequently in trauma and vascular procedures. When patients lose a certain amount of blood, they experience this syndrome, which is also called hemorrhagic or circulatory shock. The result is decreased oxygen supplied to vital organs, increased heart rate, and decreased cardiac output. This can be further complicated by the anesthetic which may enhance the effects of hemorrhage. Other indications for blood replacement include restoration of the oxygen-carrying capacity as seen in anemic patients or those with blood diseases, and to maintain clotting properties as needed in patients with hemophilia.

Trauma patients may be in critical need of blood in order to sustain vital functions. If immediate replacement is required, and the patient's blood type is known, type-specific-only RBCs (packed cells) may be administered along with fluid volume support. If the patient's blood type is unknown, O-negative blood may be administered. In either case, the surgeon must document the need for blood release without compatibility testing.

OPTIONS FOR BLOOD REPLACEMENT

There are several options available to replace blood loss in surgery; these include use of donor blood (**homologous** donation), patient donating own blood prior to surgery (**autologous** donation), patient's own blood collected and used during or after surgery (**autotransfusion**), or use of volume expanders. Each blood replacement option has indications, advantages, and disadvantages. Some of these options may not be feasible in certain cases, depending on the situation.

Homologous Donation

A common method of blood replacement is the use of donor, or homologous, blood (this is also referred to as allogenous blood). A blood bank is responsible for collecting, processing, and releasing donor blood for use. Donor blood, while carefully tested, does present some risk for transmission of blood-borne pathogens such as hepatitis B and C and human immunodeficiency virus (HIV). Thus, it is used only when clearly indicated.

Blood is separated during processing into components and then administered to treat specific needs. Component replacement therapy is an effective and efficient use of limited resources because a unit of donor whole blood, separated into components, can be used to treat several patients.

Whole Blood

Whole blood consisting of RBCs, plasma (which contains plasma proteins), stable clotting factors, and anticoagulants is rarely used for transfusion today. Whole, fresh blood is indicated only in cases of acute, massive blood loss that requires the oxygen-carrying properties of RBCs and the volume expansion provided by plasma. It is also a source of proteins and of some coagulation factors. A unit of whole blood contains enough hemoglobin to raise an anemic adult's hematocrit approximately 3 percentage points.

Packed Red Blood Cells

Most transfusions of donor blood in surgery involve the use of packed red blood cells (PRBCs), also called "packed cells." The use of PRBCs with a synthetic volume expander has proven to be as effective as whole blood, while reducing the risks of whole blood transfusion reactions. They contain hemoglobin, which transports oxygen to tissues. Packed cells are obtained by removing approximately 200 mL of plasma and most of the platelets from 1 unit (500 mL) of whole blood. The infusion of PRBCs helps restore the oxygen-carrying capacity of the patient's own circulatory system. Blood typing and cross-matching (ABO and Rh) is required. One unit of PRBCs can raise the patient's hemoglobin by 1 g/dL and the hematocrit by about 3%. Intravenous fluids are administered concurrently to restore circulating volume if needed.

Plasma

Plasma may be administered when clotting factors are needed in addition to circulating volume. This need is frequently seen when several units of blood have been replaced, because the clotting factors have been removed from donor blood. Plasma is not used for volume expansion alone, because albumin and synthetic expanders are as effective and eliminate the risk of transmission of blood-borne diseases. Plasma is stored as fresh-frozen plasma (FFP) to preserve clotting factors and thawed in a water bath prior to use. It must be administered type-specific and used within 6 hours of thawing.

Platelets

Platelets are administered in surgery when large amounts of donor blood have been used to replace the patient's volume. Because the platelets have been removed from donor blood, the result of massive transfusions may be an inability of the patient's circulatory system to clot properly. Platelets are infused to restore a more normal clotting process and to help repair damaged blood vessels. They may also be administered prophylactically in patients who have low platelet counts, such as those receiving chemotherapy or with leukemia. At room temperature, platelets must be continually gently agitated to prevent clumping (Insight 11-2).

Cryoprecipitate

Cryoprecipitate is a plasma component used in the treatment of bleeding caused by hemophilia A, von Willebrand disease, disseminated intravascular coagulation (DIC), and lack of factor XIII. Cryoprecipitate may be administered in surgery when massive amounts of blood have been replaced, severely impacting the normal coagulation process. It is usually given in 4 to 6 unit pools at a time rather than a single unit.

Autologous Donation

Patients scheduled for elective surgical procedures in which blood loss is anticipated, such as a total hip replacement, may be allowed to donate their own blood up to one month prior to surgery. This process is called autologous transfusion and usually involves two units of blood. Most patients can safely donate two units of whole blood over a period of weeks just prior to their scheduled procedure, possibly eliminating the need for donor blood. The patient's blood is collected, processed, stored, and released for surgery by the blood bank. Patients often choose this option, if available, to protect themselves from potential blood-borne disease transmission.

IN SIGHT 11-2 Platelet-Rich Plasma for Wound Healing

From a small volume of the patient's own blood, surgeons can extract a platelet concentrate suspended in plasma that contains various growth factors (cytokines). When this platelet concentrate is reintroduced into the wound, it has the potential to greatly speed up the body's natural healing response in both soft and hard tissues. This extraction of platelet-rich plasma (PRP) is the first practical application of tissue engineering. It is used for wound healing in surgery, treatment of tendonitis, cartilage repair, cardiac care, spinal disc regeneration, and dental care. It is currently being considered for skin rejuvenation. One company, Biomet, has developed a GPS III Platelet Concentrate System with an automated platelet collection process. The patient's blood is placed in the collection device, which is then placed within a centrifuge and spun for 15 minutes. The blood is separated into platelet-poor plasma, platelet-rich plasma, and red blood cells. Then, the platelet-rich plasma is collected and placed into the wound.

Autotransfusion

Another form of autologous donation used intraoperatively and postoperatively is called *autotransfusion.* Autotransfusion involves the collection, processing, and reinfusing of the patient's own blood during the surgical procedure using "cell-saver" technology with little damage to the RBCs (Fig. 11-7). There are several cell-saver machines available. Some are designed specifically for emergency procedures when rapid infusion is required. Blood can be collected in a suction-type device or via bloody sponges drained into a sterile basin of saline, then aspirated into the machine. However, blood that has been exposed to collagen hemostatic agents and some medications (such as certain antibiotics) cannot be used, because clotting in the machine may occur. Another method of autotransfusion is to use a sterile blood collection and suction canister to collect the patient's blood from the operative field. When the canister is filled, the blood is washed in a red cell washer (usually found in the blood bank) and reinfused. In this method, the blood is sent out of the surgical department to be washed and so there is time lost before reinfusion.

Autotransfusion is performed during open-heart surgery, vascular procedures, major orthopedic procedures, and some trauma procedures such as splenectomy. Autotransfusion has several advantages over the use of donor blood, including immediate replacement of blood loss without the potential for transfusion reaction or delay for blood typing and cross-matching and no risk of transmission of blood-borne pathogens. In addition, patients with religious objections to donated blood often do not object to autotransfusion. Autotransfusion is not suitable for all patients, because some trauma patients may have lost so much blood already that there is little volume left to salvage. A disadvantage of autotransfusion is that it cannot be used in the presence of cancer cells, infection, or gross contamination, for example, open gastrointestinal tract. Autotransfusion is generally contraindicated during cesarean section due to the presence of amniotic fluid. Autotransfusion is commonplace in most operating rooms today and is an effective option for replacement of blood lost during certain surgical procedures.

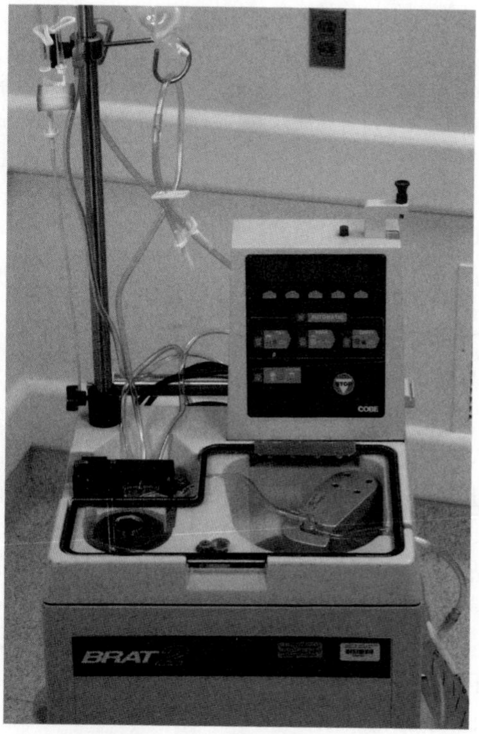

Figure 11-7 Cell-saver/autotransfusion machine.

Volume Expanders

Volume expanders are used to increase the total volume of body fluid when hypovolemia occurs. By doing so, remaining red blood cells can continue to oxygenate body tissues. One category is crystalloids, solutions that contain salts (electrolytes) and/or sugars. These include IV solutions such as Ringer solution, normal saline, and hypertonic saline. Another category of volume expanders is *colloids*, which are osmotically active and draw fluid from ECF compartments. Volume expanders can be used when donated blood or autotransfusion is not immediately available for emergency procedures. There are several colloid volume expanders available.

Albumin and plasma protein fraction (PPF) are plasma derivatives used to provide volume expansion when crystalloid solutions, such as saline and dextrose, are not adequate (as in massive hemorrhage). They are also used in the treatment of hypovolemic shock as seen in burn patients who have lost fluid volume but not RBCs. Albumin is available in concentrations of 5%, which is equal to plasma, or as a concentrated 25% in sodium chloride solution. PPF is available as a 5% solution.

Dextran expands plasma volume by drawing fluid from the interstitial space to the intravascular fluid space. It is formed by the action of a bacterium, has osmotic properties, but not oxygen-carrying capacity. Packaged as Dextran 40, it is used prophylactically for thrombosis and embolism. It improves microcirculation independent of basic volume expansion and minimizes the changes that occur in blood viscosity that accompanies shock. Dextran 70 or 75 is used to expand plasma volume in impending hypovolemic shock. It is packaged for IV administration, 6% dextran 70 in 0.9% sodium chloride (Macrodex) or 10% dextran 40 in 5% dextrose or 0.9% sodium chloride (Rheomacrodex).

Hetastarch (Hespan) is also a synthetic used for its osmotic properties. It has no oxygen-carrying capacity, but is needed to circulate red blood cells, which carry oxygen to tissues. Hetastarch is made from hydroxyethyl starch (cornstarch). It contains electrolytes (sodium, calcium potassium, and magnesium) and acts as albumin in the management of shock. When given intravenously, it expands blood volume by one to two times the amount infused. Hetastarch comes in a 6% solution in 0.9% sodium chloride.

Oxygen Therapeutics

The quest continues for blood alternatives that can transport oxygen to tissues, be given to any blood type, are safe to administer to the patient, and can be stored for long periods of time. A substitute is also needed for those with religious objections to blood transfusion. "Artificial blood" has been replaced with the more accurate term oxygen therapeutics. They are agents that enhance the oxygen-carrying capacity of the blood. They would not carry the risks associated with homologous blood transfusion and are divided into two categories: perfluorocarbon (PFC) emulsions and modified hemoglobin solutions. Perfluorocarbons are a class of chemical compound that carries and releases oxygen. Hemoglobin is derived from humans, animals, or artificially produced by recombinant technology. No product has yet been approved by the U.S. Food and Drug Administration (FDA), but several are in some phases of development or clinical trials. These include:

Hemopure is a product made from highly purified bovine hemoglobin situated in a salt solution. It is a hemoglobin-based oxygen-carrying (HBOC) solution and provides a form of hemoglobin to aid in oxygen transport to tissues. It has a shorter circulation time than blood (only 1-2 days) but does not require refrigeration. Its manufacturing process claims to rid the product of any risk of infection from viruses, including HIV, hepatitis C, and bovine spongiform encephalopathy (mad cow disease). Hemopure is stable for approximately 2 years at room temperature.

Oxygent is a solution used as an intravascular oxygen carrier. It auguments oxygen delivery to the tissues and is used to reduce the need for donor blood. It is completely man-made and its particles are removed from the blood within 48 hours by the body.

PolyHeme is a hemoglobin-based oxygen carrier that uses human hemoglobin as the oxygen carrying molecule in solution. The first step in its production is to extract and filter this hemoglobin from red blood cells. Next is a multistep process to create a polymerized hemoglobin form that avoids undesirable effects such as vasoconstriction and kidney or liver dysfunction. PolyHeme's manufacturing process eliminates blood-borne diseases and its shelf life is about 12 months under refrigeration.

Hemospan is produced in powder form, then mixed into liquid form and immediately transfused. It does not require blood typing and can be stored for years. Its technology uses coupling with polyethylene glycol to eliminate toxicity usually associated with free hemoglobin.

PROCEDURE FOR DONOR BLOOD REPLACEMENT IN SURGERY

The process for administration of donated blood products must be carefully monitored at each step to prevent transfusion of incompatible elements. Transfusion of incompatible blood or blood products can cause a fatal transfusion reaction (see Insight 11-1). The patient who needs a transfusion will be typed and cross-matched and identified with a special wrist band. A requisition slip (Fig. 11-8) with multiple carbon copies will be sent to the blood bank with patient name, identification number, amount and type (which includes blood group, Rh factor) of blood ordered. A copy of the requisition is sent back to surgery with each unit of released blood. The blood (unit) must be checked to verify its unit number and also expiration date. Meticulous records are kept in the blood bank on each unit, and the transporter will be required to verify correct information with blood bank personnel and sign out each unit released.

Once the donor units reach the surgical suite, they are to be placed in an appropriate blood refrigerator, which must have continuous temperature monitoring of 1° C to 6° C. Any units needed for immediate transfusion will be taken directly to the operating room. Both circulator and anesthesia provider will verify the patient and donor unit information prior to administration. In addition, the product itself is checked for any clots, discoloration, leaks or damage to the bag, which might result in contamination. If this occurs, the unit should not be used and must be returned to the blood bank.

When multiple units of blood are to be administered over a short period of time, or when cold blood is rapidly

BLOOD BANK REQUISITION

REGIONAL MEDICAL CENTER
ANYTOWN, USA

☐ PACKED CELLS ☐ FRESH FROZEN PLASMA ☐ PLATELETS SINGLE DONOR ☐ PLATELETS RANDOM | OTHER (SPECIFY)

DATE ______

UNIT NO. ABO & Rh	PATIENT NO. ABO & Rh	EXPIRATION DATE
		X-MATCHED BY-DATE
		☐ COMPATIBLE

PATIENT ______ BIRTH DATE ______

PHYSCIAN ______

HOSPITAL NO. ______

BLOOD BANK RELEASE	TRANSFUSION STARTING RECORD		TRANSFUSION CHECK LIST
DATE BLOOD TAKEN/TECH	TRANSFUSION ORDERED BY	TRANSFUSION STARTED DATE	☐ Order verified from chart ☐ Verbal Order
TIME TAKEN A.M. P.M.	I HAVE CAREFULLY COMPLETED THE CHECK LIST AND ATTACHED PART 1 TO PATIENT'S CHART	TRANSFUSION STARTED TIME A.M. P.M.	☐ I have established the identity of the patient. ☐ The patient's name and hospital number agree with those on the tag.
TAKEN BY	SIGNED* MD RN		☐ The blood type and Rh on the tag agree with those on the unit. ☐ Blood unit number marked on the tag agrees with the number on the unit. ☐ The blood is not outdated.
	*MUST BE SIGNED BY PERSON STARTING TRANSFUSION		

Figure 11-8 Blood requisition slip.

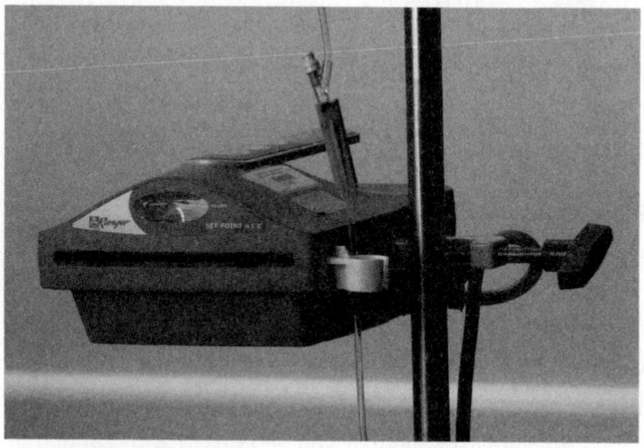

Figure 11-9 Blood warmer unit.

administered through a central venous line, the blood must be warmed to prevent transfusion complications (Fig. 11-9). If blood must be transfused rapidly, a blood pump will be used. Different types of blood pumps are available, from simple pneumatic pumps to complex electric or battery-operated units that calibrate the infusion rate precisely.

IRRIGATION SOLUTIONS

Irrigation is an essential aspect of most open and endoscopic surgical procedures. These solutions assist in clearing the surgical field of active bleeding and improving visualization during the procedures. Irrigation is gentler on tissues than sponging in preventing desiccation and dryness, which can lead to adhesion formation (Insight 11-3). Endoscopic procedures use irrigation solutions to distend hollow organs, such as the bladder and uterus, and joint spaces such as the knee and shoulder. These solutions also wash out blood, bits of resected tissue, and stone fragments while allowing for specimen collection, such as in transurethral resection of the prostate gland. However, it has been demonstrated that irrigation solutions may enter systemic circulation in large volumes, so they must be regarded as systemic medications.

CAUTION

Test the temperature of all irrigation solutions, especially those recently taken from the warmer, as too hot of a solution can cause tissue damage. If it feels hot to your gloved hand, it is too hot for the patient and should be mixed with cooler solution. Some solutions are used chilled, such as for cardiac and transplant surgery. These solutions are maintained as a "slush" for use during the procedure.

BASIC IRRIGATION SOLUTIONS

Sodium chloride 0.9% (normal saline) is traditionally the irrigation solution of choice for open surgical procedures. It is a sterile, topical, conductive, electrolyte-containing solution that is not administered by parenteral injection (there is a separately packaged sodium chloride solution for injection). Sodium chloride is used to rinse indwelling urethral catheters and surgical drainage tubes. It can be used to wash or rinse tissues, or soak surgical dressings and can serve as diluent or vehicle for administering other pharmaceutical preparations (as antibiotics in sodium chloride irrigation). Sodium chloride, if

IN SIGHT 11-3 Adhesion Barriers

Abdominal and pelvic surgery sometimes results in the formation of adhesions from scar tissue. Scar tissue forms around the incision and can cling to the surface of organs. Adhesions mature into fibrous bands, often with small calcifications and containing blood vessels. They can obstruct or distort organs causing pain, doctor's visits, the need for pain medication, subsequent surgery, and lost work time. An approach to preventing adhesion formation, in addition to excellent surgical technique, has been to use mechanical barriers and fluids. A barrier agent for prevention of adhesions should be nonreactive in tissue, maintain itself as the peritoneum and other structures regenerate (heal), and then be absorbed by the body.

Hyskon, a 32% solution of dextran 70 suspended in glucose, is used as a distention medium and has also been used as a fluid barrier to adhesions. The concept is of a viscous solution that is absorbed in 5 to 7 days and draws fluid equal to two and one-half to three times the original volume into the abdomen or pelvis. This action produces a hydro-flotation effect on internal structures to prevent adhesion formation. SprayGel is a synthetic absorbable adhesion barrier that consists of two polyethylene glycol–based liquids that are mixed during spraying. They form an adherent absorbable hydrogel, which remains intact for 5 to 7 days during the critical healing period. The agent then degrades into an absorbable, easily excreted byproduct. SprayGel is available in a laparoscopic spray system as well as an open surgery applicator.

Mechanical barriers include Interceed and Seprafilm. Interceed is derived from oxidized regenerated cellulose in a mesh form that is positioned over injured tissues. It forms a gelatinous protective layer that is absorbed within 2 weeks. Complete hemostasis is required before applying Interceed. Seprafilm is a bio-absorbable membrane derived from sodium hyaluronate and carboxymethylcellulose. Once applied, it breaks down into a hydrated gel that is absorbed within 7 days. Adept is 4% icodextrin solution that prevents adhesions by providing a physical separation of tissue surfaces during the early phases of healing.

systemically absorbed, can result in alteration of cardiopulmonary and renal function. Excessive volume of the solution or pressure during irrigation, especially in small areas or closed cavities, can result in distention or tissue disruption. If this occurs, the irrigation solution should be discontinued immediately. Sodium chloride comes in 150-mL, 500-mL, 1000-mL, 2000-mL, and 3000-mL pour bottles. It also comes in 0.45% concentration in 1500-mL and 2000-mL sizes.

TECH TIP

At the end of the surgical procedure, the surgeon will require a "wet one" and a "dry one," meaning a sponge saturated with clean, sterile sodium chloride irrigation solution and then a dry sponge. These are used to wipe off any blood from the patient's incision site, and any that has splattered or run on the patient's skin. The wet sponge also wipes any residual Betadine prep solution from the area. Then the second clean, sterile sponge is used to dry the area and prepare it for the surgical dressings. Also note to check the surgeon's face for any splattered blood, which must be removed before he or she goes out to talk with the patient's family.

⚠ CAUTION

Saline is a conductive solution and so is used with caution in the presence of the electrosurgical unit (ESU). The danger comes from the transfer of heat and current to adjacent tissues. When used in open surgical procedures, most fluid is suctioned from the field and so saline can be used with little risk. However, in endoscopic procedures the ESU is applied within the fluid, in a confined space, and so other irrigation solutions that do not have conductive properties are used.

Sterile water is used more often to rinse instruments in order to cool them after autoclaving, remove residual disinfectant before coming into contact with patient skin, soak blood from hinges and serrations before terminal cleaning and autoclaving, and cool saw blades or burrs when drilling. It is also used in splash basins to remove powder from surgical gloves immediately preoperatively and to remove blood from surgical gloves intraoperatively. It is used to dilute prep solutions (Betadine scrub solution) and to fill the balloon on Foley catheters. Like saline, sterile water can be used to cleanse indwelling urethral catheters and surgical drainage tubes and soak surgical dressings. Sterile water is nonconductive and can be used for transurethral resection of bladder tumor (TURB) because it is not absorbed through the bladder. It cannot be used for transurethral resection of the prostate (TURP) as it is not isotonic and can result in intravascular hemolysis of erythrocytes. This can also result in absorption in large amounts through vascular openings. Sterile water comes packaged in 250-mL, 500-mL, 1000-mL, 2000-mL, and 3000-mL containers. Note: there is also a sterile water packaged separately for injection.

CAUTION

Sterile water is not used for irrigation in procedures using the cell saver because it would also be suctioned up into the machine. If this occurs, hemolysis of the blood cells may result, thus they cannot be re-infused. This principle also applies in cardiovascular procedures because of the possibility of water being absorbed into the vascular system. Sterile water may not be used to irrigate in the presence of cancer cells because the solution would cause the cells to swell and possibly rupture, spilling their cancerous contents onto other tissues. However, some surgeons require sterile water irrigation for that same purpose - to destroy any free-floating cells in the area before they spread.

TECH TIP

It is good practice to remove the powder from your sterile surgical gloves before procedures, such as middle ear surgery, because it can lead to granulation tissue growth. Studies have shown that the surgical wound retains amounts of residual powder granules after surgical procedures. Use the sterile basin with water or a moistened sponge to rinse or wipe gloves, and then remove the sponge from the sterile field.

Physiosol is a balanced electrolyte solution used as sterile irrigation for wounds and also for washing and rinsing purposes. It can be used as an irrigant for body joints because its pH and electrolyte composition closely resemble that of synovial fluids. It addition, it provides a transparent fluid medium with optical properties for good visualization during arthroscopy. It is not for injection and should not be used during electrosurgical procedures. Physiosol comes in solutions of 6.0 and 7.4 pH, and is packaged in 250-mL, 500-mL, and 1000-mL pour bottles and 1000-mL flexible plastic bags.

IRRIGATION SOLUTIONS USED IN SPECIALTY PROCEDURES

Urologic irrigation solution of 3% Sorbitol is sterile, nonelectrolytic, nonhemolytic, and electrically nonconductive. It is used as an irrigating fluid for the urinary bladder because it provides a high degree of visibility without conducting heat and current from the ESU to tissues. During transurethral procedures, it removes blood and tissue fragments. During this procedure, venous sinuses may be opened and varying amounts of irrigation solutions are absorbed into the bloodstream. Thus, the patient should be monitored for altered cardiopulmonary and renal dynamics and hyperglycemia (see Insight 11-4).

CAUTION

During all procedures using a distention medium, the rate of flow and total fluid volume of the irrigation solutions must be carefully monitored. Also important is the height at which the IV pole is set, because this determines the rate of flow (via gravity) and pressure of the solution.

IN SIGHT 11-4 Transurethral Resection Syndrome

Transurethral resection syndrome is a condition that results from absorption of fluids during a transurethral resection of the prostate gland (TURP). During a TURP procedure, irrigation fluid is used to visualize the area and wash away (lavage) blood and tissue debris. As the tissue is cut by the electrocautery, bleeding occurs from the open capillaries. The irrigation fluid flow must be at a high enough pressure to clear the surgical site, so this fluid pressure is greater than or equal to the pressure of the blood flow from the tissues. The open capillaries provide an access route for the fluid to enter the bloodstream. This can result in hypervolemia with dilutional hyponatremia and acid-base imbalance (acidosis). When glycine is used as the irrigation solution, its over-absorption can lead to hyper-ammonemia. Hyper-ammonemia can lead to cerebral edema, seizures, and death.

Sorbital is sometimes used in combination with mannitol as Purisole (sorbital 2.5%, mannitol 0.54%) for transurethral procedures and in hysteroscopy. Mannitol 5% is also used in hysteroscopy when the ESU is used and is indicated to prevent hydrolysis and hemoglobin build-up during TURP.

Glycine 1.5% is a sterile nonconducting fluid used to irrigate body cavities. Its active ingredient is glycine, a naturally occurring amino acid, and like the other irrigants, is nonconductive, nonelectrolytic, and can be used with ESU. Thus is can be used in TURP and is also used in hysteroscopy. However, over absorption during this procedure can result in water intoxication with hyponatremia and acid-base imbalance (metabolic acidosis). Glycine comes packaged in 1500-mL pour bottles and 3000-mL flexible plastic bags.

Hyskon is a 32% solution of dextran 70 suspended in glucose. A water-soluble glucose polymer, it was originally used as a plasma expander. Hyskon is used to distend the uterus during hysteroscopy and to irrigate blood and tissue debris from the surgical site. It is electrolyte-free and nonconductive so it can be used with ESU. When large amounts of Hyskon are used, the possibility of systemic effects such as plasma volume expansion can occur.

SYNOVIAL FLUID REPLACEMENT

There are other body fluids that are being replaced, thanks in part to the advancement of arthroscopic surgery. Viscoseal is a 0.5% concentration, isotonic solution of hyaluronan of fermentative origin. Hyaluronan is a vital component of hyaline cartilage and synovial fluid. Viscoseal is used to irrigate joints during arthroscopic surgery, and also as a synovial fluid substitute. During arthroscopic procedures, synovial fluid is "washed away" by irrigating fluids. Viscoseal, when introduced into the joint, displaces any irrigating solutions left in the space, and leads to the re-establishment of the normal protective hyaluronan coating on the surface of the articular cartilage and synovial membrane.

IRRIGATION EQUIPMENT AND SUPPLIES

Irrigating syringes are bulb-shaped or bulb/barrel syringes (Asepto). They can also be larger standard syringes with special needle attachments for use in vascular surgery. The Asepto syringe is the most commonly used irrigator in open procedures. It is packaged sterile and holds approximately 120 cc. The regular bulb syringe, also called an ear syringe, does not have a barrel and is designed to irrigate smaller areas, such as the ear canal. It is also used to aspirate (remove) fluid from the nose and mouth of an infant, such as during cesarean sections.

TECH TIP

Keep your irrigation syringes filled and ready for use. Always note the amount of irrigation in the syringes, how much is on your table, and how much is used. This is important, because the irrigation solutions and the patient's blood will both be suctioned into the same canisters. It is impossible to measure blood loss if you do not know how much of this mixture is actually irrigation solution.

Evacuators are syringes used to insert and remove irrigation solutions in closed areas such as the bladder. Examples are an Ellik or a Toomey syringe used for TURP. The Ellik is a double-bowl shaped glass or plastic container that is filled with irrigation solution and used to "flush" the prostate area. It aspirates blood clots and resected tissue as the solution is returned back into the evacuator. The Toomey is a large syringe-type container, usually used with a metal adapter inserted onto a catheter for irrigating the bladder and prostate areas. It can also be used with an endoscope.

Continuous irrigation, such as for cystoscopy or hysteroscopy procedures, requires a closed, disposable irrigation system. Tubing is either straight as used for IVs or more commonly Y-shaped to allow attachment of two bags or bottles of irrigation solution. Continuous irrigation is also used with Coblation devices. These consist of a wand, cord for power source, tubing for suction, and tubing to be hooked up to a conductive irrigation solution such as normal saline (see Fig. 11-10 and Insight 11-5).

Irrigation for endoscopic procedures is accomplished through irrigating channels built into endoscopes, or by irrigating systems inserted into an opening or port. Irrigation solutions can also be manually inserted into endoscopes with a syringe, for small amounts; or a syringe and stopcock attached to irrigation tubing hooked up to bags of solution when larger amounts are required. There are also pumps available that supply more fluid under pressurization. With these systems, the irrigation solutions can be introduced with more force, over a longer period of time, and the pressure is adjustable (Fig. 11-11).

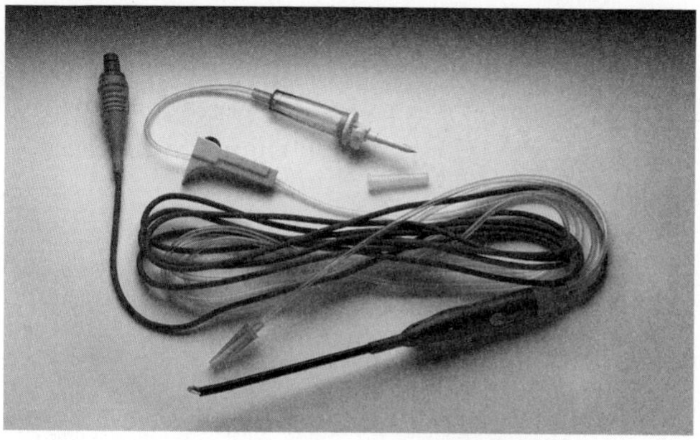

Figure 11-10 Coblator wand and tubing. *(From Nemitz R: Surgical instrumentation: an interactive approach, St. Louis, 2009, Saunders/Elsevier.)*

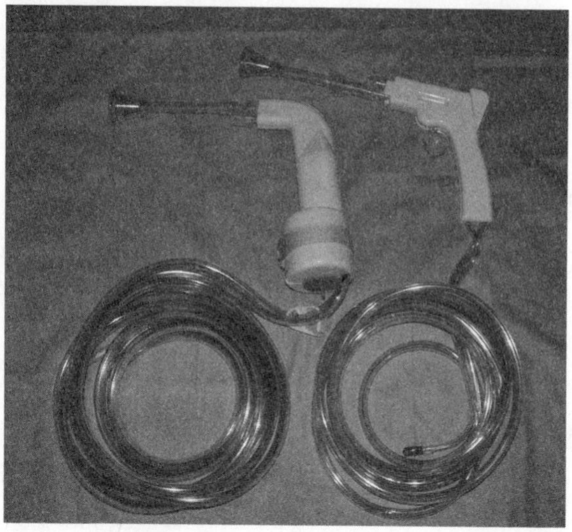

Figure 11-11 Irrigation devices.

IN SIGHT 11-5 Coblation Technology

Coblation is a trademarked term for technology that uses radiofrequency energy to excite electrolytes in a conductive irrigation medium such as normal saline. It is a controlled, non–heat-driven source of focused plasma that breaks down molecular bonds within tissue. This causes tissue to dissolve at low temperatures (usually 40° C to 70° C) and results in minimal damage to the surrounding tissues. The various devices are also designed to coagulate or seal bleeding vessels. Coblation technology is used in arthroscopy, spine and neurosurgery, otolaryngology, head and neck surgery, urology, gynecology, plastic surgery, and laparoscopy/general surgery. For videos on this technology, go to www.arthrocare.com.

ADVANCED PRACTICE FOR THE SURGICAL FIRST ASSISTANT

CHAPTER 11— Fluids and Irrigation Solutions

Key Terms

central line
hypertonic
hypotonic
osmolarity
osmosis
peripheral line
PICC line
solute
solution
solvent

When a patient's treatment necessitates intravenous medication and infusion therapy, it is the responsibility of the surgical first assistant to know why such interventions are essential and how they will affect the patient. As the surgical first assistant, you should have an understanding of the pathophysiology of fluids and how they work in the body, and be able to relate this to the need for intravenous therapy.

As mentioned earlier in the chapter, body fluids are primarily made up of water in which a variety of substances are dissolved. The total volume of water in the body is distributed between two large compartments, the intracellular and extracellular. These two compartments are separated by a semipermeable cell membrane. The extracellular compartment is subdivided into three compartments: the intravascular, interstitial, and transcellular. The compositions of the fluid contained within the two compartments are distinctive in chemical formulation. ICF is contained within the cell. Fluid found outside of the cell is extracellular (ECF). Even though the two compartments have structural differences and carry out completely different tasks, they are in constant interaction with each other in order to maintain homeostasis. **Osmosis** governs the movement of body fluids between these two compartments. Osmosis is the passage of water through a semipermeable membrane from an area with a lower concentration of **solutes** to an area with a higher concentration.

{NOTE} *In order for the cell membrane to be semipermeable it has to be more permeable to water than to solutes (thus it controls the passage of solutes). In the body, water acts as a* ***solvent****, able to hold substances as well as acting to dissolve them. Solutes are substances dissolved in water (the solvent) and the combination of the solute and the solvent forms the* ***solution****.*

EVALUATION FOR BLOOD REPLACEMENT

Evaluation of the surgical patient's blood/fluid balance begins preoperatively and is monitored intraoperatively and postoperatively. Identifying fluid and/or clotting deficiencies will help to avoid potential hemostatic risks during the surgical procedure. Assessment includes reviewing the patient's medical records and a patient interview. Preoperative laboratory tests, such as hemoglobin, hematocrit, and coagulation profile may assist in predicting the need for blood transfusion. The patient may be instructed to discontinue or modify any anticoagulant therapy; and prophylactic administration of drugs that promote coagulation and minimize blood loss (aprotinin, tranexamic acid) may be used on some procedures. Keeping blood loss to a minimum, and avoiding the need for blood transfusion, is the goal of the surgical team. The surgical first assistant contributes to minimizing intraoperative blood loss by taking immediate and accurate actions, such as immediate direct pressure to the site until bleeding is controlled, clamping or coagulating bleeding vessels, providing an unobstructed view of the surgical site for the surgeon, and using delicate tissue handling. Other methods, such as the harmonic scalpel, laser, ESU, or Coblator, may mechanically decrease blood loss. Cell savers, if appropriate, can also be used. However, it may be necessary for the surgical patient to receive fluid/blood replacement. According to the American Society of Anesthesiologists (ASA), transfusion is rarely indicated when the hemoglobin is greater than 10 g/dL, and is often indicated when the hemoglobin is less than 6 g/dL.

OSMOLARITY OF FLUIDS

In the chapter, the composition and concentration of IV fluids were discussed. The concentration of the solute in the solution will determine its **osmolarity** (tonicity, measured in osmoles [Osm] per liter of solution [Osm/L]). Normal saline (0.9% sodium chloride) is an isotonic solution. This is defined as occurring when fluid that surrounds the cell membrane has the same tonicity and osmotic pull as inside the cell. Therefore the cell remains unchanged. A **hypotonic** solution is when the fluid on the outside of the cell membrane has a lesser tonicity and osmotic pull than the fluid on the inside of the cell membrane. Therefore more fluid will flow into the cell causing it to swell and possibly burst. The opposite of this is a **hypertonic** solution in which fluid on the outside of the cell membrane has a greater tonicity and osmotic pull than on the inside of the cell membrane. Thus more fluid will be pushed out of the cell causing it to shrink and shrivel. (See Fig. 11-12 and Table A.)

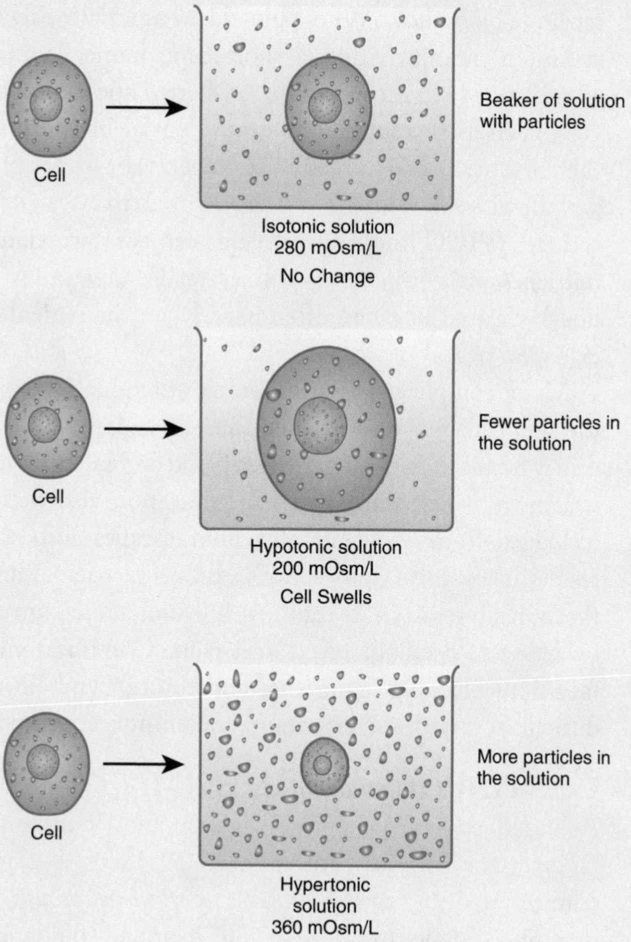

Figure 11-12 Osmotic solutions.

Table A Osmolarity of Sodium Chloride Solution

Solutions	Concentration	Treatment
Hypertonic	3% and 5%	Cerebral edema and hyponatremia
Isotonic	.09%	IV fluids
Hypotonic	0.225%, 0.33%, 0.45%	Dehydration and hypernatremia

INTRAVENOUS SITES AND COMPLICATIONS

The surgical first assistant is not responsible for starting IVs (without additional, verified training) but should be aware of IV sites, protocols, and terminology to assist in patient comfort and safety. IV fluids may be administered via a **peripheral line**, as into a vein in the arm, leg, or scalp (of an infant). The blood circulation through these veins can dilute the components in the IV fluids and the rate of infusion should not exceed 200 mL in 1 hour. Most transparent IV fluids can flow safely and smoothly through peripheral veins. If blood transfusion or replacement is administered, a larger vein is preferred to facilitate blood flow. Whole blood and especially packed cells can be viscous and are often infused within a short time frame. Intravenous fluids can also be administered via a **central line**, where a special catheter is placed into a large vein, such as the subclavian vein. Central lines are accessed directly (through the chest wall) or indirectly via a neck vein or peripheral vein in the arm. If a peripheral vein is used, this is referred to as a peripherally inserted central catheter (**PICC line**). Larger veins can accommodate higher concentrations of nutrients and components with faster IV flow rates (greater than 200 mL in 1 hour). Central lines are often used when the patient needs IV therapy over an extended period of time.

ASSISTANT *ADVICE*

The surgical first assistant should constantly monitor the patient's tissue status. Irrigation fluids (i.e., normal saline) is applied to prevent drying during the procedure and to prevent overheating of saw blades and burrs, which can cause thermal damage to surrounding tissues. In addition, anytime the incision and/or tissues are exposed to room air, drying occurs. The surgical first assistant should dampen (irrigate) the tissues on a regular basis and/or place a wet sponge over the areas if possible to prevent desiccation.

Major complications of IV therapy are phlebitis, infiltration, and infection at the site. Phlebitis results when the vein becomes red, irritated, or painful. If the vein is fragile, it may rupture with blood and IV fluids leaking into the tissue. This is known as "blowing a vein." Infiltration also occurs when the IV catheter dislodges from the vein and fluid escapes into the surrounding tissue. It results in coolness and pallor to the skin, edema, and swelling. Any break in the skin's integrity can result in infection. Infection at the site is characterized by redness, swelling, fever, and pain. Complications of central lines include infection, bleeding, gangrene, and thromboembolism. Central lines are more difficult to insert and maintain, and complications can result in septicemia.

CONTINUOUS AND INTERMITTENT IRRIGATION

As described in the chapter, irrigation and IV fluids are used for a multitude of tasks in the surgical setting. Both IV fluids and irrigation solutions can be administered by two methods: *continuous* or *intermittent*. Continuous IV therapy is done to replace and maintain fluids in the body. Continuous irrigation is fluid instilled into an area of the body through a steady flow. An example of this is distending the bladder for TURP or to ensure visualization during an arthroscopy. Intermittent infusions are used for medication administration and secondary fluid replacement. Examples of intermittent administration are IV piggybacks, IV push (bolus), and heparin or saline locks. Intermittent irrigation is also introduced onto an area or into a cavity of the body that is then suctioned or sponged. This is done to remove blood and debris from the site as during a débridement using the Pulsavac, or following a laparotomy by pouring irrigation from the sterile pitcher into the abdomen.

Advanced Practices Bibliography

Mosby's medical dictionary, ed 8, St. Louis, 2009, Mosby/Elsevier.

Olsen JL, Giangrasso AP, Shrimpton D, et al: *Medical dosage calculations*, ed 9, Upper Saddle River, New Jersey, 2008, Pearson Prentice Hall.

Pickar G, Abernethy AP: *Dosage calculations*, ed 8, New York, 2008, Thomson Delmar.

Rothrock JC, Seifert PC: *Assisting in surgery: patient-centered care*, U.S., 2010, CCI.

Advanced Practices Internet Resources

Abbott Laboratories: www.abbott.com.

Baxter: www.baxter.com.

Drugs.com: *Ionosol and Dextrose*. www.drugs.com/pro/ionosol-and-dextrose.html.

Drugs.com: *Isolyte P in Dextrose*. www.drugs.com/pro/isolyte-p-in-dextrose.html.

Drugs.com: *Plasma-Lyte 56*. www.drugs.com/pro/plasma-lyte-56.html.

eMedicine from WebMD: *Hypernatremia*. www.emedicine.com/emerg/topic263.htm.

MayoClinic.com: *Dextrose (Intravenous Route)*. www.mayoclinic.com/health/drug-information/DR603083.

Practice Guidelines for Perioperative Blood Transfusion and Adjuvant Therapies. http://www.asahq.org/publicationsAndServices/BCTGuidesFinal.pdf.

Advanced Practices: Learning the Language (Key Terms)

Using your textbook or a standard medical dictionary, look up and write the definitions of each term.

- central line
- hypertonic
- hypotonic
- osmolarity
- osmosis
- peripheral line
- PICC line
- solute
- solution
- solvent

Advanced Practices: Review Questions

1. Why is normal saline considered an isotonic solution?
2. Which type of solution will make the cell shrink? Why?
3. What is the difference between continuous and intermittent IV administrations? Give examples of each.

KEY CONCEPTS

- The human body's make-up includes fluid electrolytes and nonelectrolytes distributed into intracellular and extracellular fluid compartments.
- Blood and fluid replacement to normal levels are essential for survival.
- Major electrolytes are sodium, chloride, potassium, calcium, phosphate, and magnesium.
- Too much of the electrolyte in the blood is hyper-, too little is called hypo-; such as too much potassium is hyperkalemia, too little is hypokalemia.
- Most all surgical patients receive an IV to administer and maintain fluids and to establish a direct access to the circulatory system for medication administration.
- Common IV fluids used in surgery are sodium chloride, dextrose in water and sodium chloride, and lactated Ringer solution.
- Normal saline, which is 0.9% sodium chloride, is the most common IV fluid used in surgery.
- Blood serves many functions in the body such as transports oxygen, nutrients, waste, hormones, and enzymes; and maintains the acid-base balance, temperature, and water content.
- In the average adult, circulating blood volume is approximately 70 mL/kg of body mass.
- Blood consists of formed elements (RBCs, WBCs, platelets) and plasma.
- Hemoglobin is a protein responsible for carrying oxygen and carbon dioxide between the lungs and the cells.
- Hematocrit is the volume of erythrocytes in a given volume of blood expressed as a percentage.
- The most common indication for blood replacement in surgery is hypovolemia.
- Options for blood replacement include homologous donation, autologous donation, autotransfusion, volume expanders, and—in the future—oxygen therapeutics.
- There is a specific hospital protocol to follow when obtaining blood from the blood bank for the surgical patient.
- Irrigation is used to clear the surgical field of blood and tissue debris, distend hollow organs, allow for specimen collection, and act as a diluent or vehicle for the administration of other pharmaceutical preparations.

- The irrigation solution of choice for most surgical procedures is 0.9% sodium chloride (normal saline).
- Normal saline is conductive and not to be used in the presence of the electrosurgical unit (ESU).
- Sterile water is used for a variety of functions including instrument care and handling, glove cleaning, cooling of instruments during surgical cases, and cleansing of urethral catheters.
- There are special irrigation solutions used for specific surgeries.
- Irrigation equipment includes: bulb syringes, Asepto syringes, large standard sized syringes, irrigating systems, and pump-irrigators.

Bibliography

Eppley BL, Woodell JE, Higgins J: Platelet quantification and growth factor analysis from platelet-rich plasma: implications for wound healing, *Plast Reconstr Surg* 114(6): 1502–1508, 2004.

Fuller JK: *Surgical technology: principles and practice,* ed 5, Philadelphia, 2010, Saunders/Elsevier.

Mosby's medical dictionary, ed 8, St. Louis, 2009, Mosby/Elsevier.

Pickar G, Abernethy AP: *Dosage calculations,* ed 8, New York, 2008, Thomson Delmar.

Olsen JL, Giangrasso AP, Shrimpton D, et al: *Medical dosage calculations,* ed 9, Upper Saddle River, New Jersey, 2008, Pearson Prentice Hall.

Pamphlets.

GPS II Platelet Concentrate System: CFT Cell Factor Technologies, Inc. Biomet Manufacturing Corp. Form No. Y-BMT-871R/111504/K.

Internet Resources

Abbott Laboratories: www.abbott.com.

Adler-Storthz K, Newland JR, Tessin BA, et al: Human papillomavirus Type 2 DNA in oral verrucous carcinoma, *J Oral Pathol Med* 15(9):472–475, 2006. Available at www3.interscience.wiley.com/journal/119500029/abstract. Accessed July 23, 2010.

American Red Cross: *Blood Types*. www.redcrossblood.org/learn-about-blood/blood-types.

ArthroCare ENT: www.arthrocareent.com/wt/page/index.

Bhagwat VM, Ramachandran BV: Malathion A and B esterases of mouse liver-I, *Biochem Pharmacol* 24(18):1713–1717, 1975. Available at www.ncbi.nlm.nih.gov/entrez/query.fcgi?cmd=Retrieve&db=PubMed&list_uids=14. Accessed July 23, 2010.

Drugs.com: *Hespan*. www.drugs.com/mtm/hespan.html.

Drugs.com: *Sorbitol*. www.drugs.com/pro/sorbitol.html.

eMedicine from WebMD: *Hypernatremia*. www.emedicine.com/emerg/topic263.htm.

Genzyme Corp: *SEPRAFILM Adhesion Barrier*. www.seprafilm.com.

Hospira, Inc: *1.5% Glycine Irrigation, USP*. http://dailymed.nlm.nih.gov/dailymed/fdaDrugXsl.cfm?id=523.

Hospira, Inc: Home Page www.hospira.com.

Hospira, Inc: *Physiosol Irrigation*. http://dailymed.nlm.nih.gov/dailymed/fdaDrugXsl.cfm?id=1107&type=display.

Internet Scientific Publications, LLC: www.ispub.com/ostia/index.php?xm1filepath=journals/ija/vol3n1/turp.xml.

Maharaj D: World Laparoscopy Hospital: *Postoperative Adhesion Prevention: A Sticky Problem*. www.laparoscopyhospital.com/post_operative_adhesion_prevention_in_laparoscopy.html.

Mayo Clinic: *Blood Transfusion*. www.mayoclinic.org/blood-transfusion/.

www.emedicine.medscape.com/article/432650-overview.

www.emedicine.medscape.com/article/827930-overview.

www.oucom.ohiou.edu/dbms-witmer/Downloads/Klabunde-08-10-00.pdf.

http://www.sinclairbioresources.com/Downloads/Report-Series/Hemorrhagic%20Shock%20Models%20in%20Swine.pdf.

Medications.com: *Macrodex information*. www.medications.com/drugs/macrodex.

Ortho-Clinical Diagnostics, Inc: *RhoGAM*. www.rhogam .com.

Rein MS, Hill JA: 32% dextran 70 (Hyskon) inhibits lymphocyte and macrophage function in vitro: a potential new mechanism for adhesion prevention, *Fertil Steril* 52 (6):953–957, 1989. Available at www.ncbi.nlm.nih.gov/pubmed/2480251. Accessed July 24, 2010.

ShoulderDoc: www.shoulderdoc.co.uk/patient_info/viscoseal.asp.

Singh IL, Chow WL, Chablani L: Synovial reaction to glove powder, *Curr Orthop Pract* 99:285–292, 1974. Available at http://journals.lww.com/corr/citation/1974/03000/Synovial_Reaction_to_glove_powder.31.aspx.

doi.wiley.com/10.1111/j.1600-0714.1986.tboo657.x. Accessed July 24, 2010.

Vaughns ABO Blood Group Chart: www.vaughns-1-pagers.com/medicine/blood-type.htm.

LEARNING THE LANGUAGE (KEY TERMS)

Using your textbook or a standard medical dictionary, look up and write the definitions of each term.

agglutination
antibody
antigen
arrhythmia
autologous
autotransfusion
electrolyte
hematocrit
hemoglobin
hemolysis
homologous
hypercalcemia
hyperkalemia
hypernatremia
hypocalcemia
hypokalemia
hyponatremia
hypovolemia
intravenous
isotonic
metabolic acidosis

REVIEW QUESTIONS

1. What are the basic functions of blood?
2. What is the average circulating blood volume in an adult?
3. Which surgical patients may require blood replacement?
4. What are the formed elements of blood? What is the main purpose of each?
5. What is hemoglobin? Hematocrit? What are the normal ranges in adults?
6. What are two electrolytes that have particular importance to the surgical patient? Why?
7. What common IV fluids are used in surgery? What is the purpose of each?
8. List two reasons to "start" an IV on the surgical patient preoperatively.
9. What is the primary reason for the surgical patient to receive blood replacement?
10. What is the difference between homologous and autologous donation?

CRITICAL THINKING

1. Sodium chloride 0.9% is said to be isotonic. Why is it the irrigation solution of choice for most surgical procedures?
2. What should be considered when giving a dextrose IV solution to a diabetic patient?
3. What are some of the risks involved when giving the patient a transfusion of whole blood?
4. What should the surgical technologist consider and be prepared for when the surgical patient is given large amounts of donor blood?

Scenario

You are assigned to the GU room for the day. The first procedure is a TURP on a 55-year-old man with an enlarged prostate gland.

1. What type of irrigation solution will be used?
2. Why is this solution used on this procedure?
3. Why must the rate of flow and the total volume of the solution used be carefully monitored?

CHAPTER 12

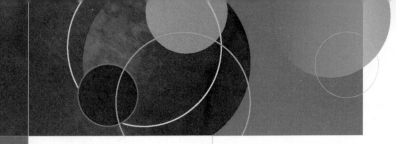

Antineoplastic Chemotherapy Agents

OBJECTIVES *After completing this chapter, you should be able to:*

1. Define terms and statistics related to cancer.
2. Discuss different types of abnormal cell growth.
3. List the classifications of antineoplastic agents.
4. Define targeted cancer therapy.
5. Describe biologic response modifiers.
6. Describe gene therapy in the treatment and prevention of diseases.
7. Discuss the epidemiology of cancer and the most prevalent carcinogen in the United States.
8. Discuss nanotechnology and its application in medicine and pharmacology.
9. List new types of agents being researched for cancer therapy.

KEY TERMS

antineoplastic agents
benign
cancer
carcinogen
cytotoxic
epidemiology
etiology
malignant
metastasis
neoplasm
palliative
primary site
remission
secondary site

The term **cancer** (sometimes referred to as carcinoma or CA) is a common one in the surgical setting. It is actually a group of diseases characterized by an uncontrolled growth of cells. This mass of cells has no useful function for the body; rather, it causes dysfunction and alters the structures of the surrounding cells. There are more than 100 different types of cancer that have been identified. In the United States, cancer is the second leading cause of death, with heart disease being first. Nearly one third of all Americans are affected by some type of cancer during their lives and it accounts for nearly one of every four deaths. Cancer may be found in any age group, but is often seen in older people. As the years of human life expectancy continue to increase, there is more evidence of cancer. The rate of occurrence for certain types of neoplastic disease, including breast, lung, and skin cancers, continues to increase, and these cases are seen frequently (along with colon cancers) for surgical intervention (Box 12-1).

The exact cause of cancer remains a mystery. It is known that cancer is caused by both internal and external factors. Internal factors include such things as inherited gene mutations, hormones, and strength of the immune system. External factors are use of tobacco, infectious organisms, and exposure to chemicals and radiation, which includes sun exposure (Box 12-2). It is understood that before cancer can start, a disruption (possibly in the cell's genetic material) must occur that transforms normal cells into malignant ones. Normal body cells divide and multiply, replacing dying ones. When this rate of cell division is disrupted and not controlled, an abnormal growth of cells is formed. This abnormal growth is called a tumor, or **neoplasm**. Neoplasms may be **benign**, which means they resemble normal tissue, grow slowly, are highly organized cells, and do not normally spread into surrounding tissue. These tumors may be surgically removed if they disrupt normal body functions or cause pain. Neoplasms may also be **malignant**, or cancerous. These cells are unorganized and immature, multiply rapidly, and invade surrounding tissues. The original site of the tumor is called the **primary site**. When malignant cells travel through the circulatory or lymphatic systems and spread to other areas of the body, they form another tumor called a **metastasis**. Each of these new locations of cancer is referred to a **secondary site**. Many times, surgery is performed to diagnose or remove cancerous tumors. However, surgery may not be the only treatment available to the patient with cancer.

CHEMOTHERAPY AGENTS

Pharmaceutical agents play an important role in the treatment of cancer outside the surgical setting. **Antineoplastic agents**, those that fight cancer, can be used as systemic treatment in the primary or main tumor, and in its metastases. This is often in addition to surgical treatment. These agents are **cytotoxic** and thus harm normal cells as well as malignant ones. They are often given intravenously in high doses on an established schedule. This regimen allows normal cells to recover in between chemotherapy medication doses. Antineoplastic agents are used for **remission**, **palliative** effects, and/or to prolong life. Remission is the abatement (stopping) of symptoms and possible cure of the disease. Palliation (as already discussed in the text) means the relief of symptoms without cure. Antineoplastic agents are classified according to their mechanism of actions: alkylating agents, antimetabolites, mitotic inhibitors (plant alkaloids), antineoplastic antibiotics (anthracyclines), hormones, and hormone antagonists. Steroids and antiemetics are also used along with antineoplastics to fight certain types of cancers and to help prevent nausea and

Box 12-1 SEVEN WARNING SIGNS OF CANCER: CAUTION

Change in bowel or bladder habits
A sore that will not heal
Unusual bleeding or discharge
Thickening or a lump in the breast or elsewhere
Indigestion or difficulty swallowing
Obvious change in a wart or mole
Nagging cough or hoarseness

Box 12-2 ABCs FOR DETECTING SKIN CANCER

Asymmetry: A mole that looks different on one half as compared with the other half
Border: The edges of the mole are jagged, blurry, or irregular
Color: The color of the mole changes (as it darkens, loses color, or has multiple colors)
Diameter: The mole is greater than ¼ inch or 6 mm in diameter (the size of a pencil eraser)
Elevation: The mole is raised above the skin and has an uneven surface (sometimes listed as evolving and referring to any change)

vomiting—common side effects of chemotherapy. Other chemotherapy side effects include diarrhea, bone marrow depression, rashes, alopecia (hair loss), and scaling or dryness of the skin. Antineoplastic agents are contraindicated in pregnancy and in patients with renal or hepatic disorders.

Alkylating drugs are the largest group of anticancer agents and are toxic to tissues that grow rapidly. They include the first antineoplastic drug, nitrogen mustard, which was introduced for this purpose in the 1940s (mustard gas was used in chemical warfare in World War I). Alkylating agents kill by directly damaging the DNA strands and keeping the cancer cells from reproducing. These agents affect all phases of the cell cycle. Thus, they are highly toxic and effective against many types of cancers such as acute and chronic leukemias, lymphomas, multiple myeloma, and solid tumors of the breast, ovaries, uterus, lungs, bladder, and stomach. Examples of alkylating agents include cyclophosphamide (Cytoxan) and carboplatin (Paraplatin). The newer medications in this drug category are called nitrosoureas. They are used to treat tumors of the brain, testes, and ovary, and include temozolomide (Temodar) and carmustine (BiCNU).

Antimetabolites are the oldest group of anticancer agents (except for the original nitrogen mustard). They disrupt the cells' metabolic processes by interfering with DNA and RNA growth. Thus, the neoplastic cell is unable to divide, resulting in cell death. Antimetabolites are used in the treatment of many cancers such as leukemias, tumors of the ovaries, lung, bladder, breast, and intestinal tract. Examples include the more commonly known agents methotrexate (Folex, Mexate) and 5-fluorouracil (5-FU, Adrucil).

{NOTE} *Many of these anticancer drugs have other applications. For example, methotrexate is also used in confirmed ectopic pregnancy when the ectopic mass is still small. It is injected into the muscle and reaches the embryo via the bloodstream, killing the cells that are developing in the placenta. The embryo is reabsorbed into the body, and the fallopian tube is not damaged. The drug 5-fluorouracil is used in ophthalmic surgery. It is injected beneath the outer eye membrane following glaucoma surgery to impede growth of scar tissue that could interfere with the surgical outcome.*

Mitotic inhibitors are derivatives of plant extracts. They block cell division by preventing chromosomes from dividing and migrating to the ends of the cells (the M phase or the metaphase stage of the cell cycle). These agents can be used as single medications or in combination drug therapy. Uses of mitotic inhibitors include treatment of advanced breast and ovarian, colon, pancreatic, and lung cancers, and squamous cell cancers of the head and neck. Examples include the medications paclitaxel (Taxol) and docetaxel (Taxotere), which are derived from the bark and needles of the European yew tree. Others are vinblastine (Velban), and vincristine (Oncovin) from the periwinkle plant and etoposide (Toposar) derived from the May apple.

Antineoplastic antibiotics (anthracyclines) are different from those used for treating infections. These antibiotics target specific types of cancers by inhibiting protein and RNA synthesis and binding DNA, which causes fragmentation of the cell. They, like most antineoplastic agents, have toxic effects. The first antibiotic used in this manner, dactinomycin, was in the treatment of animal tumors in the 1940s. The antibiotics differ and are used to treat a variety of cancers such as leukemia, squamous cell cancers, Wilms tumor, testicular cancer, and ovarian, lung, breast, and bladder cancers. Examples include bleomycin sulfate (Blenoxane) and doxorubicin (Adriamycin).

Mitomycin (Mutamycin, MTC, Mitomycin-C) is an anti-tumor antibiotic that is used to prevent recurrence of an eye growth called a pterygium. It can also be used to treat or shrink cancerous growths on the eye.

Hormones and hormone antagonists are the least toxic of the anticancer drugs and are used in combination therapy for treating various cancers. Drugs in this category are the sex hormones (hormone-like drugs) that influence the production or action of female and male hormones. They include androgens and antiandrogens, estrogens and antiestrogens, and progestins. These agents act as antagonists that inhibit tumor cell growth and compete with endogenous hormones. One example is the use of androgens, which promotes regression of breast tumors. Hormone antagonists exert beneficial effects by altering the hormonal environment that promotes cancer growth, for example, as when sex hormones such as estrogen are used to treat prostate cancers. Estrogens suppress androgen production by acting in the pituitary gland to decrease interstitial cell–stimulating hormone. This results in the decreased production of androgens by the testes, which helps to decrease the progression of prostatic cancer. Hormones (corticosteroids) also act as anti-inflammatory agents to suppress the tissue's inflammatory process and prevent severe allergic reactions. When used in this way, they are considered as steroids. When they are used to kill cancer cells or slow their growth, they fall into the chemotherapy category. These corticosteroids are primarily used for treating cancers of the breast, endometrium, and prostate. Examples include leuprolide (Lupron) and tamoxifen (Nolvadex). Those used as steroids are prednisone, methylprednisolone (Solu-Medrol), and dexamethasone (Decadron).

TARGETED THERAPY

Targeted cancer therapies involve the use of drugs or other substances that interfere with specific molecules involved in a tumor's growth. Scientists sometimes call these "molecularly targeted drugs." Targeted therapies are more effective than other types of treatments because they focus on molecular and cellular changes specific to cancers, and they are less harmful to the body's normal cells. Many targeted cancer therapies have been approved by the U.S. Food and Drug Administration (FDA) to treat specific types of cancers such as estrogen receptor (ER)-positive breast cancer, certain types of leukemia, and lung cancers. Examples include tamoxifen and toremifene (Fareston), imatinib mesylate (Gleevec), and gefitinib (Iressa).

BIOLOGIC RESPONSE MODIFIERS

Biologic response modifiers (BRMs) are agents that have been developed through biochemical technology to boost, or enhance, the body's immune system. Immunotherapy uses BRMs to help the body fight cancer. They can be used in conjunction with chemotherapy agents. As previously discussed, chemotherapy agents destroy not only cancer cells but also normal cells such as white blood cells (WBCs), which are essential in protecting the body from infections. The main functions of BRMs are to enhance the body's immunologic function and to destroy or interfere with tumor activities. Further indications for BRM uses are being investigated. Two agents are used to treat chemotherapy side effects by stimulating specific bone marrow production of blood cells. The first is erythropoietin (Epogen, Procrit), which is used to treat patients with anemia by stimulating red blood cell (RBC) production. The second is filgrastim (Neupogen), which binds to bone marrow cells and stimulates the growth of neutrophils—key components of the immune system (Insight 12-1).

Other BRM agents are alpha interferon and interleukin-2. They are natural proteins (called cytokines) produced in small amounts primarily by cells of the immune system called T cells. When given in greatly increased concentrations, alpha interferon boosts immune cells so they are better able to attack cancerous cells. It can also change the structure of cells to make them more normal in their behavior and less like cancer. Alpha interferon is used to treat a specific type of leukemia and for use in an acquired immunodeficiency syndrome–related tumor called Kaposi sarcoma. It is also being used to treat hepatitis C. Interleukin-2 has been found to contain antitumor effects, and it strengthens the body's natural defense mechanism. It causes some cancer cells to be

IN SIGHT 12-1 Cancer Vaccines

Vaccines are medicines that act to boost the immune system to defend the body against infection and to protect it from damaged or abnormal cells, such as those found in cancer. Vaccines used to fight cancer are classified as biological response modifiers. There are two broad types of cancer vaccines:

- Preventative or prophylactic vaccines, which prevent cancer from developing, and
- Therapeutic vaccines, which treat already existing cancers by strengthening the body's own natural defenses to recognize and attack cancer cells.

The FDA has approved two cancer preventative vaccines. These work by targeting infectious agents that can contribute to the development of cancer. One is against the hepatitis B virus, which can cause liver cancer, and the other is against the human papillomavirus types 16 and 18, which are responsible for cervical cancer. At this time, there is no FDA approved cancer treatment vaccine. An effective cancer treatment of this type is difficult to produce, because cancer is hard to detect, even by the body. It can escape the immune system or weaken the natural immune responses. However, there is ongoing research to develop cancer treatment vaccines. Active clinical trials are progressing for cancer of the bladder, brain, breast, kidney, lung, and prostate . . . just to name a few.

recognized and eliminated by immune cells. It is used especially in renal cell cancers and malignant melanoma.

GENE THERAPY

Gene therapy is an experimental technique that uses genes to treat or prevent disease. This concept is easy to understand, but difficult to implement. In the past two decades, gene therapy resulted in patient deaths and so was almost discontinued. However, medical advances have once again brought this therapy to the forefront of science. In the future, gene therapy may allow doctors to treat a disorder or disease by inserting a gene into a patient's cell rather than using chemicals, radiation, drugs or surgery. There are several approaches being tested such as to replace a mutated gene with a healthy copy to prevent disease, inactivate a mutated gene that is functioning improperly, or introduce a new gene into the body to help fight infection or disease. While gene therapy is very promising in its theory, the technique to accomplish it remains risky and is still undergoing study and research. A "vehicle" is needed to carry the good genes into a human cell. At this time, scientists are looking at specific viruses to accomplish the task. This approach still requires significant research to not only find the proper virus, but also to understand the virus' genes in order to use it. The research must also consider the patient's own immune system and its response to the virus and the new gene.

Another possible vehicle being researched is surface-modified nanodiamond particles. These particles result from detonating diamonds into dust, down to 5 nanometers in size. It is hoped that gene therapy will become medicine's next "big breakthrough" and it is currently being tested for treatment of diseases that have no other cures.

SEARCH FOR A CURE

Epidemiology is the science that studies factors that determine and influence the frequency, distribution, and cause of disease, and seeking to find a cure. The epidemiology of cancer reflects patterns based on gender, age, geographic location, and socioeconomic status. In the United States for example, lung cancers are equally likely to occur in men and women. In women, the leading sites of fatal cancers are the lung, breast, colon, and rectum. In men, leading sites are the lung, prostate, colon, and rectum. **Etiology** is the cause of disease. As previously stated, the exact cause of cancer (its etiology) is not known. Evidence suggests that cellular genes (which are responsible for cellular metabolism, division, and growth) convert to malignant oncogenes (these are genes found in chromosomes of tumor cells) that cause uncontrolled cell growth and replication. We do know there are cancer-causing substances, or external factors as previously mentioned. These are known as **carcinogens**. For example, tobacco is the most important known carcinogen in the United States. It is estimated that 30% of all cancer deaths could be avoided by eliminating tobacco. More than 400,000 people die each year as a result of tobacco usage, making this the leading cause of preventable deaths.

Research is ongoing regarding the uses of antineoplastic agents. Relatively few agents have been discovered in the past decade; however, new combinations of agents and higher doses have shown promise for positive results in cancer treatment. One of the newest classes of antineoplastic agents is angiogenesis inhibitors. These medications work to block the construction of new capillaries (i.e., blood supply) to cancerous tumor cells. This prevents the cells from receiving nutrients, and the tumor stops growing or in some cases regresses, or shrinks, to a microscopic dormant lesion. The FDA has approved bevacizumab (Avastin) for use with other drugs to treat colorectal cancer that has spread to other parts of the body (metastasized), some small cell lung cancers, and some breast cancers that have metastasized. This drug was the first angiogenesis inhibitor proven to delay tumor growth.

Another area of science and technology that focuses on atomic- and molecular-scale structures is nanotechnology. To measure these supersmall particles, a nanometer is used. A nanometer is one billionth of a meter, so nanoscale particles and devices can enter most cells. Nanomedicine is the application of nanotechnology to medicine. Nanomedicine uses these tiny nanoparticles to target specific tissues and organs. They can serve as diagnostic, therapeutic, antiviral, antitumor, or anticancer agents. With the ability to manipulate on this level, researchers want to use nanoparticles as image contrast agents, and for diagnostic purposes. One application would be to coat gold shells onto nanoparticles and use these nanoshells in the circulatory system. The nanoshells would absorb light and could be used for deep tissue imaging. Other potential applications include blood testing, optical triggered medication delivery, and targeting cancer cells in the body for destruction. By modifying nanoshells, they could seek out abnormal cells, or tumors, that could then be imaged, biopsied, and targeted with light to provoke the cell's death. Nanopharmacology is the use of nanotechnology for pharmaceutical applications such as creating and then matching medicinal compounds to the patient for maximum effect. As technology continues to advance, nanodevices and perhaps nanorobots will be developed to perform many medical tasks. Nanorobotic artificial phagocytes called "microbivores," which would patrol the bloodstream in search of unwanted pathogens such as bacteria or viruses and then digest them, are being researched (Figure 12-1).

Early forms of surgical nanorobots, which have been used to cut dendrites from single neurons without damaging cell viability, are being explored. Future applications include equipping nanorobots with operating instruments and the mobility to perform precise intracellular surgeries and even minimally invasive eye surgery. Scientists envision biocompatible surgical nanorobots that find and eliminate cancerous cells, remove microvascular obstructions, and perform tissue and organ transplants.

Currently, there is research on the enzyme telomerase, which is found in all cancers. This enzyme helps the human body reach adulthood and then shuts off. In cancer patients, telomerase is turned back "on," which causes uncontrolled cell growth. Scientific studies are being performed to decode and translate the structure of this enzyme. If scientists can see what telomerase looks like, perhaps they can find a molecule that can "turn off" its damaging effects. Another area being researched is customizing drugs. This concept matches patients with drugs that will work best for them. Among tests gaining acceptance are those that show how well the patient's body may absorb certain drugs, such as tamoxifen in the treatment of breast cancer. Discovering these variations among patients will assist physicians in deciding which drugs to prescribe, what dose to use, and what side effects will occur.

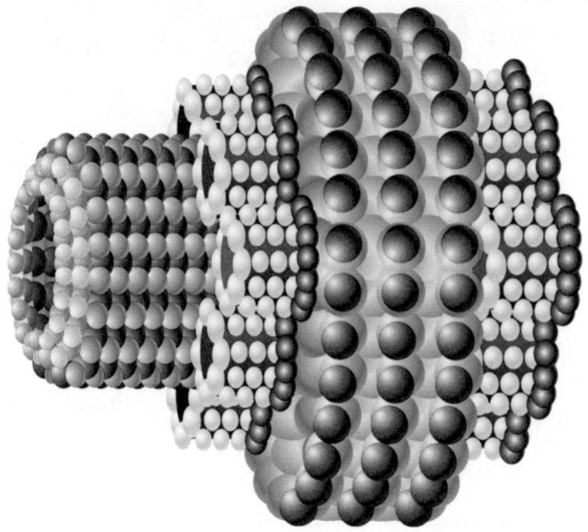

Figure 12-1 Nanorobots may be used to patrol the bloodstream for unwanted pathogens.

ADVANCED PRACTICES FOR THE SURGICAL FIRST ASSISTANT

CHAPTER 12—Antineoplastic Chemotherapy Agents

Key Terms

anaplastic
brachytherapy
differentiated
in situ
proliferate
radioisotopes
teletherapy
teratogenic

When antineoplastic chemotherapy agents are administered to treat malignant tumors, the size, site, grade, and stage of the tumor is considered. Tumors are classified by their stage of invasion and the degree of metastasis (grade) to show the extent of the cancer's spread (Tables A and B). Cancer staging can be defined in two ways: the clinical stage, which is based on all information before surgery, and the pathological stage, which adds additional information once the tumor has been excised and examined microscopically by a pathologist. For solid tumors such as breast, cervical, ovarian, colon, kidney, laryngeal, lung, bladder, and melanoma, the TNM staging is used. TNM stands for *tumor*, *nodes*, and *metastases* (Table C).

Table A Tumor Classification

Grade	Description
0	Normal tissue
1	Most **differentiated**, like parent tissue, least malignant
2	Moderately well differentiated, some structural change from normal
3	Poorly differentiated and extensive change from normal
4	Loss of cell differentiation—**anaplastic** changes

Table B Tumor Staging

Stage	Description
0	Cancer in situ without invasion of surrounding tissue
I	Limited to site of origin
II	Local spread
III	Extensive local and regional spread
IV	Widespread body metastasis

Table C TNM Staging

Primary Tumor (T)	
TX	Primary tumor cannot be evaluated
T0	No evidence of primary tumor
Tis	Carcinoma **in situ**
T1, T2, T3, T4	Size or extent of primary tumor
Regional Lymph Node Involvement (N)	
NX	Regional lymph nodes cannot be evaluated
N0	No cancer found in the lymph nodes
N1, N2, N3	Lymph node involvement, number and extent of spread
Distant Metastasis (M)	
MX	Distant metastasis cannot be evaluated
M1	No distant metastasis
M2	Distant metastasis is present

Chemotherapy may be the primary treatment, or it may be combined with radiation therapy and surgery. If the tumor is extensive and/or metastatic, chemotherapy may be used to reduce its size followed by surgical excision and then further use of chemotherapy and possibly radiation. This second course of chemotherapy is administered to destroy any remaining cancer cells that the body's immune system cannot destroy. Antineoplastic agents have the ability to interrupt cell growth or replication of normal and malignant cells as they go through the phases of cell replication. For example, antimetabolites interfere with DNA synthesis; mitotic inhibitors (plant alkaloids) interfere with cell reproduction. The alkylating gents, antibiotics, and hormones interfere with various stages of the cell cycle. Cancers that **proliferate** rapidly and have a short cell replication cycle are the most affected by antineoplastic agents. It is common practice to give antineoplastic agents in combinations of two or more at a time. Many of these drugs also contain immunosuppressive properties that decrease the patient's ability to fight off infections. Antineoplastic agents are cytotoxic and, as with all drugs, have side effects. The most serious of these are found in cells that normally replicate rapidly, such as bone marrow, epithelium of the gastrointestinal (GI) tract, hair follicles, and sperm-forming cells.

- Bone marrow suppression can lead to bleeding, anemia, and infection.
- GI tract epithelium is very sensitive to these agents, which leads to stomatitis and diarrhea.
- Hair follicles are affected, which results in alopecia.
- Women should be advised not to become pregnant during treatment with antineoplastic agents as fetal malformations may occur due to **teratogenic** effects on the fetus. Men should be advised these agents can cause sterility, due to the effects on the germinal epithelium of the testes.
- Nausea and vomiting can be severe and antiemetics are often given along with the antineoplastic agents.
- Weight loss and malnutrition may occur and nutritional supplements and increased fluids are normally advised.

It is not unusual to administer radiation therapy to shrink the tumor and chemotherapy to discourage the growth of metastatic cells. Radiation therapy is the medical use of ionizing radiation as part of cancer treatment to destroy malignant cells, either for curative or palliative effect. This form of cancer therapy uses radioactive isotopes, or **radioisotopes,** to damage the DNA of cancer cells. The isotopes may be administered as seeds or pellets directly into the tumor (**brachytherapy**), as radiation therapy via a machine (**teletherapy**), or systemically as capsules or intravenous solutions. For example, radium 426 and iridium 192 needles are used for intrauterine cancer. Cobalt 60 is used for many varieties of cancerous tumors. Radioiodine (I-131) is used to treat hyperthyroidism and thyroid cancer.

Advanced Practices Bibliography

Fulcher E, Fulcher R, Soto C: *Pharmacology principles and applications*, ed 2, 2009, Saunders/Elsevier.

Mosby's medical dictionary, ed 8, St. Louis, 2009, Mosby/Elsevier.

Advanced Practices Internet Resources

MedicineNet: *Chemotherapy and Cancer Treatment, Coping with Side Effects.* www.medicinenet.com/script/main/art.asp?articlekey=21716.

MedicineNet: *Image Collection, Skin Problems.* www.medicinenet.com/script/main/art.asp?articlekey=107539.

MedicineNet: *Precancerous Skin Lesions and Skin Cancer Pictures Slideshow.* www.medicinenet.com/skin_cancer_pictures_slideshow/article.htm.

National Cancer Institute: *Breast Cancer Treatment and Pregnancy (PDQ)*. www.cancer.gov/cancertopics/pdq/treatment/breast-cancer-and-pregnancy/Patient/page3.
RadiologyInfo.org: *Radioiodine (I -131) Therapy for Hyperthyroidism*. www.radiologyinfo.org/en/info.cfm?pg=radioiodine.
Skin Cancer Foundation: www.skincancer.org.
Staging: Questions and Answers: www.nci.nih.gov/cancertopics/factsheet/Detection/staging.
World Nuclear Association: *Radioisotopes in Medicine*. www.world-nuclear.org/info/inf55.html.

Advanced Practices: Learning the Language (Key Terms)

Using your textbook or a standard medical dictionary, look up and write the definitions of each term.

- anaplastic
- brachytherapy
- differentiated
- in situ
- proliferate
- radioisotopes
- teletherapy
- teratogenic

Advanced Practices: Review Questions

Define each key term using complete sentences.

1. What is the difference between clinical and pathologic staging of cancer?
2. Define TNM staging.
3. What would a TNM staging of T1N0M0 signify?
4. List six possible side effects from antineoplastic agents.
5. Define radiation therapy and explain how it works against cancer.

KEY CONCEPTS

- Cancer is also called carcinoma or CA.
- Cancer is the second leading cause of death in the United States.
- The exact cause, or etiology, of cancer is unknown.
- The term malignant describes cancer cells that have disrupted cell division and have uncontrolled growth.
- The term benign describes cells that resemble normal tissue and do not normally spread to surrounding areas.
- The term metastasis describes a tumor that has spread to other areas of the body.
- Chemotherapy is the use of pharmaceutical agents to treat cancers.
- Chemotherapeutics, or antineoplastic agents, are divided into classifications according to their mechanism of actions: alkylating agents, antimetabolites, mitotic inhibitors, antineoplastic antibiotics, hormones, and hormone antagonists.
- Targeted cancer therapies are drugs or substances that affect cancer by interfering with specific molecules involved in the tumor's growth and progression.
- BRMs are agents used to enhance the body's immune system.
- Gene therapy is being researched as a way to use genetics to treat or prevent diseases.
- Epidemiology is the science that studies factors that influence the frequency and distribution of disease.
- Carcinogens are cancer-causing substances; an example is tobacco.
- Angiogenesis inhibitors are antineoplastic agents that target the tumor's blood supply to shrink or stop tumor growth.
- Nanomedicine is nanotechnology being applied to medical diagnostics, medication delivery, and treatment of neoplasms.
- Nanopharmacology is nanotechnology for pharmaceutical applications.
- Research is ongoing in the fight against cancer, such as studies that look at enzymes that are common in all cancers, and the development of drugs customized to the patient.

Bibliography

Freitas RA Jr: Nanotechnology, nanomedicine and nanosurgery, *Int J Surg* 3(4):243–246, 2005. Available at http://www.nanomedicine.com/Papers/IntlJSurgDec05.pdf. Accessed July 28, 2010.

Fulcher E, Fulcher R, Soto C: *Pharmacology principles and applications,* ed 2, 2009, Saunders/Elsevier.

Greider CW, Blackburn EH: Telomeres, telomerase and cancer, *Sci Am* 274(2):92–97, 1996. Available at www.mdconsult.com/das/journal/view/0/N/651926?issn=&source=MI. Accessed July 28, 2010.

Mosby's medical dictionary, ed 8, St. Louis, 2009, Mosby/Elsevier.

Moscou K, Snipe K: *Pharmacology for pharmacy technicians,* St. Louis, 2009, Mosby/Elsevier.

Neimark J: The second coming of gene therapy, *Discover: Science, Technology, and The Future,* September 2009. Available online at http://discovermagazine.com/2009/sep/02-second-coming-of-gene-therapy/article_view?b_start:int=2&-C=. Accessed July 24, 2010.

Panda A, Mandeep S, Bajaj R, et al: Topical mitomycin C for conjunctival-corneal squamous cell carcinoma, *Am J Ophthalmol* 135(1):122–123, 2003.

Internet Resources

American Cancer Society: www.cancer.org.

American Lung Association: *Smoking.* http://action.lungusa.org/site/Search?query=Smoking&x=0&y=0.

BabyCenter: www.babycenter.com.

BreastCancer.org: *New Chemotherapy Agents Cut Advanced Breast Cancer Mortality in Half.* www.breastcancer.org/treatment/chemotherapy/new_research/20081209.jsp.

Chemotherapy.com: *Treating Cancer with Chemotherapy.* www.chemotherapy.com/treating_with_chemo/treating_with_chemo.jsp?src=ppc&WT.srch=1.

Drugs.com: *Blenoxane.* www.drugs.com/blenoxane.html.

Drugs.com: *Epogen.* www.drugs.com/epogen.html.

Drugs.com: *Lupron.* www.drugs.com/lupron.html.

Emory University, Cancer Quest: *Cancer Treatment: BRM.* www.cancerquest.org/index.cfm?page=186.

Glaucoma Research Foundation: *Glaucoma Surgery.* www.glaucoma.org/treating/surgery.php.

National Cancer Institute Fact Sheet: *Angiogenesis Inhibitors Therapy.* www.cancer.gov/cancertopics/factsheet/therapy/angiogenesis-inhibitors.

National Cancer Institute Fact Sheet: *Cancer Vaccines.* www.cancer.gov/cancertopics/factsheet/cancervaccine.

National Cancer Institute Fact Sheet: *Targeted Cancer Therapies.* www.cancer.gov/cancertopics/factsheet/Therapy/targeted.

National Eye Institute: *News and Events.* www.nei.nih.gov/neitrials/static/study21.asp.

Reporter, Vanderbilt University Medical Center's Weekly Newspaper, Forum Encourages 'Small Thinking' Through Nanotechnology Research May 2, 2003, *www.mc.vanderbilt.edu/reporter/?ID=2666.*

WebMd: *Methotrexate for Ectopic Pregnancy.* www.webmd.com/baby/methotrexate-for-ectopic-pregnancy.

Women's health: *Methotrexate for Ectopic Pregnancy.* www.womens-health.co.uk/mtx.asp.

LEARNING THE LANGUAGE (KEY TERMS)

Using your textbook or a standard medical dictionary, look up and write the definitions of each term.

antineoplastic agents
benign
cancer
carcinogen
cytotoxic
epidemiology
etiology
malignant
metastasis
neoplasm
palliative
primary site
remission
secondary site

REVIEW QUESTIONS

1. The most important known external factor for causing cancer is
a) Alcohol
b) Tobacco
c) Radiation
d) Pollution

2. Another name for a tumor is ______________________.
3. If a tumor is benign, this means its cells
   a) Multiply rapidly
   b) Are unorganized
   c) Are highly organized
   d) Can invade surrounding tissues
4. Cytotoxic is defined as ______________________.
5. The abatement or stopping of symptoms and possible cure of the disease is called ______________________.
6. The relief of symptoms without cure is termed ______________________.
7. The first antineoplastic drug(s) was/were
   a) 5-Fluorouracil
   b) Nitrogen mustard
   c) Methotrexate
   d) Hormone antagonists
8. The antineoplastic drug used for ectopic pregnancy is ______________________.
9. Corticosteroid hormones used in antineoplastic therapy act as
   a) Antibiotics
   b) Enzyme inhibitors
   c) Tumor cell inhibitors
   d) Anti-inflammatory agents
10. How do interferons and interleukins work?
11. The term for "the cause of a disease" is ______________________.
12. The technology used on a molecular scale is called ______________________.
13. The antineoplastic agents that attack the tumor's blood supply are called ______________________.

CRITICAL THINKING

1. Why would a chest radiograph be performed preoperatively on a patient with cancer of the larynx?
2. Why is it so difficult to find a cure for cancer?

UNIT 3

ANESTHESIA

As a surgical technologist, you'll observe the administration of anesthesia in the operating room nearly every day. Why is it necessary to learn about anesthesia? After all, administration of anesthetic agents is far outside the realm of the technologist's clinical practice. The fact is, understanding the terminology, methods, and agents of anesthesia will give you a more complete picture of surgical patient care. You will be a more effective member of the surgical team if you know the names and classification of anesthetic and supplemental agents, as well as their purposes. As team members, you'll be asked to obtain medications with whose generic and trade names you must be familiar. And to facilitate smooth flow of patient care, you'll need to understand preoperative and intraoperative anesthesia routines and medications. In both routine and emergency situations, all team members must contribute maximum effort to achieve the best possible patient outcome. For the surgical technologist, part of that effort includes learning the rudiments of pharmacology as it relates to anesthesia.

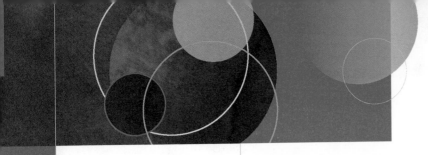

CHAPTER 13 Preoperative Medications

OBJECTIVES *After completing this chapter, you should be able to:*

1. Define terminology related to preoperative medications.
2. Identify the purpose of preoperative anesthesia evaluation.
3. List sources of patient information used for preoperative evaluation.
4. List the components of a preoperative evaluation.
5. Identify classification of preoperative medications.
6. Identify the purpose of each group of preoperative medications.
7. State examples of medications in each classification.

KEY TERMS

amnestic
analgesia
anterograde
anticholinergic
antisialagogue
anxiolysis
aspiration
benzodiazepine
NPO
opioid
vagolysis

Preoperative preparation is necessary to maximize the safety and comfort of every surgical patient. The surgical technologist may, on occasion, work in a preoperative care unit or assist in preoperative preparation of patients requiring elective or emergency surgery. To effectively assist the anesthesia care team, surgical technologists should understand the classifications, purposes, and common pharmacologic agents used to prepare the patient for surgery.

PREOPERATIVE EVALUATION

A preoperative anesthesia evaluation, or assessment, is performed on all surgical patients and is conducted by the anesthesia provider. The anesthesia provider may be an anesthesiologist, an anesthesiologist assistant (AA), or a certified registered nurse anesthetist (CRNA). The purpose of a preoperative anesthesia evaluation is to gather pertinent patient information to determine the optimal anesthetic plan. Information is gathered from several sources, including the patient's medical records, a preoperative patient interview, physical examination, and preoperative testing results. The preoperative anesthesia evaluation is used to confirm the patient's surgical diagnosis and to assess concurrent medical conditions that might increase the risk of anesthesia-related complications. It also identifies any medications the patient may be taking (including herbal and other over-the-counter [OTC] medications) and any allergies the patient may have.

The evaluation usually consists of a questionnaire (Fig. 13-1) to be completed by the patient and a follow up interview with the anesthesia provider (Fig. 13-2), who completes a pre-anesthesia evaluation form (Fig. 13-3). The pre-anesthesia physical examination is a complete assessment of the patient's physical status. Special emphasis is placed on assessment of diabetes and diseases of the cardiovascular and respiratory systems. In addition, the patient's upper airway is evaluated to assess the potential risk of difficult airway management. The airway is evaluated for all patients, even when a local or regional anesthesia plan is intended.

Additional preoperative testing may be ordered depending on the findings of the preoperative evaluation. A panel of routine preoperative tests for all patients has not been shown to accurately predict anesthesia-related complications, so tests are ordered only when the patient's condition or conditions indicate a necessity. For example, a potassium level is assessed for patients taking diuretics (see Chapter 7) and a blood glucose level is determined for patients with diabetes. Examples of other preoperative tests that may be indicated for select patients include electrocardiogram (ECG), pulmonary function studies, hemoglobin and hematocrit measurements, coagulation studies, and serum chemistry panels. When all the necessary information is obtained, the patient's preoperative physical status is classified according to criteria established by the American Society of Anesthesiologists (Table 13-1).

PREOPERATIVE MEDICATIONS

During the preoperative evaluation, the anesthesia provider will determine the patient's need for preoperative medications. Preoperative medications are given as needed to prepare the patient for surgery, both psychologically and physically. Preoperative medications can be classified by action, each group having a specific purpose.

SEDATIVES

Sedatives are given to relieve anxiety, which is common in surgical patients. In most patients, these drugs produce a mild drowsiness, and they may have **amnestic** (pertaining to amnesia) and antiemetic effects. The most common sedatives used preoperatively are the **benzodiazepines**, a chemical classification of drugs used to control anxiety. In low doses, benzodiazepines produce **anxiolysis** (relief of anxiety) and at higher doses produce sedation and **anterograde** amnesia.

> **MAKE IT SIMPLE**
>
> Use medical terminology to help understand the terms anterograde and retrograde amnesia. The prefix "retr/o" means backward or behind, so people with retrograde amnesia don't remember events that led up to a particular event—such as the time immediately before a motor vehicle accident. Those events occurred backward in time. The prefix "anter/o" means in front of, so patients with anterograde amnesia don't remember events that occur from a point forward—forward in time.

The patient will remain conscious, but may not remember events that occur once the sedative is administered. This effect may explain why some patients have the perception that they were anesthetized in the preoperative preparation area.

The benzodiazepine family of drugs includes diazepam (Valium), lorazepam (Ativan), and midazolam (Versed). One characteristic of benzodiazepines is high lipid solubility, which means that the chemicals are absorbed quickly and completely and are easily able to cross the blood-brain barrier to exert their effects. Benzodiazepines are highly bound to plasma proteins (see Chapter 1). These three agents vary in their affinity for receptor binding sites, which accounts for differences in potency. Benzodiazepines are administered intravenously in weight-dependent dosages (mg/kg) for preoperative sedation.

An adverse effect of benzodiazepines is respiratory depression, so patients must be continuously monitored after administration of these agents. Benzodiazepines also cause some systemic vasodilation, which may lead to cardiovascular depression in patients who are hemodynamically unstable. This effect is minimal in otherwise healthy patients.

Midazolam (Fig. 13-4) is the most common benzodiazepine administered preoperatively. See Table 13-2 for a comparison of benzodiazepines.

ANALGESICS

Some patients may require **analgesia** (pain relief; literally "without pain") preoperatively. Examples include trauma patients and those patients who will require insertion of invasive monitors (see Chapter 14) prior to surgery. When indicated for analgesia, **opioids** may be administered preoperatively. The term *opioid* refers to all drugs, natural, semisynthetic, or synthetic, having morphine-like actions.

Preanesthesia Questionnaire

The information you supply below assists in the development of your anesthesia care.
Please complete this questionnaire accurately and completely.

Patient Name ______________________________

Age ________ **Weight** ______ **Height** ________ **Date** ________

Allergies ______________________________

____

Current Medications (Prescription and Nonprescription)______________________________

____

Prior Operations ______________________________

____

Preanesthesia Questionnaire

Please answer the following questions. These responses will help us provide the anesthetic that is best for you.

Yes	No	Question
[ ]	[ ]	Have you recently had a cold or the flu?
[ ]	[ ]	Are you allergic to latex (rubber) products?
[ ]	[ ]	Have you experienced chest pain?
[ ]	[ ]	Do you have a heart condition?
[ ]	[ ]	Do you have hypertension (high blood pressure)?
[ ]	[ ]	Do you experience shortness of breath?
[ ]	[ ]	Do you have asthma, bronchitis, or any other breathing problem?
[ ]	[ ]	Do you (or did you) smoke? Packs/day _____. Number of years _____. Date you quit ___________.
[ ]	[ ]	Do you consume alcohol? Drinks/week ________.
[ ]	[ ]	Do you take or have you taken recreational drugs?
[ ]	[ ]	Have you taken cortisone (steroids) in the last six months?
[ ]	[ ]	Do you have diabetes?
[ ]	[ ]	Have you had hepatitis, liver disease, or jaundice?
[ ]	[ ]	Do you have a thyroid condition?
[ ]	[ ]	Do you have or have you had kidney disease?
[ ]	[ ]	Do you have ulcers or other stomach disorders?
[ ]	[ ]	Do you have a hiatal hernia?
[ ]	[ ]	Do you have back or neck pain?
[ ]	[ ]	Do you have numbness, weakness, or paralysis of your extremities?
[ ]	[ ]	Do you have any muscle or nerve disease?
[ ]	[ ]	Do you or any of your family have sickle cell trait?
[ ]	[ ]	Have you or any blood relatives had difficulties with anesthesia?
[ ]	[ ]	Do you have bleeding problems?
[ ]	[ ]	Do you have loose, chipped, false teeth, or bridgework?
[ ]	[ ]	Do you have any oral piercings (such as studs or rings) in your tongue or lip?
[ ]	[ ]	Do you wear contact lenses?
[ ]	[ ]	Have you ever received a blood transfusion?
[ ]	[ ]	(Women) Are you pregnant? Due date ___________.

Figure 13-1 Sample preoperative patient questionnaire. (*Copyright 2010 AANA. Available at* www.aana.com/ForPatients.aspx?id=775, *accessed July 26, 2010.*)

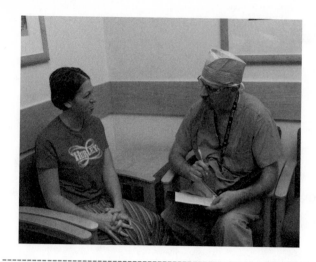

Figure 13-2 The anesthesia provider conducts a preoperative interview with the patient.

Opioids cause analgesia and mild sedation in usual doses and may reduce the amount of anesthesia needed for the surgical procedure. Nausea and vomiting may occur and are thought to be a result of opioid-induced stimulation of the nausea trigger zone in the medulla. Slowing of respiration and reduced intestinal motility are expected. Because of slowed respiration, the patient is monitored with a pulse oximeter (see Chapter 14) and supplemental oxygen may be given. Respiratory depressant effects of opioids are significantly enhanced when benzodiazepines are administered. The patient's level of consciousness should be assessed frequently when opioids are administered. Preoperative use of opioids may be contraindicated for outpatient surgery because of the prohibitively intense patient monitoring required. The sedative effect of benzodiazepines may preempt the need for opioids in some instances.

Morphine (Astramorph, Duramorph) is a natural opioid that may be used preoperatively. Morphine may be indicated for patients experiencing significant pain who are expected to be admitted as inpatients after surgery. Morphine is given intravenously in doses of 5 to 15 mg for average adults, depending on the patient's ability to tolerate the drug. Onset of action is expected in 2 to 5 minutes, with peak in 10 to 15 minutes, and effects often last 2 to 4 hours or more.

The most common synthetic opioids are meperidine (Demerol) and fentanyl (Sublimaze). Meperidine is administered intravenously in doses of 75 to 100 mg to provide preoperative analgesia. Onset of effect occurs in 1 to 3 minutes, peaks at 5 to 20 minutes, and provides analgesia for 2 to 4 hours. Fentanyl is 75 to 125 times more potent than morphine; it is characterized by rapid onset (30 seconds) and short duration (30 to 60 minutes). It is administered in doses of 1 to 2 micrograms per kilogram (mcg/kg) for preoperative analgesia. See Table 13-3.

{NOTE} *Opioids are covered under federal and state controlled substances acts (see Chapter 2) and must be handled according to hospital policy. The surgical technologist must be thoroughly familiar with institutional procedures regarding controlled substances.*

ANTICHOLINERGICS

Anticholinergics are agents that block the action of the neurotransmitter acetylcholine, inhibiting the transmission of parasympathetic nerve impulses. Acetylcholine (ACh) is a key neurotransmitter in the autonomic nervous system, so these agents exert systemic effects.

Anticholinergics are not routinely used preoperatively, but may be indicated in specific instances to inhibit mucous secretions of the respiratory and digestive tract (**antisialagogue** effect). Most anesthetic agents in use today do not cause significant salivation, so anticholinergics are less frequently indicated. Decreased oral secretions may be desired when an endotracheal tube is in place for a general anesthetic or for intra-oral procedures such as bronchoscopy or maxillofacial surgery. These medications may also be administered preoperatively to block certain receptors on the vagus nerve (**vagolysis**). A common side effect is an increased heart rate, which is an example of the systemic effects of anticholinergics.

When indicated, anticholinergics most frequently used preoperatively are atropine, glycopyrrolate (Robinul), and scopolamine. Glycopyrrolate is twice as potent an antisialagogue as atropine and has a longer duration. Scopolamine is 3 times more potent an antisialagogue than atropine and is given when both antisialagogue effect and sedation are desired. Atropine is administered intravenously in doses of 0.4 to 0.6 mg; onset is almost immediate and duration is 15 to 30 minutes. Glycopyrrolate is administered intravenously in doses of 0.1 to 2 mg, onset occurring within 1 minute and lasting 2 to 3 hours. Scopolamine is given intravenously in doses of 0.3 to 0.6 mg; onset is immediate and effects are seen for 30 to 60 minutes. See Table 13-4.

PREANESTHESIA EVALUATION

Age	Sex M F	Height in/cm	Weight lb/kg

Proposed procedure

Pre-procedure vital signs B/P P R T

Previous anesthesia/operations — None ☐

Current medications — None ☐

Family history of anesthesia complications — None ☐

Allergies — NKDA ☐

AIRWAY/TEETH/HEAD AND NECK

History from: ☐ Patient ☐ Significant other ☐ Parent/guardian ☐ Chart

☐ Communication//language problems
☐ Poor historian

SYSTEM	WNL	COMMENTS
RESPIRATORY: Asthma, Bronchitis, COPD, Dyspnea, Orthopnea, Pneumonia, Productive cough, Recent URI, SOB, Tuberculosis	☐	Tobacco use: ☐ Yes ☐ No ______ packs/day for ______ years
CARDIOVASCULAR: Abnormal EKG, Angina, ASHD, CHF, Dysrhythmia, Exercise tolerance, Hypertension, MI, Murmur, Pacemaker, Rheumatic fever, Valvular disease	☐	
HEPATO/GASTROINTESTINAL: Bowel obstruction, Cirrhosis, Hepatitis/Jaundice, Hiatal henia/reflux, Nausea and Vomiting, Ulcers, Muscle weakness, Neuromuscular Dis., Paralysis, Paresthesia, Syncope, Seizures	☐	Ethanol use: ☐ Yes ☐ No Frequency ______ "Street drug" use: ☐ Yes ☐ No Frequency ______
NEURO/MUSCULOSKELETAL: Arthritis, Back problems, CVA/Stroke/TIAs, DJD, Headaches/↑ ICP, Loss of consciousness	☐	
RENAL/ENDOCRINE: Diabetes, Renal failure/dialysis, Thyroid disease, Urinary retention, Urinary tract infection, Weight loss/gain	☐	
OTHER: Anemia, Bleeding tendencies, Cancer, Chemotherapy, Dehydration, Hemophilia, Immunosuppressed, Pregnancy, Sickle cell dis./trait, Recent steroids, Tranfusion history		

DIAGNOSTIC STUDIES

EKG

Chest X-ray

Pulmonary studies

Other

LABORATORY STUDIES

Hgb/Hct/CBC

Electrolytes

Urinalysis

Other

Problem list/diagnoses

Planned anesthesia/special monitors

PHYSICAL STATUS 1 2 3 4 5 E

POSTANESTHESIA NOTE

Signed ______ Date______ Time______

PATIENT IDENTIFICATION

Pre-anesthesia medications ordered

Evaluator signature — Date — Time

Figure 13-3 Sample preanesthesia evaluation. (*From American Association of Nurse Anesthetists: Preanesthesia Evaluation. 1991,* www.aana.org. *Available at* www.aana.com/uploadedFiles/Resources/Practice_Documents/preeval_form_jpg.pdf. *Accessed July 26, 2010.*)

{NOTE} *Recall from Chapter 1 that drugs (such as scopolamine) that exert systemic effects have multiple indications and so may be classified in several therapeutic categories. Scopolamine is an antisialagogue, a sedative, and an antiemetic. As such, it is discussed in this section in its physiologic action classification as an anticholinergic. Scopolamine will also be presented in the discussion of gastric agents (body system category) in its therapeutic classification as an antiemetic.*

Table 13-1 AMERICAN SOCIETY OF ANESTHESIOLOGISTS' PHYSICAL STATUS CLASSIFICATION SYSTEM

Classification	Definition
P1	A normal healthy patient
P2	A patient with mild systemic disease
P3	A patient with severe systemic disease
P4	A patient with severe systemic disease that is a constant threat to life
P5	A moribund patient who is not expected to survive without the operation
P6	A declared brain-dead patient whose organs are being removed for donor purposes

(From American Society of Anesthesiologists, www.asahq.org/clinical/physicalstatus.htm*. Accessed July 24, 2010.)*

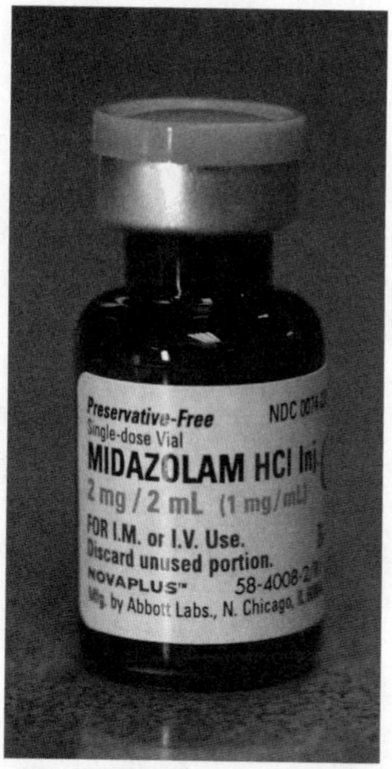

Figure 13-4 Vial of midazolam.

TECH TIP

Anticholinergics may also be used intraoperatively to block the vagal response (called reflex bradycardia) to certain stimuli such as stretching the peritoneum during open abdominal procedures, bowel manipulation, cervical traction in gynecologic cases, carotid artery dissection, or stretching eye muscles during retinal procedures. Alert the anesthesia provider when you are about to increase retraction pressure on any of those structures. Pay close attention to ECG sounds during those types of procedures to detect reflex bradycardia.

GASTRIC AGENTS

Anxiety and fear, so often seen in surgical patients, initiates a stress response mediated by the sympathetic nervous system, which may slow down or stop the digestive process (Insight 13-1). The presence of food in the stomach, as may be found in trauma patients, and the acidic nature of gastric contents may present significant risk to patients requiring general anesthesia. During

Table 13-2 COMPARISON OF BENZODIAZEPINES USED PREOPERATIVELY

Generic Name	Trade Name	Dosage	Onset (min)	Peak (min)	Duration (hrs)
midazolam	Versed	1-2 mg	0.5-1	3-5	0.25-1.25
lorazepam	Ativan	1-4 mg	1-2	20-30	6-10
diazepam	Valium	5-10 mg	1	3-4	1-6

Table 13-3 COMPARISON OF ANALGESICS USED PREOPERATIVELY

Generic Name	Trade Name	Dosage	Onset (min)	Peak (min)	Duration (hrs)
morphine	Astramorph	5-15 mg	2-5	10-15	2-4
meperidine	Demerol	75-100 mg	1-3	5-20	2-4
fentanyl	Sublimaze	1-2 mcg/kg	0.5	5-15	0.5-1

Table 13-4 COMPARISON OF ANTICHOLINERGICS USED PREOPERATIVELY

Generic Name	Trade Name	Dosage	Onset (min)	Duration (hrs)
atropine	None	0.4-0.6 mg	Immediate	0.25-0.5
glycopyrrolate	Robinul	0.1-2 mg	1	2-3
scopolamine	None	0.3-0.6 mg	Immediate	0.5-1

IN SIGHT 13-1 Gastric Physiology Review

The digestive system is responsible for intake and processing of nutrients and elimination of nutrient waste. The stomach, which is part of the digestive system, processes food by two means—mechanical and chemical. The mechanical process of digestion is due to the peristaltic motions of the muscles and folds (rugae) of the stomach, which mix food with gastric secretions. This mixture becomes a thin liquid, called chyme, which is propelled in small amounts through the pylorus into the duodenum. The chemical process of digestion is due to the action of an enzyme called pepsin. In the presence of hydrochloric acid (HCl), pepsin becomes active and breaks down protein contained in the ingested food. Hydrochloric acid is produced by the parietal (oxyntic) cells of the stomach and is the chemical responsible for the acidic nature of gastric contents. It is interesting to note that the stomach contains 1 billion parietal cells, each capable of secreting 3.3 billion hydrogen ions per second. Secretion of these chemicals is controlled by both the nervous system and the endocrine system. The nervous system regulates production of gastric chemicals via stimulation of the parasympathetic fibers of the vagus nerve. The sight and smell of food also initiate stimulation of gastric glands to produce digestive chemicals. Ingestion of food causes stretching of the stomach, which is transmitted through the nerves, and a response is generated that produces more stimulation of gastric glands. For further explanation of digestion, consult a physiology textbook.

induction of general anesthesia, the lower esophageal sphincter may relax to an extent that a reflux of gastric contents may occur. In addition, some agents administered at this time may cause nausea, with an increased risk for vomiting. If the patient vomits or gastric reflux occurs during induction of anesthesia, gastric contents can enter the lungs, causing mild to severe damage. This complication is called **aspiration**, which may result in aspiration pneumonitis. While the estimated occurrence of aspiration is low (1 in 3200 operations), the potential for patient harm is significant. When the lungs are damaged by aspiration, it is implicated in 10% to 30% of anesthesia deaths.

Even though elective surgical patients are **NPO** (*nil per os*, or nothing by mouth) (Insight 13-2), gastric secretions are still present. Patients at increased risk for aspiration include those with gastrointestinal (GI) obstruction, history of gastroesophageal reflux disease (GERD), diabetes, obesity, or pregnant patients in labor or scheduled for cesarean section. In addition, patients

IN SIGHT 13-2 "NPO After Midnight" or Fasting Before Elective Surgery

It has long been assumed that if we reduced gastric fluid volume we would reduce the risk of pulmonary aspiration of stomach contents upon induction of anesthesia. However, gastric emptying times vary by what is in the stomach (solid food versus clear liquids). Recommendations have been modified so that clear liquids (such as water, carbonated beverages, clear tea, or black coffee) are allowed up to 2 hours before induction of anesthesia. Oral medications can now be taken with up to 150 mL of water in the hour preceding induction. Gum-chewing is not allowed preoperatively due to resulting increases in gastric fluid volume.

presenting with a need for emergency surgery may have a full or partially full stomach. When indicated in patients with risk factors for gastric reflux and possible aspiration, several different agents may be used for preoperative prophylaxis, alone or in combination with other agents.

Antacids

Antacids are used to chemically neutralize gastric acid already present in the stomach. Several antacids are available OTC, such as Tums. Preoperative administration of an antacid is intended to minimize damage to the lungs from gastric acid should aspiration occur. Sodium citrate with citric acid (Bicitra) is a nonparticulate liquid antacid that may be administered preoperatively to neutralize the acidity of stomach contents. Gastric acid normally has an acidity, or pH, of 2 to 3. Sodium citrate is metabolized to sodium bicarbonate—a base that chemically neutralizes gastric acid. When indicated, sodium citrate is given orally in a dose of 15 to 30 mL. Effects are immediate and the duration is approximately 2 hours.

H_2 Receptor Antagonists

Histamine (H_2) receptor antagonists are antacids named for their physiologic action on the receptors found on parietal cells in the stomach. By blocking H_2 receptors, these agents temporarily interfere with the production of gastric acid by parietal cells. These agents are not used in emergency surgery because they do not change the acid already present in the stomach.

The most common H_2 blockers given preoperatively are cimetidine (Tagamet), famotidine (Pepcid), and ranitidine (Zantac). Cimetidine is given intravenously as a preoperative medication in a dose of 2 to 4 mg/kg. Effects occur within 4 to 5 minutes and last approximately 4 hours. Famotidine may be given orally in a dose of 20 to 40 mg the night before or the morning of surgery or intravenously in a dose of 20 mg. Onset of effects is noted in 20 to 45 minutes, and effects last for 7 to 9 hours. Ranitidine is administered intravenously preoperatively, 50 mg, with effects occurring within 15 minutes and lasting 6 to 8 hours.

Proton Pump Inhibitors

Proton pump inhibitors (PPIs) are medications that bind irreversibly with the acid pump of parietal cells and prevent the release of hydrochloric acid (gastric acid). These agents are examples of *prodrugs* (see Chapter 1) because they are administered in an inactive form and are converted by the body into active drug molecules. Proton pump inhibitors are unique in that they are not converted to active drugs in the liver, but in the parietal cell canaliculus (tubular canals into which hydrochloric acid is secreted). These drugs prevent the final step of gastric acid production by interfering with hydrogen (H^+) and potassium (K^+) ion exchange in the H^+/K^+-ATPase proton pump, which is located on the surface of parietal cells.

The prototype drug in this category is omeprazole (Prilosec), but it is not commonly used preoperatively because it takes days to become fully effective. In some situations, omeprazole may be given in a high dose of 40 mg orally the evening before and again 2 to 6 hours before surgery to reduce both the volume and acidity of gastric contents. Other drugs in this category are lansoprazole (Prevacid), esomeprazole (Nexium), pantoprazole (Protonix), and rabeprazole (AcipHex). Prevacid IV, Nexium IV, and Protonix IV are available in freeze-dried powder form that must be reconstituted prior to IV administration. Intravenous administration of 40 mg of pantoprazole (Protonix IV) will reduce gastric acid in 20 minutes.

Antiemetics and Gastrointestinal Prokinetics

Antiemetics are agents administered preoperatively to reduce nausea and minimize the possibility of postoperative nausea and vomiting (PONV) in at-risk patients.

The types of patients most at risk for PONV are pediatric (especially preadolescents); those patients who have or will receive opioids, barbiturates, or etomidate; and female patients (females are two to three times more likely to experience PONV than males, particularly after intra-abdominal surgery). Obesity has been assumed to be associated with increased risk of PONV, but a systematic review of research failed to demonstrate significant influence of body weight on PONV. Recent evaluation also failed to demonstrate obesity as a predictor of PONV.

Certain procedural factors also contribute to the incidence of PONV, such as length of procedure (longer procedures increase the risk for PONV) and type of procedure. Types of procedures associated with a greater risk of PONV include abdominal procedures (especially female laparoscopic) and procedures usually performed on children, such as strabismus correction, tonsillectomy and adenoidectomy, orchiopexy, and middle ear procedures. Research studies continue to better determine which patients are most likely to benefit from the administration of preoperative antiemetics.

Three main categories of medications are used to prevent PONV:

- GI prokinetics (metoclopramide)
- Neuroleptics (droperidol)
- Serotonin antagonists (ondansetron)

Metoclopramide (Reglan) is classified as a GI prokinetic agent and is used to reduce gastric fluid volume in at-risk patients such as diabetic patients with gastroparesis, pregnant patients, those with anticipated difficult airway, and emergency patients who have not been NPO. It stimulates motility of the upper GI tract (and thus, gastric emptying) without stimulating gastric acid secretion, but administration of metoclopramide does not assure complete emptying of the stomach. Additionally, metoclopramide reduces the risk of postoperative nausea because it also works as a peripheral and central dopamine receptor antagonist. It is administered intravenously, 10 mg (adult dose), with onset expected in 1 to 3 minutes and duration of 1 to 2 hours. See Table 13-5.

Droperidol (Inapsine) is an antiemetic drug with sedative properties that is less frequently used in current practice. The U.S. Food and Drug Administration (FDA) requires a "Black Box" warning on droperidol, the most serious warning for an FDA-approved drug. Indications for use of droperidol have been limited, and its use is restricted to second-line only, because of an increased risk of fatal cardiac arrhythmias. When indicated, droperidol is administered intravenously, 15 mcg/kg, with effects seen in 3 to 10 minutes and duration of 2 to 4 hours.

The most commonly used antiemetic agent used preoperatively is ondansetron (Zofran). It is classified as a serotonin antagonist, also known as a 5-HT3 receptor antagonist. This category of medications also includes granisetron (Kytril) and dolasetron (Anzemet), which

Table 13-5 GASTRIC AGENTS USED PREOPERATIVELY

Generic Name	Trade Name	Dosage	Onset (min)	Duration (hrs)
ANTACID				
sodium citrate	Bicitra	15-30 mL	Immediate	2
H_2 BLOCKERS				
cimetidine	Tagamet	2-4 mg/kg	4-5	4
famotidine	Pepcid	20-40 mg	20-45	7-9
ranitidine	Zantac	50 mg	15	6-8
PROTON PUMP INHIBITORS				
pantoprazole	Protonix IV	40 mg	15-30	12
ANTIEMETICS				
ondansetron	Zofran	4 mg	5-10	12-24
metoclopramide	Reglan	10 mg	1-3	1-2

are most often used to manage chemotherapy-induced nausea and vomiting. Dolasetron (Anzemet) is a prodrug (see Chapter 1) that must be metabolized or broken down to an active metabolite, hydrodolasetron, to exert its effect. These agents are relatively free from side effects compared with metoclopramide and droperidol, but they are more costly.

Ondansetron (Zofran) is given intravenously in a dose of 4 mg over a period of 2 to 5 minutes immediately before induction. Its effects last from 12 to 24 hours, and it has been very effective in reducing the incidence of PONV, especially in patients undergoing ambulatory gynecologic or middle ear procedures. Ondansetron may also be given in combination with dexamethasone, (Decadron) 8 mg, for an additive effect noted in the first 3 hours after surgery.

Another drug that may be given to prevent PONV is scopolamine. In some reports, it has been shown to be as effective as ondansetron in preventing PONV. It is usually administered by dermal patch, which may be applied the night before or just before surgery. Side effects include visual disturbances, dizziness, and dry mouth. The patch contains 1.5 mg of scopolamine, which is absorbed at a rate of 5 mcg per hour for approximately 72 hours.

ADVANCED PRACTICE FOR THE SURGICAL FIRST ASSISTANT

CHAPTER 13—Preoperative Medications

Key Terms

bowel prep
convulsions
hypertension

MEDICATIONS FROM THE MEDICAL SETTING TO THE SURGICAL SETTING

In addition to the preoperative medicines described earlier in the chapter, there are others that must be considered before the patient undergoes a surgical procedure. Medications are prescribed either for surgical preparation or as part of a current therapy for an unrelated condition. One of the most common preparations for all patients undergoing elective GI procedures is the "bowel prep." Healthcare workers often discount this procedure, even though it affects the patient systemically. Other medicines that patients may be taking preoperatively would be antihypertensive or anticonvulsive drugs. Patients may remain on these medicines throughout the surgical procedure, usually under the advice of the anesthesia provider. The surgical first assistant should be aware of these medicines and preparations and their effects upon the surgical patient.

Bowel Preparations

All patients undergoing abdominal surgical procedures where the small bowel, colon, or rectum may be involved will be required to perform a preoperative bowel preparation. A thorough bowel prep will eliminate any bowel content before surgery to provide a clear view of the colon. The prep includes instructions for a clear liquid diet and drinking a bowel prep solution so many hours before the procedure. At one time the bowel prep was a two-phase procedure: a mechanical phase of emptying the bowel and a chemical phase using an antibiotic. It was thought the antibiotic would help to eliminate resident bacteria (*Escherichia coli*, or *E. coli*) from the bowel. This is no longer common practice; however, prophylactic antibiotics may be given before the procedure to patients with hip or knee prostheses, vascular stints, or artificial heart valves. Vancomycin (Vancocin) or gentamicin (Garamycin) may be used for this purpose. The mechanical phase of the prep is done by the patient, at home, usually the day before the procedure. It consists of medications to evacuate all feces from the colon. An example of one such medication is the administration of 2 liters of polyethylene glycol-electrolyte solution (PEG-ES), sodium chloride, sodium bicarbonate, and potassium chloride in an oral solution called HalfLytely. This solution is combined in a kit with two bisacodyl (Dulcolax) laxative tablets, and is taken by mouth, at home, and begins working within an hour. Polyethylene glycol-electrolyte solution is available in the pharmacy under trade names such as Colyte, NuLYTELY, and GoLYTELY. These may be prescribed without the bisacodyl tablets and are called MoviPreps. These preps increase the amount of water in the intestinal tract, which stimulates bowel movements. They contain potassium, sodium, and other minerals, which replace the electrolytes that are eliminated from the body during the bowel evacuation. They can also be used before a barium x-ray or other intestinal procedures. (Note: there are also medications given in tablet form, as enemas, or as bowel suppositories to achieve the same purpose.) As these preparations cause diarrhea in order to evacuate fecal material, patients undergoing a bowel prep will experience a significant fluid loss. This fact combined with the patient's NPO status will require administration of more fluids intraoperatively and postoperatively. Patients with other medical problems may not tolerate this fluid shift and will require hospitalization to complete the prep. The PEG-ES preparation may cause nausea in some patients. Metoclopramide (Reglan), 10 mg orally, may be prescribed to alleviate the nausea in order to retain the prep.

Anticonvulsants

Convulsions affect approximately 0.5% to 2% of the population and are treated with medication referred to anticonvulsants. These medications act on the neurons in the brain by depressing their discharge and preventing seizure activity. Patients require a continuous level of anticonvulsants to prevent a seizure event. Therefore, surgical patients may need to remain on this therapy throughout the procedure and postoperatively. Anticonvulsants can be placed in several categories, which include benzodiazepines, barbiturates, hydantoins, oxazolidinediones, and succinimides. There are also several miscellaneous anticonvulsants that are available. Examples of specific medicines are found in Table A: Anticonvulsants.

Table A Anticonvulsants

Category	Examples
Benzodiazepines	Diazepam, clonazepam, clorazepate, lorazepam
Barbiturates	Phenobarbital, mephobarbital, primidone
Hydantoins	Fosphenytoin, phenytoin
Oxazolidinediones	Paramethadione, trimethadione
Succinimides	Ethosuximide, methsuximide, phensuximide
Miscellaneous	Valproic acid, carbamazepine, gabapentin, lamotrigine

HYPERTENSION MEDICINES

Hypertension is defined as a blood pressure greater than 140/90, and affects about 25% of the population. The vast majority of hypertensive patients require an antihypertension drug therapy to control the blood pressure. Any interruption of this therapy will cause the patient's blood pressure to rise and may have an adverse effect on the outcome of the surgical procedure. Therefore, patients being treated for hypertension are instructed to take their daily medications the morning of surgery. Physicians today have many medicines in their arsenal to control hypertension. These medicines are grouped according to their effects on the body. There are six groups: diuretics, β-blockers, angiotension converting enzyme (ACE) inhibitors, calcium channel blockers, and α-blockers. The sixth is a new group of medications now being used called angiotensin-receptor blockers (ARBs). They are similar to ACE inhibitors because they help dilate arteries. This action lowers blood pressure and makes it easier for the heart to pump blood throughout the body. Also, like ACE inhibitors, ARBs can improve congestive heart failure (CHF) symptoms and prolong life. Ongoing studies are comparing the effects of ARBs with the ACE inhibitors and are investigating the use of both in patients with heart failure.

Patients may require a combination of several medications to control the hypertension. When treating hypertension it is best to take the staged approach. The patient is prescribed one type of medicine while monitoring the blood pressure. Additional medications from other groups are added until the blood pressure returns to normal level.

Advanced Practices Bibliography

Fulcher E, Fulcher R, Soto C: *Pharmacology principles and applications*, ed 2, 2009, Saunders/Elsevier.

Moscou K, Snipe K: *Pharmacology for pharmacy technicians*, St. Louis, 2009, Mosby/Elsevier.

Advanced Practices Internet Resources

About.com, High Blood Pressure: *Tips for Lowering Your Salt and Sodium Intake.* http://highbloodpressure.about.com/od/prevention/tp/lower-your-salt-intake.htm.

Drugs.com: *MoviPrep*. www.drugs.com/moviprep.html.

EndoNurse: *Bowel Preps*. www.endonurse.com/articles/07augfeat5.html.

EndoNurse: *BOWEL PREPS: The Good, the Bad and the Ugly.* www.endonurse.com/articles/bowel-preps.html.

Google: *Definitions of Hypertension*. www.google.com/search?q=define: hypertension&aq=0&oq=hypertension definition&aqi=l1g4.

Healthcommunities.com: *High Blood Pressure Medication. www.cardiologychannel.com/hypertension/pharm.shtml.*

HealthSquare.com: *High Blood Pressure: Drugs that Bring Pressure Down.* http://www.nhlbi.nih.gov/health/public/heart/hbp/hbp_low/hbp_low.pdf.

http://www.brighamandwomens.org/departments_and_services/womenshealth/hearthealth/your-care-explained/medications/blood-pressure-drugs/.

MayoClinic.com: *High Blood Pressure (hypertension), Symptoms.* www.mayoclinic.com/health/high-blood-pressure/DS00100/DSECTION=symptoms.

NYU Medical Center: *NuLYTELY Bowel Prep for Colonoscopy.* www.med.nyu.edu/crs/patient/preop/nulytely.html.

Palo Alto Medical Foundation: *Colyte/Trilyte Colonoscopy Preparation*. Patient Instructions (1). www.pamf.publicationsAndServices/gastroenterology/ColyteColon.pdf.

Palo Alto Medical Foundation: *Colyte/Trilyte Colonoscopy Preparation.* Patient Instructions (2). www.pamf.publicationsAndServices/gastroenterology/FrColyteColon.pdf.

Salix Pharmaceuticals, Inc: *MoviPrep - Bowel Prep.* www.salix.com/products/moviprep/index.aspx.

Advanced Practices: Learning the Language (Key Terms)

Using your textbook or a standard medical dictionary, look up and write the definitions of each term.

- bowel prep
- convulsions
- hypertension

Advanced Practices: Review Questions

1. Which procedures will require a preoperative bowel prep? Why?
2. How does the patient cleanse the bowel before the procedure?
3. Name two preparations for bowel cleansing.
4. How do anticonvulsants work?
5. Name the groups of medications used to treat hypertension.

KEY CONCEPTS

- A preoperative assessment is made by the anesthesia team to determine the appropriate anesthesia method.
- A preoperative evaluation consists of a patient interview, physical examination, and medical records review.
- Several general categories of medications may be used to prepare the patient both physically and psychologically for surgery. These include sedatives, analgesics, anticholinergics, and several types of GI drugs.
- To assist the anesthesia care team, the surgical technologist should be familiar with drugs administered preoperatively and their purposes.

Bibliography

American Society of Anesthesiologists Task Force on Preoperative Fasting: Practice guideline for preoperative fasting and the use of pharmacologic agent to reduce the risk of pulmonary aspiration: application to healthy patients undergoing elective procedures, *Anesthesiology* 90(3):896–905, 1999. Available at www.asahq.org/publicationsAndServices/NPO.pdf. Accessed July 25, 2010.

Evers A, Maze M: *Anesthetic pharmacology: physiologic principles and clinical practice,* St. Louis, 2004, Churchill Livingstone/Elsevier.

Fulcher E, Fulcher R, Soto C: *Pharmacology principles and applications,* ed 2, 2009, Saunders/Elsevier.

Kester M, Karpa K, Quraishi S, et al: *Elsevier's integrated pharmacology,* St. Louis, 2007, Mosby.

Moscou K, Snipe K: *Pharmacology for pharmacy technicians,* St. Louis, 2009, Mosby/Elsevier.

Nagelhout J, Plaus K: *Nurse anesthesia,* ed 4, St. Louis, 2010, Saunders/Elsevier.

Nagelhout J, Zaglaniczny K, Haglund V: *Handbook of Nurse Anesthesia,* ed 2, Philadelphia, 2001, Saunders/Elsevier.

Stoelting R, Miller R: *Basics of anesthesia,* ed 5, St. Louis, 2007, Churchill Livingstone/Elsevier.

Internet Resources

American Association of Nurse Anesthetists: *Consent for Anesthesia Services.* www.aana.com/practicedocuments.aspx.

American Association of Nurse Anesthetists: *Preanesthesia Evaluation.* www.aana.com/uploadedFiles/Resources/Practice_ Documents/preeval_form_jpg.pdf.

American Association of Nurse Anesthetists: *Pre-Anesthesia Questionnaire.* www.aana.com/ForPatients.aspx?id=775.

Medical Pharmacology and Disease-Based Integrated Instruction: *Preoperative Medication: Sedative Hypnotics and Other Agents and Issues.* www.pharmacology2000.com/Central/sedhyp/shobj4.htm.

Neuroscience for Kids: *The Autonomic Nervous System.* http://faculty.washington.edu/chudler/auto.html.

Pathology of the Digestive System: *The Parietal Cell: Mechanism of Acid Secretion.* www.vivo.colostate.edu/hbooks/pathphys/digestion/stomach/parietal.html.

LEARNING THE LANGUAGE (KEY TERMS)

Using your textbook or a standard medical dictionary, look up and write the definitions of each term.

amnestic
analgesia
anterograde
anticholinergic
antisialagogue
anxiolysis
aspiration
benzodiazepine
NPO
opioid
vagolysis

REVIEW QUESTIONS

1. Why is a preoperative evaluation conducted?
2. What are the categories of preoperative medications?
3. What is the purpose of each category of preoperative medications?
4. Can you state an example of a medication in each category of preoperative medications?

CRITICAL THINKING

Scenario

Mr. O'Neill is a very nervous, obese 61-year-old man with a history of diabetes and GERD. He is scheduled for an open reduction and internal fixation of a distal tibial fracture. He received a preoperative dose of 2 mg of midazolam (Versed) 15 minutes before being brought into the operating room. As he is settled on the operating room bed, the circulator begins to explain the importance of postoperative wound care to Mr. O'Neill.

1. In addition to midazolam, which other categories of preoperative medications do you think Mr. O'Neill will have received and why?
2. Is this the appropriate time to instruct Mr. O'Neill regarding his wound care? Why or why not?

CHAPTER 14

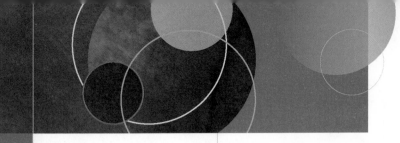

Patient Monitoring and Local and Regional Anesthesia

OBJECTIVES *After completing this chapter, you should be able to:*

1. Define terminology related to patient monitoring and anesthesia.
2. Describe types of patient-monitoring devices.
3. Compare and contrast local and regional anesthesia.
4. List surgical procedures that may be performed under local or regional anesthesia.
5. Identify common agents used in local anesthesia and regional anesthesia.
6. Discuss the use of epinephrine in local anesthetic agents.
7. Describe types of regional blocks.

KEY TERMS

auscultation
blood pressure
capnometry
electrocardiography
epidural
exsanguination
intrathecally
local anesthesia
monitored anesthesia care (MAC)
pulse oximetry
regional anesthesia

Surgical intervention and administration of anesthetic agents are complex and challenging processes that place enormous physiologic stress on the patient. The administration of anesthesia requires continuous monitoring of the patient's vital signs. Intraoperative monitoring has become more comprehensive and precise, enabling continuous assessment of critical indicators. The surgical technologist must become familiar with the various types of patient monitoring, components of the devices, and purposes. Although the primary focus of the scrubbed surgical technologist is at the surgical site, it is crucial that each team member be aware of the patient's well-being at all times and be prepared to provide support to the anesthesia provider and patient when necessary.

Both the American Society of Anesthesiologists (ASA) and the American Association of Nurse Anesthetists (AANA) have published standards of care regarding patient monitoring.

In addition, the Council on Surgical and Perioperative Safety (CSPS), an incorporated multidisciplinary coalition of professional organizations whose members are directly involved in the care of surgical patients, has published a Safe Surgery Principle regarding patient monitoring. It states:

{NOTE} *The CSPS endorses perioperative monitoring of patient physiologic parameters appropriate to patient co-morbidities, the anesthetic technique employed and the complexity of the procedure. Physiologic alarms should be audible.*

In the second part of this chapter, we begin a discussion of anesthesia. The term *anesthesia* literally means "without sensation." The patient may be conscious or unconscious, but while receiving any type of anesthesia, he or she should not perceive pain. The precise chemical and physiologic means by which anesthetics work are not yet fully clear; but we do know that the mechanism depends on the type of agent being administered. Some drugs, for instance, induce amnesia, whereas others induce unconsciousness or change the perception of pain. There are four major types of anesthetic techniques: local, regional, sedation/monitored anesthesia care (MAC), and general. This chapter presents basic information on local and regional anesthesia and a brief description of sedation/MAC. Basic concepts of general anesthesia are covered in Chapter 15.

PATIENT MONITORING

Each of the patient's vital signs is continuously monitored during surgical intervention. Continuous monitoring provides a means to rapidly identify changes in the patient's physiologic status. The first line of patient monitoring is direct observation of the patient by the anesthesia provider and its importance cannot be underestimated. The patient's oxygen saturation is monitored by direct observation and by use of the pulse oximeter. Respiration is monitored by patient observation and, when under heavy sedation or general anesthesia, by measuring levels of expired carbon dioxide. Circulation is monitored by continuous electrocardiography (rate and rhythm) and by frequent measurement of blood pressure. Temperature is assessed by various methods as indicated by patient situation. During general anesthesia, the patient's neuromuscular function and level of awareness are monitored when indicated. Certain patient conditions and some particular surgical procedures may require advanced or invasive monitoring methods such as placement of arterial or central venous pressure lines. See Box 14-1 for a summary of the most common physiologic functions monitored in the surgical patient.

MAKE IT SIMPLE

The complex nature of surgical patient monitoring can be simplified by applying the principles of cardiopulmonary resuscitation (CPR): **a**irway, **b**reathing, and **c**irculation (ABC). While under local or regional anesthesia the patient maintains his or her own airway (oxygenation) and it is confirmed by pulse oximetry. Under general anesthesia, the airway is secured with an endotracheal tube or laryngeal masked airway. In some instances of general anesthesia, the patient's airway is controlled via bag/mask ventilation by the anesthesia provider. Breathing (respiration) is monitored by direct observation, confirmed with the pulse oximeter and capnography, and controlled or assisted by an anesthesia provider when the patient is under general anesthesia. Circulation is monitored by electrocardiography and blood pressure.

ELECTROCARDIOGRAPHY

The patient's heart rate and rhythm will be continually assessed using **electrocardiography**. Electrocardiography is the process of recording the electrical impulses of the heart. Electrodes that sense the electrical activity of the heart are placed on the patient's skin and attached to leads, which transmit those electrical impulses to the electrocardiogram (ECG) device. The electrical activity of the heart is recorded and displayed on a screen. The ECG may be set to record a tracing of the electrical activity on a strip of paper. The ECG device is also set to emit an audible signal to indicate heart rate and rhythm.

CAUTION

For patient safety, the audible ECG signal must be set loud enough to be heard by the anesthesia provider over extraneous operating room noise.

Box 14-1 SUMMARY OF THE MOST COMMON PHYSIOLOGIC FUNCTIONS MONITORED IN SURGICAL PATIENTS

Function	Value
Electrocardiogram (ECG)	Adult resting: 60-100 bpm Children 1 to 10 years: 70–130 bpm Infants (1-11 months old): 80-120 bpm Newborns (0-30 days old): 70-190 bpm
Pulse oximetry	oxygen saturation should be above 95% in healthy patients
Blood pressure	Less than 120 mm Hg systolic and less than 80 mm Hg diastolic
Temperature	37° C or 98° F
Capnometry	sustained carbon dioxide waveform greater than 30 mm Hg indicates correct placement of endotracheal tube
Consciousness	A scaled number between 45 and 60 indicates an appropriate depth of general anesthesia
Neuromuscular function	Zero of the four twitches indicates complete muscle relaxation.
Arterial pressure	Establish patient baseline waveform and monitor changes; digital values range 90-140/60-90 mm Hg
Central venous pressure	Establish patient baseline waveform and monitor changes; digital values are inconsistent and less reliable than waveform analysis
Pulmonary artery pressure	Establish patient baseline waveform and monitor changes; digital values range 15-25/8-15 mm Hg but are less reliable than waveform

The ECG may be recorded using three-lead or five-lead systems. The surgical technologist in the circulating role may assist the anesthesia provider in placing the electrodes, which should be securely adhered to areas of clean, dry skin. The electrodes should be protected from prep solutions and placed so that a change in the patient's position (e.g., supine to lateral) will not disrupt electrode contact. In a five-lead system, electrodes are placed on each shoulder, each hip, and in the fifth intercostal space near the left anterior axillary line. A baseline reading is obtained, and the ECG is used to monitor changes in the heart rate and rhythm during surgery.

The ECG is supplemented by **auscultation** (listening to the sounds of the chest, e.g., the heart rate, rhythm, and pulmonary sounds) with a precordial stethoscope. A modified version of a standard stethoscope, the precordial stethoscope is taped onto the patient's chest at the left sternal border or in the suprasternal notch. Alternatively, an esophageal stethoscope may be used, particularly if the chest is prepped into the sterile field. A long piece of tubing extends from the stethoscope to a specialized earpiece placed in the anesthesia provider's ear, thus enabling continuous auscultation. Auscultation is also used to assess respiratory rate and lung sounds as well as to verify placement of airway devices used in general anesthesia.

TECH TIP

A review of basic physiology of the electrical conduction system of the heart is highly recommended. The surgical technologist should be able to interpret a normal ECG cycle, including the meaning of the P wave, QRS complex, and T wave. By listening to the audible ECG in the background noise of the operating room, the surgical technologist should be able to appreciate various types of dysrhythmias, including bradycardia, tachycardia, and asystole. Additionally, the surgical technologist should be able to identify a premature ventricular contraction (PVC) and the presence of an active pacemaker by its characteristic spike. Each of these abilities contributes to the surgical technologist's value as a surgical team member. The ability to recognize and appreciate the importance of changes in heart rate and rhythm enables the surgical technologist to provide assistance to the anesthesia provider and patient when necessary.

PULSE OXIMETRY

Pulse oximetry is a noninvasive measure of the oxygen saturation of blood. A two-sided sensor probe is attached to a finger, toe, or earlobe (Fig. 14-1). The probe emits red and infrared light, which is absorbed while passing through tissue. Remaining light is detected by the opposite side of the sensor probe and used to calculate the saturation of peripheral oxygen (Spo_2). Ideally, the saturation should be above 95%. When indicated, pulse oximetry readings are confirmed with a measurement of arterial blood gases. Readings may be affected by administration of intravenous dyes such as methylene blue (see Chapter 6), but most devices used today are capable of adjusting to such conditions. Vasoconstriction due to hypothermia can affect readings when using a finger sensor.

An audible signal reflects pulse rate and the signal tone indicates saturation. A deeper tone indicates lower oxygen saturation. For patient safety, this audible signal must be loud enough to be heard by all members of the operating room team.

TECH TIP

Even while cleaning up the back table after a procedure, the surgical technologist should be alert to the rate and tone of the pulse oximeter. A slow pulse or dropping oxygen saturation during emergence from anesthesia may signal an emergency situation such as laryngospasm (see Chapter 16). The surgical technologist must be able to identify such a situation, stop cleanup duties, and turn full attention to the patient and the needs of the anesthesia provider until the crisis has been resolved.

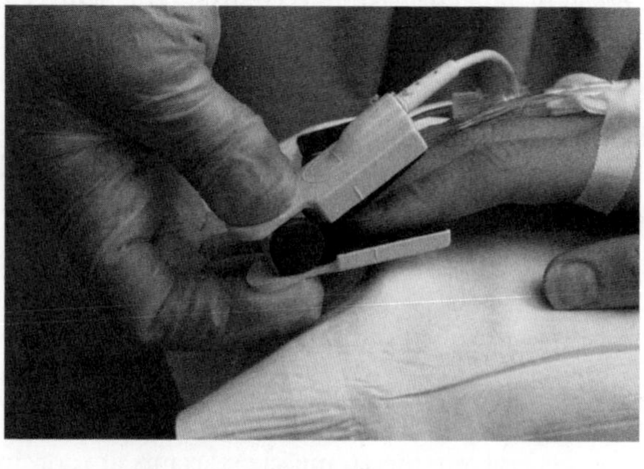

Figure 14-1 A sensor probe clip for the pulse oximeter is attached to the patient's finger.

BLOOD PRESSURE

Blood pressure (BP) is a measure of the force of blood against the vessel walls. Blood pressure is typically measured at the brachial artery. An inflatable cuff is placed on the patient's upper arm. The cuff is inflated to a pressure that occludes the pulse and the pressure is gradually released. The point at which the pulse is first detected is the systolic pressure and the point at which the pulse can no longer be detected is the diastolic pressure. Automated blood pressure devices have replaced the old mercury-based sphygmomanometers, but readings are still reported in millimeters of mercury (mm Hg). To obtain an accurate reading of blood pressure, the cuff must be an appropriate size for the patient. The cuff should be long enough to cover the circumference of the patient's upper arm plus about 40%. The width of the cuff is important too. A cuff that is too narrow may record higher pressure and a cuff that is too wide may record lower than the accurate pressure.

Normal blood pressure in a healthy adult is considered to be less than 120 mm Hg systolic and less than 80 mm Hg diastolic. Opinions are changing regarding what is considered a normal blood pressure measurement. In adults over age 50, a measurement that was once accepted as normal blood pressure is now considered pre-hypertensive. Multiple variables affect blood pressure, including ventricular contraction strength, capillary resistance, vessel wall elasticity, and blood volume.

The blood pressure cuff is placed on the patient's arm that does *not* have the IV cannula in place whenever possible. The cuff is connected to a device that automatically measures blood pressure at specified intervals, usually every 5 minutes. During induction of general anesthesia, blood pressure is monitored more frequently. The machine may be set to emit an audible alarm if blood pressure is not within preset parameters.

An invasive measure of blood pressure may be obtained through placement of an arterial line, discussed later in this section.

TEMPERATURE

All patients are at risk for mild to significant hypothermia and, when under general anesthesia, there is a risk for the rare event of malignant hyperthermia, so temperature monitoring is indicated. Temperature may be assessed from any number of locations, including skin, axilla, bladder, esophagus, and ear. Simple liquid crystal temperature strips can be placed on the patient's forehead for basic monitoring of skin temperature. More precise measurements of core temperature are indicated in some patients and for some types of surgical procedures. In such cases a lower esophageal probe may be used because it offers the most accurate reading of core temperature with the least risk of patient injury. Normal body temperature varies from patient to patient and it also varies by the time of day. Oral temperature is usually within a limited range near 98° F (approximately 37° C). A patient's baseline temperature measurement is obtained and changes are monitored and assessed. Core temperatures lower than 36° C indicate hypothermia. Hypothermia alters several normal body functions and it is associated with an increased risk of surgical site infections. Pediatric and geriatric patients are particularly vulnerable to a drop in temperature. Several precautions are taken to minimize heat loss such as a forced-air warmer or a hypo/hyperthermia unit, and the patient's body temperature is continually monitored to verify the effectiveness of those precautions.

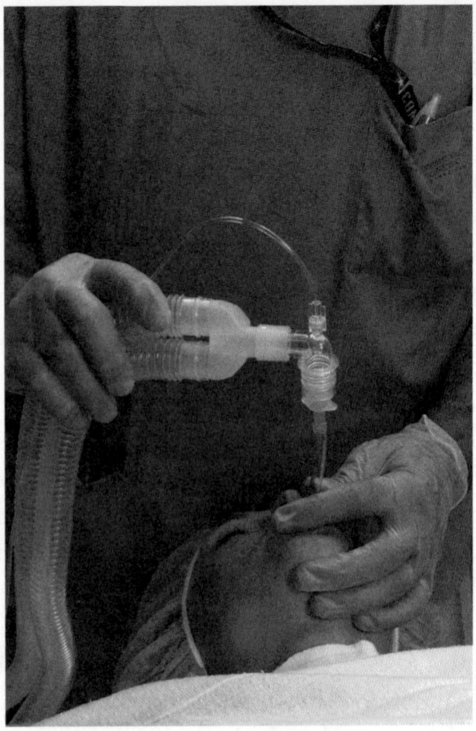

Figure 14-2 Tubing extends from an adapter on the ventilator circuit to the respiratory analyzer to measure expired CO_2.

CAPNOMETRY

Capnometry is a measurement of carbon dioxide (CO_2) exhaled by the patient, called end-tidal CO_2. This monitor is used to verify adequate ventilation whenever the patient is under heavy sedation or general anesthesia. In general anesthesia, an adapter is connected to the breathing circuit and a small-diameter piece of tubing extends from the adapter to the analyzer (Fig. 14-2). An oxygen cannula with a CO_2 sampling tube is available to monitor the sedated patient. The concentration of expired CO_2 is measured and displayed as a continuous graph and in numerical value. An audible alarm is set to indicate when preset levels are exceeded. Capnometry is an extremely valuable tool in the assessment of respiratory function and can serve a critical role in early detection of problems such as an esophageal intubation, compromised ventilation, or malignant hyperthermia (see Chapter 16). Other types of respiratory analysis devices also measure levels of oxygen and inhaled anesthetic agents. Mass spectrometry such as the system for anesthetic and respiratory analysis (SARA) is not frequently used in current practice. The large system analyzers have been largely replaced by infrared spectrometry multi-gas analyzers.

MONITORING CONSCIOUSNESS

Traditionally, the depth of various components of general anesthesia has been monitored in several ways, including basic vital signs and nerve stimulation. However, traditional monitoring methods may not have been sufficient in some patients to adequately assess the level of patient awareness under anesthesia. Patient awareness while under anesthesia is a rare but significant concern (see Chapter 15) estimated to occur in approximately 1 to 2 of 1000 patients undergoing general anesthesia. In an effort to assist the anesthesia provider in assessing the depth of consciousness under anesthesia, a modified electroencephalogram (EEG) may be used to determine the level of consciousness by recording electrical activity in the brain. It provides a direct measure of the effect of general anesthetic agents on the brain. EEG information is obtained from a sensor placed on the patient's forehead. The monitor interprets the information and displays a reading between 0 and 100, a scale used to indicate the patient's level of consciousness. A number near 100 indicates that the patient is fully awake and responsive and a number between 45 and 60 indicates an appropriate depth of general anesthesia with a low probability of explicit recall (see Chapter 15).

NEUROMUSCULAR FUNCTION

During general anesthesia, muscle relaxants are administered to facilitate endotracheal intubation and a relaxed surgical site (see Chapter 15). A nerve stimulator is used to assess neuromuscular function and the extent of blockade. A stimulus is delivered to the nerve from a surface electrode or probe, often placed at the ulnar nerve or a branch of the facial nerve. Four stimuli (called a "train of four," or TOF) are administered, and the extent of the block is estimated based on the twitch response. The presence of four of the four twitches indicates no muscle relaxation, whereas zero of the four twitches indicates complete muscle relaxation. Nerve stimulation is used to determine if the patient's jaw and vocal cords are adequately relaxed for intubation and to determine when additional muscle relaxants should be administered during a surgical procedure. Nerve stimulation is also used to assess the extent to which muscle relaxants are wearing off and the patient is becoming ready to breathe on his or her own after surgery.

ADVANCED MONITORING

Certain patient conditions and surgical procedures may require additional monitoring. These invasive monitoring techniques include arterial catheterization and pressure monitoring, central venous catheterization and pressure monitoring, and pulmonary artery catheterization (Swan-Ganz catheter). An arterial pressure–monitoring catheter (often referred to as an arterial line or "art-line") is usually placed in the radial artery and connected to a transducer that records continuous, immediate, and highly accurate measurement of blood pressure. Placement of an arterial line is indicated for a number of reasons, including potential for rapid changes in blood pressure, frequent sampling of arterial blood for blood gas analysis (ABGs), or when routine blood pressure measurement is inaccurate.

When indicated, a central venous pressure–monitoring catheter (CVP line) is positioned in the superior vena cava and is used to assess the volume of blood returning to the heart. A CVP line is also used to assess the need for fluid replacement and to prevent fluid overload.

A pulmonary artery (PA) catheter (such as a Swan-Ganz catheter) is guided through the heart into a branch of the pulmonary artery to obtain measurements of central venous pressure, pulmonary artery pressure, pulmonary capillary wedge pressure, and cardiac output. PA catheters are most frequently used in adult patients during cardiac surgery, lung transplantation, and liver transplantation.

During heart surgery, transesophageal echocardiography (TEE) may be used to assess cardiac function. A probe is placed into the esophagus and high-frequency sound waves are emitted through the tissue. An image of the heart is obtained and interpreted. TEE can be used to observe cardiac wall motion and valve function, assess intravascular fluid volume, and to identify the presence of air in the heart. Blood flow through the heart can be assessed using echocardiography and pulse-wave, continuous, or color Doppler technology.

When the patient has been admitted to the operating room and all the appropriate basic monitoring devices are in place, baseline measurements are recorded and the patient is ready for administration of anesthesia. Invasive monitoring devices may be placed prior to or after the administration of general anesthesia.

LOCAL AND REGIONAL ANESTHESIA

To accomplish anesthesia, transmission of the sensation of pain through nerve impulses can be interrupted at several locations, including nerve endings, groups of nerves, or at the level of the brain. **Local anesthesia** is the administration of an anesthetic agent to nerve endings in the surgical site. **Regional anesthesia** is accomplished by the administration of the same type of agents, but at a group of nerves called a plexus. Regional anesthesia typically provides both sensory and motor block to an entire area of the body, because a group of nerves is anesthetized. General anesthesia (see Chapter 15) interferes with the brain's ability to interpret pain impulses coming from anywhere in the body.

LOCAL ANESTHESIA

A local anesthetic is administered to the immediate surgical site. Whether injected (infiltrated) into tissue or applied topically to mucosal membranes, it affects a small, circumscribed area. Local anesthetics, such as lidocaine, interfere with sensory nerve endings in the operative area; thus, they block transmission of pain impulses to the brain. When local anesthesia is used without an anesthesia provider present, it is imperative that a registered nurse be assigned to monitor the patient's vital signs during the surgical procedure. The registered nurse assesses the patient's physical condition and psychological status so that appropriate measures can be taken to maintain patient safety and comfort. Heart rate and rhythm is measured by ECG, and BP, respirations, and oxygen saturation are also monitored continuously. The registered nurse may administer sedatives as ordered by the surgeon. Only physically healthy and psychologically stable patients undergoing brief, uncomplicated surgical procedures are appropriate candidates for local anesthesia without monitoring by an anesthesia provider.

A specialized type of local infiltration is called tumescent anesthesia and it is widely used in aesthetic surgery such as liposuction. Tumescent anesthesia is a technique that involves injection of a large volume of a dilute solution into subcutaneous tissues to facilitate fat suctioning, provide local anesthesia, and reduce blood loss. The solution commonly contains 0.05% to 0.1% lidocaine, epinephrine 0.5 to 1.5 mg/L, and normal saline. Sodium bicarbonate may be added to increase absorption and shorten onset time. Glucocorticoids such as triamcinolone may also be added to reduce inflammation and potential scarring.

Applications for Local Anesthesia

Local anesthesia without anesthesia provider monitoring has several applications. In general surgery, local injections are appropriate for excision or biopsy of small soft tissue masses such as lipomas, nevi, or other skin lesions. In orthopedic surgery, local anesthesia is used for limited work on digits, such as repair of finger lacerations or toenail excisions. Local anesthesia is used in plastic surgery for limited facial procedures, such as excision of lesions or minor scar revisions. In urology, cystoscopy may be performed with a topical anesthetic agent. Because local anesthesia blocks sensory nerve impulses only at the site of injection or application, the patient cannot feel pain in that area but is still able to move muscles and feel pressure.

Agents Used for Local Anesthesia

Local anesthetic agents are chemically classified as either aminoesters or aminoamides. The pharmacokinetic action of local anesthetics is significantly different from that of other drugs and it differs between the two chemical classes of agents (Insight 14-1). The duration of action of local anesthetics is due to the differences in their individual lipid-binding affinity, which also accounts for variations in duration depending on the area of the body to be anesthetized.

The first local anesthetic agents, topical cocaine and injectable procaine (Novocain), were aminoesters.

Cocaine is a naturally occurring alkaloid derived from coca leaves. It has long been known to have anesthetic effects when used topically on mucous membranes. It may be used in nasal surgery, but is less frequently used today because acceptable alternatives are available.

CAUTION

Cocaine is for topical use only; it is never injected.

INSIGHT 14-1 Pharmacokinetics of Local Anesthetic Agents

It may be helpful to review the processes of pharmacokinetics applied to local anesthetics. It is interesting to note that pharmacokinetics is quite different for local anesthetics than it is for other medications. Recall that absorption is the process in which medications are taken into the body and the process of distribution takes the drug to its site of action. Local anesthetics are different in that they are injected or applied topically *directly to* the intended site of action. The pharmacokinetic processes of absorption and distribution by the circulatory system actually cause a reduction in the intended effect of local anesthetics at the site of action. Dilute epinephrine may be added to a local anesthetic to cause vasoconstriction and thus slow the absorption of the agent into systemic circulation.

The pH of tissues at the site of action also affects the action of local anesthetics. When an infection is present, the tissue is slightly acidic, which reduces the ability of these agents to exert their effects.

Plasma protein binding is another important aspect of the distribution phase of pharmacokinetics. Local anesthetic agents vary widely in the extent of plasma protein binding, which impacts availability for metabolism and excretion. Procaine (Novocain, an aminoester) is only 6% bound, lidocaine is 64% bound, mepivacaine is 77% bound, and ropivacaine is 94% bound to plasma proteins.

Because the chemical structures are different, the two types of local anesthetic agents are also metabolized in different ways. Aminoester local anesthetics are metabolized in the blood. These chemicals are hydrolyzed by enzymes circulating in the plasma (plasma cholinesterase) and are rapidly excreted in urine. Aminoamides are almost completely metabolized by hepatic enzymes in the liver and very little of the unchanged drug molecules is excreted in urine.

Cocaine comes in 4% and 10% solutions; thus it may be administered on cotton applicators or nasal packing, or it may be sprayed directly on the mucosal surface. In addition to its anesthetic properties, cocaine is also a powerful vasoconstrictor. This means it reduces bleeding and helps shrink mucous membranes. Thus it was particularly useful in nasal surgery because it allowed better visualization in the nasal cavity. Dosages are carefully calculated to the patient's age and physical condition, and the lowest dose necessary is used to achieve the required anesthetic effect. Concentrations greater than 4% increase potential for systemic toxic reactions. The maximum safe dose is 1.5 mg/kg. Adverse effects are seen primarily in the central nervous system (CNS). These include excitement and depression, and may lead to respiratory arrest. Because of these complications, cocaine is less often used in nasal surgery today. Nasal local anesthesia is currently more commonly accomplished with injection of lidocaine (Xylocaine) and the topical application of either phenylephrine (Neo-Synephrine) or the nasal spray oxymetazoline (Afrin) to shrink mucous membranes.

CAUTION

Cocaine is a controlled substance. It should never be left unattended in the operating room, and any cocaine solution dispensed but unused should be returned to the pharmacy or destroyed. At least two people should witness the destruction of unused cocaine to verify that it has not been used for illicit purposes.

Two other aminoester local anesthetic agents are also used in surgery. Benzocaine (14%, contained in Cetacaine spray) is a topical agent with rapid onset and a duration of 30 to 60 minutes. It may be applied prior to bronchoscopy or fiberoptic endotracheal intubation. Tetracaine (Pontocaine) is a potent and long acting local anesthetic. A 0.5% solution may be used for topical anesthesia prior to cataract surgery. Tetracaine may also be used in spinal anesthesia, a type of regional anesthesia, because it provides rapid onset and excellent motor and sensory block lasting 90 to 120 minutes.

The most common local anesthetic agents used in surgery are aminoamides: lidocaine (Xylocaine), bupivacaine (Marcaine; Fig. 14-3), and ropivacaine (Naropin). A less commonly used local anesthetic agent is mepivacaine (Carbocaine). All of these agents, except ropivacaine, may be combined with dilute epinephrine (see Chapter 8). Most local anesthetics (except ropivacaine) cause some vasodilation, which speeds absorption. Recall that epinephrine is a potent vasoconstrictor. When combined with a local anesthetic agent, epinephrine causes local vasoconstriction, slowing the absorption of the agent into the circulatory system. This action keeps the local anesthetic in the surgical site longer, thus increasing the duration of effect. Some manufacturers will call attention to local anesthetic agents mixed with epinephrine by adding red print or a red band on the vial label for rapid identification. Local anesthetics without epinephrine may have a blue band on the label. This practice helps staff visually identify the correct formulation, but it is not a substitute for thorough reading of the entire label prior to delivery to the sterile field.

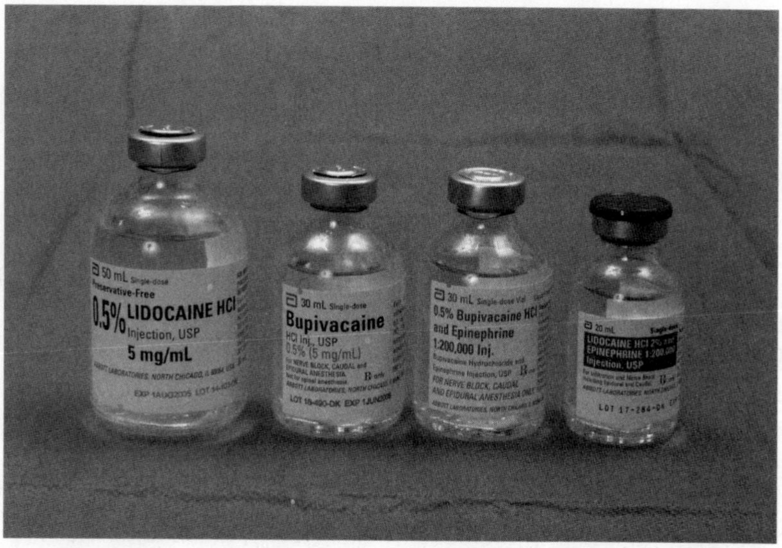

Figure 14-3 Lidocaine and bupivacaine are available with and without epinephrine.

CAUTION

Local anesthetic agents with epinephrine should NOT be used for peripheral infiltration anesthesia on fingers, toes, external ear, external nose, or penis because of vasoconstriction caused by epinephrine.

CAUTION

Epinephrine premixed in a local anesthetic agent is present in very tiny amounts (most commonly one part of epinephrine to 100,000 or 200,000 parts of solvent). The surgical technologist must be aware that epinephrine is also available separately in the very high concentration of 1:1000, 100 times or 200 times stronger than the dose intended for injection (see Chapter 8 and Insight 14-2). It is vital to administer epinephrine in the correct concentration for the correct purpose and by the correct route. If the high 1:1000 concentration of epinephrine is inadvertently injected, severe tachycardia (rapid heart rate) and hypertension will result, increasing the potential for cardiac arrest (see Insight 8-2). All medications present on the sterile field must be correctly labeled (name and dose) and identified when passing to the surgeon to avoid medication administration errors.

The most common local anesthetic agent in use today is lidocaine. Lidocaine is fast acting and rapidly metabolized. The duration of anesthesia with infiltrated lidocaine is approximately 30 to 60 minutes. If epinephrine is added to a lidocaine solution, the duration of effect is increased by approximately 50%. The prolonged effect occurs because epinephrine slows systemic absorption, keeping more of the drug at the site of action. Lidocaine is available for injection in solutions of 0.5%, 1%, 1.5%, and 2%, with and without epinephrine 1:100,000 and 1:200,000. It is also available in a 4% solution for topical application.

{NOTE} *Some people may mistakenly refer to lidocaine as "Novocain," which is a completely different agent. Novocain is the trade name for procaine, which was used by dentists for many years, but is seldom used currently. Procaine is classified chemically as an aminoester-type anesthetic. Aminoester-type anesthetics cause more allergic reactions than aminoamide-type anesthetics. Patients who are allergic to Novocain do not usually have allergies to lidocaine, because these agents have different chemical structures and metabolic pathways.*

Bupivacaine (Marcaine, Sensorcaine) is an aminoamide anesthetic, which is about four times more potent than lidocaine and has a longer duration, from 4 to 8 hours. Bupivacaine is available in solutions of 0.25%, 0.5%, and 0.75%, with and without epinephrine 1:200,000. Bupivacaine is more highly bound to plasma proteins than lidocaine and it is more lipid soluble, which help account for

IN SIGHT 14-2 Practical Math and Lidocaine with Epinephrine Dosages

Basic mathematics is used in the calculation of strength, dosage, and ratios of medications. Local anesthetics, with and without epinephrine, are examples of the daily use of math in the operating room.

For example, lidocaine is available in a 1% solution. This means that 1 g of solute (the medication) is contained in 100 mL of solvent (the diluent). Multiply this dose by 10 and the result is 10 g/1000 mL or 10 g/L. Or this figure can be divided by 1000 to obtain the equivalent, which is 10 mg/mL, If the patient receives an injection of 20 mL of 1% lidocaine, the dosage of lidocaine is 200 mg (20 mL times 10 mg).

Epinephrine dosages are expressed as a ratio. For example, dilute epinephrine (1:100,000 or 1:200,000) may be added to lidocaine. The ratio indicates a solution of 1 part epinephrine (the solute) to 100,000 or 200,000 parts of solvent (the diluent). A 1:1 solution means there is 1 g of solute per gram (mL) of solvent. Thus, a 1:100,000 solution of epinephrine contains 0.01 mg/mL or 10 mcg/mL. In contrast, epinephrine is also available separately in a 1:1000 solution, that is, 1 g/1000 mL or 1 g/1 L. Divided by 1000, it can be expressed as 1 mg/1 mL. The dosage is dramatically different if 1:1000 (1 mg/mL) solution is used instead of the 1:100,000 (0.01 mg/mL) solution. Inject 30 mL of epinephrine 1:100,000 and the dose is 0.3 mg, but inject 3 mL of 1:1000 epinephrine and the dose is 30 mg—a 100-fold increase.

Understanding principles of basic mathematics can make a significant difference in protecting the surgical patient from medication errors.

its longer duration. Unlike other local anesthetics, bupivacaine's duration of action is not prolonged by the addition of epinephrine, but adding epinephrine to bupivacaine does limit vascular uptake and peak serum concentrations. Bupivacaine also binds to cardiac muscle, so its chief adverse effect is cardiotoxicity. Bupivacaine 0.75% is no longer used for obstetric surgery because of the increased risk for cardiotoxicity. It is also contraindicated for intravenous regional anesthesia because of toxicity.

Ropivacaine (Naropin) is an aminoamide local anesthetic agent released for use in 1996. It is similar in duration to bupivacaine, but is generally less cardiotoxic. It is available in concentrations of 0.2%, 0.5%, 0.75%, and 1% in polypropylene ampules (Fig. 14-4) of 10 mL and 20 mL and in 30-mL single dose vials.

Mepivacaine (Carbocaine, Polocaine) is another aminoamide anesthetic that has a similar potency to lidocaine, with slightly longer duration (45-90 minutes). Mepivacaine is available in solutions of 1%, 1.5%, 2%, and 3% solution and may be combined with epinephrine. It is not available for topical use. Mepivacaine is used less often because it doesn't have a significant advantage over lidocaine, which is used more frequently and thus is more readily available. See Table 14-1 for a comparison of common local anesthetic agents.

MAKE IT SIMPLE

The names of all the local anesthetic agents end in "-caine." It is easy to identify the amide anesthetics when you remember the "*i*." The letter *i* occurs in am*i*de and in the first part of the name of each amide agent—l*i*docaine, bup*i*vacaine, rop*i*vacaine, and mep*i*vacaine. The letter i does not occur in the first part of the names of ester anesthetics—cocaine, benzocaine, and tetracaine.

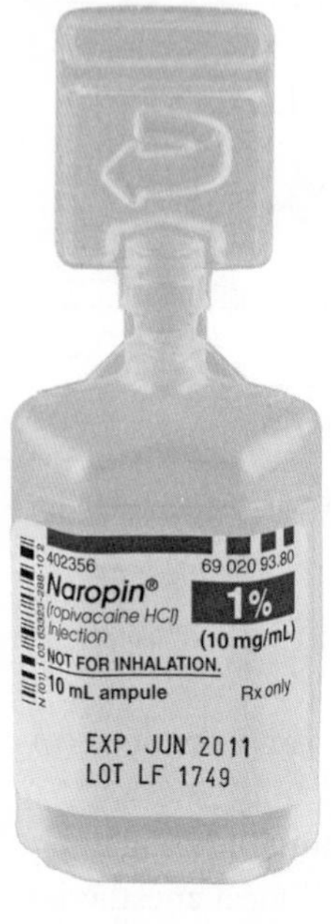

Figure 14-4 The medication labeling on polypropylene ampules of ropivacaine can be difficult to read. *(Courtesy of APP Pharmaceuticals, LLc., A Company of the Fresenius Kabi Group, Schaumburg, Ill.)*

Adverse reactions to amide local anesthetics are primarily dose-related and affect both the CNS and the cardiovascular system. See Table 14-2 for a comparison of maximum dosages of local anesthetics. Adverse CNS effects are variable, from drowsiness at low doses to excitement or agitation at higher doses. Excitement may or may not occur, and the patient may go from a drowsy state to unconsciousness and into respiratory arrest. Nausea and vomiting may also occur. Other CNS adverse effects include visual disturbances, tingling, slurred speech, and excitability, which can lead to seizures. Cardiovascular adverse effects are also dose-related and include hypotension, bradycardia, and

Table 14-1 COMPARISON OF COMMON LOCAL ANESTHETIC AGENTS

Generic Name	Trade Name	Solutions Available	Duration (hours)
bupivacaine	Marcaine, Sensorcaine	0.25%, 0.5%, 0.75%	4-8
cocaine	N/A	4%, 10%	0.5-2
lidocaine with epinephrine	Xylocaine	0.5%, 1%, 1.5%, 2%	0.5-1.5
mepivacaine	Carbocaine, Polocaine	1%, 1.5%, 2%, 3%	0.75-1.5
ropivacaine	Naropin	0.2%, 0.5%, 1%	2-6

Table 14-2 COMPARISON OF APPROXIMATE MAXIMUM DOSAGES OF LOCAL ANESTHETICS FOR INFILTRATION

Agent	Concentration (%)	Volume (mL)	Dose (mg/kg)
bupivacaine	0.25	up to 70	up to 2
lidocaine	0.5		
without epinephrine		up to 60	up to 4.5
with epinephrine		up to 100	up to 7
mepivacaine	1	up to 40	up to 7
ropivacaine	0.5	up to 40	up to 2

Note: This table is intended for comparison only and not for use as clinical dosage recommendations.

ventricular arrhythmias leading to possible cardiac arrest. Systemic toxicity of local anesthetics is most commonly due to inadvertent intravascular injection during peripheral nerve infiltration.

REGIONAL ANESTHESIA

Regional anesthesia blocks nerves (not just nerve endings) at specific locations; thus, it provides a larger anesthetized area. Whereas local anesthesia involves injection of a local anesthetic at the operative site, regional anesthesia involves injecting a local anesthetic into the nerves that supply the operative region. Regional blocks can affect sympathetic, sensory, and motor nerve supply, so an anesthetized limb may be immobile as well as numb. Regional blocks are effective for many types of surgical procedures, but frequently take more time to administer than a general anesthetic. Various types of regional anesthetic techniques are usually named for the nerves or areas of the body to be blocked. Although nearly any group of nerves can be blocked, we discuss only the most frequently used regional anesthetic techniques in this text. The most commonly used regional blocks are spinal and epidural, collectively referred to as central neuraxial blockade (CNB).

Any type of regional anesthesia requires continuous monitoring of the patient's vital functions, including heart rate and ECG, BP, respirations, and oxygen saturation.

Spinal Anesthesia

For spinal anesthesia, agents are injected **intrathecally**, that is, through the dura mater into the subarachnoid space and cerebrospinal fluid in the lumbar area of the spine (Fig. 14-5). Injection is at the end of the spinal cord, usually not higher than L3 to L4. This technique anesthetizes the entire lower body. Preoperative preparation may include administration of anxiolytics (see Chapter 13) and analgesics to minimize discomfort. The circulator commonly assists the anesthesia provider during injection of a spinal anesthetic by helping the patient to get into optimum position (Fig. 14-6). The patient may be positioned laterally to facilitate correct needle placement. That is, patients may lie on the side, with knees bent and chin on chest. Thus, the patient is usually instructed to curl up as much as possible, pushing his or her lower back out toward the anesthesia provider. This position spreads the vertebral bodies apart so the spinal needle may be more easily inserted. It is, however, difficult for some patients, especially the elderly, to curl their backs. These patients may be assisted gently into position, using caution to avoid injury. Alternatively, patients may be in a sitting position for administration of a spinal anesthetic (Fig. 14-7). The patient may sit on the operating bed with his or her back to the anesthesia provider.

Skin around the injection site area is prepped with an antiseptic agent and a small fenestrated sterile drape is placed over the area. Local anesthesia is injected through skin and subcutaneous tissue prior to insertion of a spinal needle through the ligaments and dura. The spinal needle is correctly placed when a drop of cerebral spinal fluid (CSF) appears. A syringe containing anesthetic agent is attached to the spinal needle and a small amount of CSF is aspirated to reconfirm placement. The agent is injected, the needle and syringe are withdrawn and the patient is placed in supine position. The level of anesthesia is verified, often with the use of an alcohol wipe. Alcohol will feel cold on an unblocked area of skin

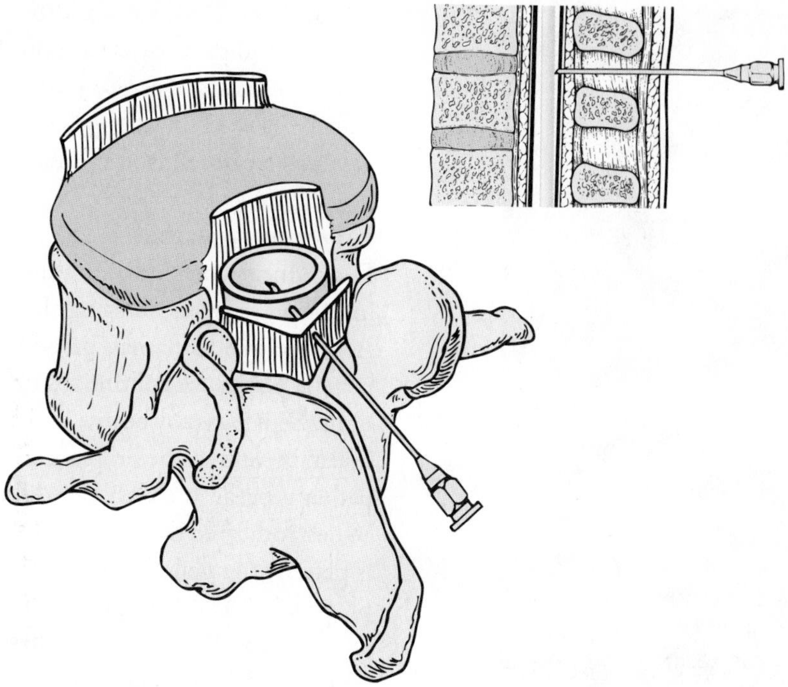

Figure 14-5 Location of spinal anesthesia injection.

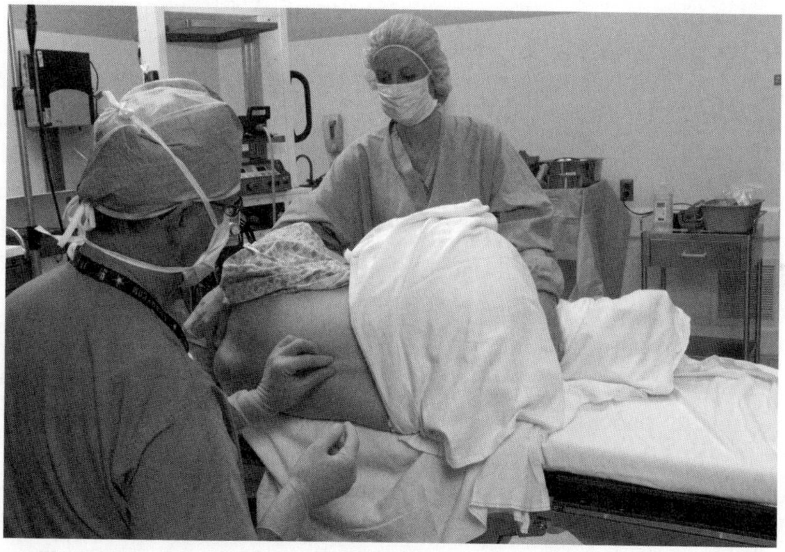

Figure 14-6 Patient positioned laterally for spinal administration.

and warm or neutral on a blocked area. Another technique that is commonly used to assess the level of spinal anesthesia is pinprick. The patient feels a sharp pinprick on an unblocked area of skin and a dull sensation on a blocked area.

Spinal anesthesia is usually quicker to administer than an epidural and provides more intense sensory and motor blockade. In addition, proper needle placement is clearly verified by the appearance of CSF. If continuous spinal anesthesia is indicated, a small catheter is placed for repeated dosing.

The most common local anesthetic agents used for spinal anesthesia include tetracaine and bupivacaine (both lasting 90-120 minutes). Epinephrine may be added to prolong blockade, but it may also delay postoperative urination during recovery so epinephrine is less frequently used for outpatient surgery. Instead, an opioid such as fentanyl (10-25 mcg) or sufentanil (10 mcg)

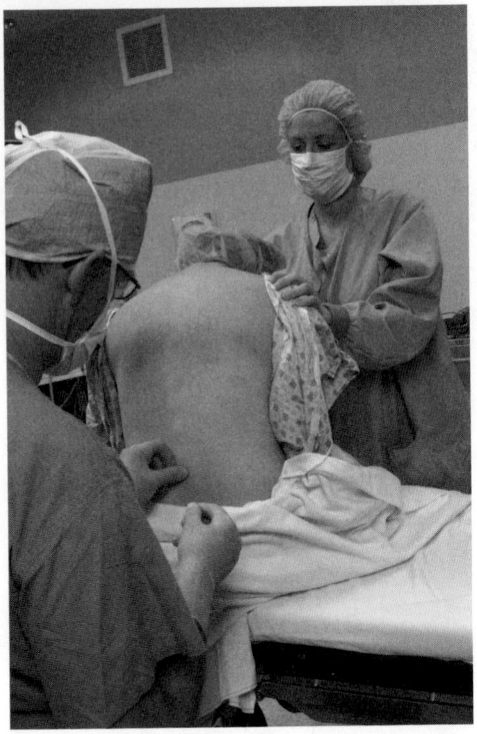

Figure 14-7 Patient in a sitting position for spinal administration.

may be added to prolong duration of spinal anesthesia without prolonging recovery time.

Spinal anesthesia is used for procedures of the lower abdomen, perineum, and lower extremities. It is often used for transurethral resection of the prostate gland or bladder tumors, for lower leg vascular procedures such as embolectomy, for select orthopedic procedures such as total knee arthroplasty, and for cesarean sections.

A drop in blood pressure may occur with administration of a spinal or epidural anesthetic because of vasodilation. Younger, more athletic patients with lower resting heart rates have a higher risk for significant bradycardia under spinal anesthesia. Another complication of spinal anesthesia is postdural puncture headache, which can be severe and is thought to be associated with the creation of a persistent tear or slit in the dura. Severe postdural puncture headaches may be treated by administration of a "blood patch," that is, an injection of 10 to 15 mL of the patient's blood at the original spinal injection site. An extreme manifestation of neurotoxicity attributed to the use of 5% lidocaine in spinal anesthesia is cauda equina syndrome, a paralysis of nerves resulting in lower extremity muscle weakness and impaired bowel and bladder function. Lidocaine in high concentrations (5%) is not used in spinal anesthesia because of the potential for neurotoxicity.

Intrathecal catheters and pumps are used to deliver analgesics to patients with various types of chronic pain. These devices are not used for surgical anesthesia, but may be placed in the surgical setting as part of the patient's treatment for chronic pain issues.

Epidural Anesthesia

In **epidural** anesthesia, an anesthetic agent is injected into the space surrounding the dura mater (Fig. 14-8). A single injection may be administered, or a catheter may be placed for continuous infusion or repeated injections. Sedation may be given to help relieve discomfort of injection and catheter placement (except in pregnant patients because sedation would also affect the baby). When indicated for use in pediatric patients, an epidural is placed after general anesthesia is induced. Positioning, prepping, and draping for administration of an epidural anesthetic is identical to that described for a spinal anesthetic. Local anesthesia is administered at the injection site and an epidural needle is placed. A catheter is advanced through the needle and the needle is withdrawn. The catheter is taped in place on the patient's back and an empty 3 mL syringe is attached. Correct placement is verified when CSF does *not* enter the syringe. A test dose of agent is administered, followed by small doses at intervals over a 1 to 3 minute period. Common agents used for epidural anesthesia include lidocaine, bupivacaine, and ropivacaine. Dilute epinephrine (1:200,000) may be added to prolong duration and small doses of opioids may be used to reduce the concentration of the local anesthetic agent.

Epidural anesthesia is used to relieve the pain of labor and vaginal delivery, as well as to provide anesthesia for cesarean section. Bupivacaine (0.25% and 0.5%) is an excellent choice for obstetric epidural anesthesia. A motor block will almost always be obtained with a bupivacaine concentration of 0.5%. In obstetric anesthesia, concentrations of 0.125% plus very low doses of fentanyl are used to provide "walking epidurals" (i.e., sensory block without motor block).

Epidural blocks may also be used as an adjunct to general anesthesia in select patients to minimize the amount of agents needed; they may also be used for postoperative pain control after such procedures as thoracotomy.

Epidural anesthesia has some advantages over spinal anesthesia including reduced risk of hypotension, less incidence of postdural puncture headache (because the dura is not intentionally punctured) and epidural

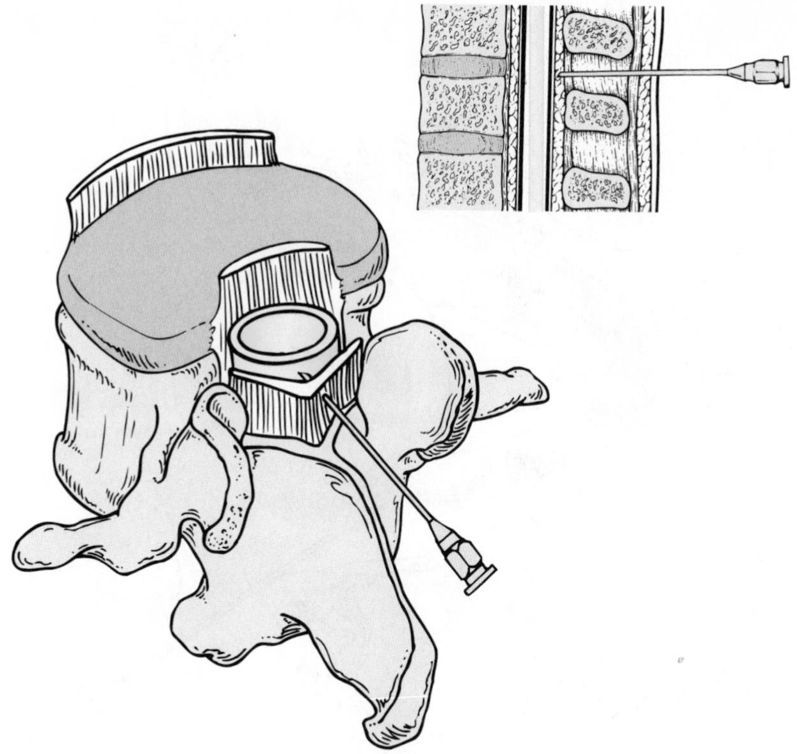

Figure 14-8 Location of epidural anesthesia injection.

anesthesia may be administered at levels above L3 to L4. Epidural anesthesia requires greater volume of agent (typically 20 mL) than spinal (typically 1-2 mL) and has a longer onset of action. But, epidural is preferred over spinal anesthesia when the surgical procedure duration is variable or extended or when prolonged postoperative analgesia is necessary.

Caudal Block

Caudal anesthesia is a type of epidural block injected into the epidural space via the sacral canal (Fig. 14-9). Caudal blocks used for vaginal childbirth are administered in the obstetrical unit rather than in the surgical suite. Caudal blocks may also be used in conjunction with general anesthesia for urologic and lower-extremity surgical procedures in children and for postoperative pain management.

Retrobulbar Block

Retrobulbar blocks are injected behind the eye into the muscle cone (Fig. 14-10) to block branches of the oculomotor nerve. These blocks may be used for procedures requiring a motionless, anesthetized eye. Retrobulbar blocks may be administered by an ophthalmologist or an anesthesia provider. A typical injection is made up of equal parts of 0.5% to 0.75% bupivacaine and 2%

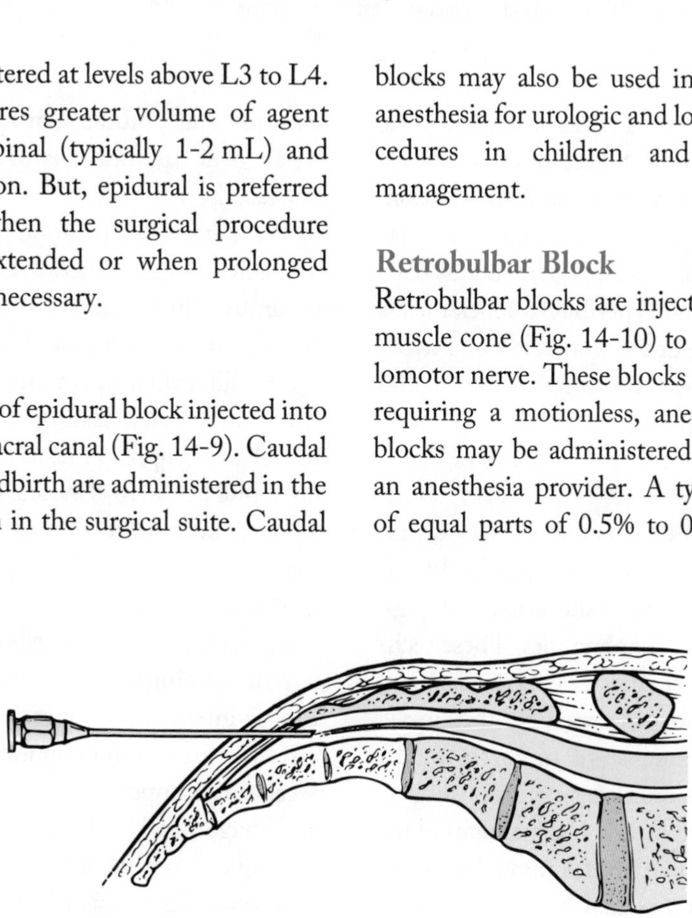

Figure 14-9 Location of caudal block.

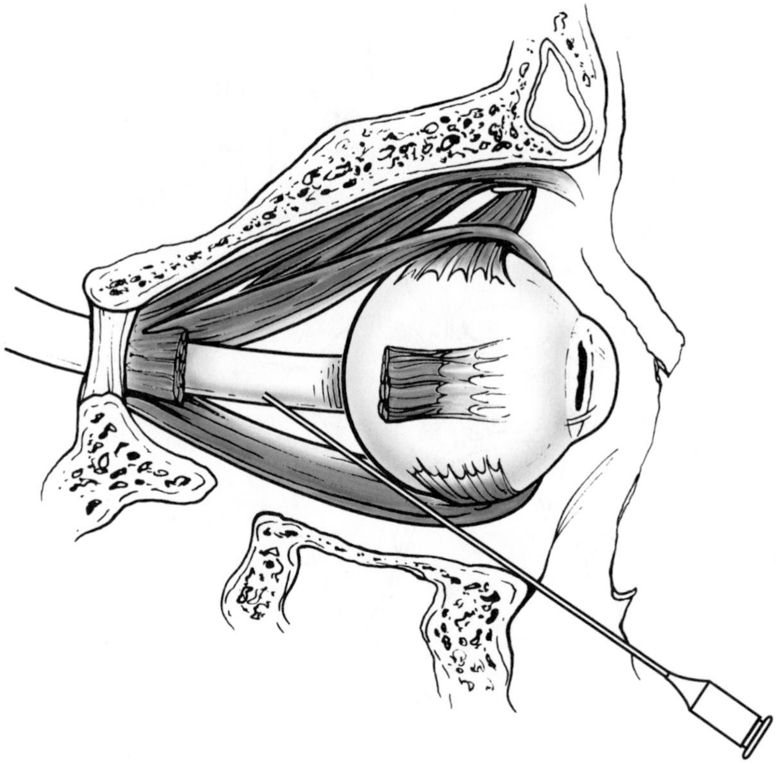

Figure 14-10 Location of retrobulbar anesthesia injection.

lidocaine with 150 units of hyaluronidase (see Chapter 10). To minimize patient discomfort, a sedative may be given intravenously prior to retrobulbar injection. Once the most common anesthesia technique for cataract extraction, retrobulbar blocks are less frequently used today. A similar technique called peribulbar block injects the anesthetic agent outside of the muscle cone to avoid the optic nerve, but it requires more anesthetic agent and has a slower onset of action.

Extremity Block

There are several techniques for extremity block, also called peripheral nerve block. These types of blocks may be used for procedures on distal arms and legs, and the hand and fingers, and foot and toes. These techniques vary depending on the anesthesia provider's expertise and preference, but in practice the upper extremities (arm, hand, fingers) are more frequently blocked than the lower extremities. For most surgical procedures on the lower extremities, a spinal or epidural is preferred rather than using several nerve blocks to achieve equal blockade. The arm may be blocked at several locations—including the brachial plexus, median, radial, and ulnar nerves—whereas the leg may be blocked at the femoral, obturator, or sciatic nerves. Depending on the surgical site, portions of the hand, foot, and digits may also be blocked.

Preoperative preparation for extremity block includes premedication with anxiolytics and analgesics to lessen discomfort during administration of the block. One of the anesthetic agents used for extremity blocks is 1% to 1.5% lidocaine, which provides onset in 10 to 20 minutes and a block lasting 2 to 3 hours. Ropivacaine (0.5%) and bupivacaine (0.375%-0.5%) have a slower onset but last 6 to 8 hours. The nerves to be blocked are identified with a nerve stimulator or ultrasound probe.

A brachial plexus block may be used for procedures on the hand, forearm, or elbow. A brachial plexus block may be administered in several different locations including interscalene, supraclavicular, and infraclavicular, but the most common approach is axillary (Fig. 14-11). Because it is important not to penetrate the nerve sheath or damage nearby blood vessels when performing this technique, a needle attached to a nerve stimulator may be inserted first. This allows the anesthesia provider to precisely locate the nerves of the brachial plexus. Approximately 30 to 40 mL of local anesthetic is

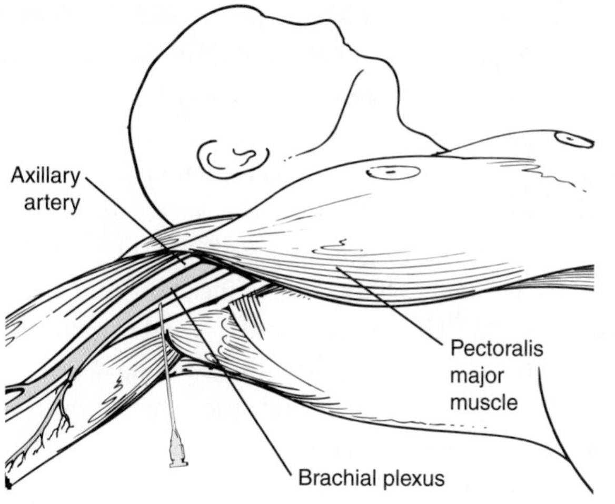

Figure 14-11 Location of axillary block injection.

injected around the nerves that are adjacent to the axillary artery, which makes the entire arm both numb and immobile. This technique may be used for manipulation and casting of fractures in patients who present a high risk for complications of general anesthesia; thus, it's a favored technique for use in alcohol-intoxicated patients whose CNS is already depressed.

Most regional extremity blocks have one primary disadvantage—it takes time for them to take effect. This means they may delay surgery. Extremity blocks may therefore be administered in the preoperative holding area. Some institutions have a separate "block room" where the anesthetic agent is administered and the block is allowed time to fully take effect prior to transport to the operating room. However, it is sometimes difficult to time the block so that the patient is ready when the operating room becomes available.

Intravenous Regional Anesthesia

One of the most common extremity blocks is intravenous regional anesthesia (IVRA), also called Bier block. IVRA is faster and easier to administer than brachial plexus block and onset is immediate. This technique can be employed for procedures on upper and lower distal extremities, although it is most frequently used for procedures on hands. It is particularly useful for soft tissue procedures lasting 1 hour or less such as release of carpal tunnel, trigger finger, or moderate Dupuytren contracture.

Lidocaine is the most common agent used for IVRA. For upper extremity procedures, 50 mL of 0.5% lidocaine provides 45 to 60 minutes of anesthesia. Epinephrine is not used with lidocaine to prolong effect because IVRA duration is dependent upon tourniquet time rather than an agent's particular duration. Bupivacaine is not generally used for IVRA because of the risk of cardiotoxicity.

For a procedure on the hand, for example, a pneumatic or electric double-cuffed tourniquet is placed around the patient's proximal (upper) arm. An intravenous catheter is inserted in a dorsal vein of the hand and blood is forced from the distal limb (**exsanguination**) by elevating the arm and wrapping it tightly with an Esmarch rubber bandage (Fig. 14-12). The proximal tourniquet cuff is inflated to 100 mm Hg greater than the patient's systolic blood pressure and the bandage is removed. Approximately 40 to 50 mL of 0.5% lidocaine is injected into the catheter and the catheter is removed. The arm may present with a blotchy appearance due to incomplete exsanguination. The tourniquet remains inflated throughout the procedure to keep the anesthetic agent in the area. If the cuff pressure becomes too uncomfortable for the patient, the distal cuff is inflated and the proximal cuff is deflated, which provides a measure of relief. IVRA is both rapid and effective; but there may be some discomfort caused by exsanguination and tourniquet use. Often the patient requires mild sedation.

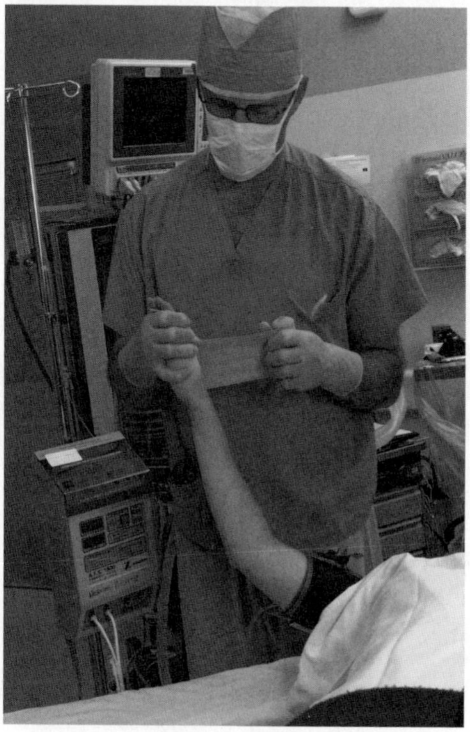

Figure 14-12 Patient's extremity is exsanguinated prior to administration of an intravenous regional (Bier) block.

Once the surgical procedure is completed, the tourniquet cuff is released slowly to avoid rapid infusion of the anesthetic into the systemic circulation. The most significant risk of IVRA is tourniquet failure, which could cause a toxic volume of anesthetic agent to rapidly enter systemic circulation. Discomfort caused by tourniquet pressure generally precludes use of IVRA for procedures lasting more than an hour. IVRA is not usually the technique of choice for fracture reduction because of discomfort caused by exsanguination and because IVRA does not provide postoperative analgesia. Another contraindication to IVRA is traumatic laceration, which may allow uncontrolled release of the agent from the limb.

SEDATION AND MONITORED ANESTHESIA CARE

The American Society of Anesthesiologists (ASA) has defined the term **monitored anesthesia care (MAC)** as a specific anesthesia service for a diagnostic or therapeutic procedure that includes all aspects of anesthesia care—before, during, and after the procedure. According to the ASA Position on Monitored Anesthesia Care (as updated September 2, 2008), MAC may include varying levels of sedation, analgesia, and anxiolysis as needed. The levels of sedation for diagnostic or therapeutic procedures range on a scale from minimal sedation (anxiolysis) to moderate sedation/analgesia (conscious sedation) to deep sedation/analgesia to general anesthesia. The anesthesia provider monitors all vital signs including the patient's heart rate and ECG, BP, respirations, and oxygen saturation continuously during these procedures.

Indications for MAC include the nature of the procedure, the patient's clinical condition, and/or the potential need to convert to a general or regional anesthetic. There are many diagnostic and/or therapeutic procedures that are conducted using MAC. Some common applications for MAC include colonoscopy, cataract extraction, pacemaker insertion, venous access port or catheter insertion, or placement of a dialysis access graft. Agents that may be administered during MAC include midazolam (Versed), fentanyl (Sublimaze), alfentanil (Alfenta), meperidine (Demerol), and propofol (Diprivan).

ADVANCED PRACTICES FOR THE SURGICAL FIRST ASSISTANT

CHAPTER 14—Monitoring Local Anesthesia and Regional Anesthesia

Key Terms

- circumoral
- erythema
- para-aminobenzoic acid (PABA)
- pain threshold
- pain tolerance
- tinnitus
- urticaria

CLASSIFICATIONS OF LOCAL ANESTHETICS

Local anesthetics are classified into two groups: aminoesters (esters) and aminoamides (amides). The structural difference of these two agents is the pathway in which they are metabolized and their allergic potential. Esters are relatively unstable in solution and are rapidly hydrolyzed in the body by acetylcholinesterase at the neuromuscular junction. One of the metabolic products of hydrolysis is **para-aminobenzoic acid (PABA)**, which is associated with hypersensitivity and allergic reactions. Ester agents include cocaine, procaine, tetracaine, and chloroprocaine.

Amides are relatively stable in solution, and are slowly metabolized by the enzymes in the liver. Allergic reactions are extremely rare and so amides are more commonly used in current clinical practice. Amides include lidocaine, prilocaine, bupivacaine, ropivacaine, and mepivacaine. A simple way to remember which local anesthetics are amides is to look at their generic spelling: the letter "i" appears twice.

CAUTION

Because amides are metabolized in the liver, care should be used in patients with severe liver disease or patients taking medication that interferes with the metabolism. Monitoring for signs of toxicity is critical.

ADVERSE EFFECTS OF LOCAL ANESTHETICS

In the surgical first assistant role, it is imperative to understand that the principal adverse effects of local anesthetics are allergic reactions and systemic toxicity. Keep in mind that aminoamides are less allergenic than aminoesters (due to the metabolic product PABA) and, although rare, allergic reactions can be life-threatening.

Allergic reactions are classified into two categories: local and systemic. A local allergic reaction (hypersensitivity) is similar to allergic contact dermatitis. Clinical signs may include **erythema**, **urticaria**, and edema. Systemic allergic reactions (anaphylactic signs) may include generalized erythema, urticaria, facial edema, wheezing, bronchoconstriction, cyanosis, nausea, vomiting, hypotension, and cardiovascular collapse. Treatment is symptomatic and supportive (see Chapter 16).

Systemic toxicity of local anesthetics is due to excess concentration of the medication in the blood. This effect is most often encountered after an accidental intravascular injection, administration of an excessive dose or rate of injection of the anesthetic, delayed drug clearance, or administration into vascular tissues. See Table A for maximum dosages of common local agents.

Systemic toxicity of local anesthetics involves the CNS and the cardiovascular system. Signs and symptoms of CNS toxicity may include **tinnitus**, **circumoral** numbness, metallic taste in the mouth, lightheadedness, visual disturbances, nausea and/or vomiting, slurred speech, muscular twitching, drowsiness, seizures, and coma. Cardiovascular toxicity can produce reduced cardiac contractility, vasodilation, and dysrhythmias. Peripheral effects include vasoconstriction at low doses and vasodilation at higher doses, which results in hypotension. Signs and symptoms of cardiovascular toxicity include chest pain, shortness of breath, palpitations, lightheadedness, diaphoresis, and syncope. Severe systemic toxicity is treated by maintaining the patient's airway, and administering oxygen and fluids. Seizures are controlled with diazepam, thiopental, or succinylcholine. Cardiac instability may be managed with vasodilators, antiarrhythmics, and inotropes. Systemic absorption of the anesthetic can be reduced by one third with the addition of a vasoconstrictor such as epinephrine.

CONCENTRATION OR DOSAGE

Local anesthetics are presented in percent of concentration or percent of strength. They are calculated as the number of grams of medication in 100 mL of solution. Therefore, a 2% lidocaine solution is 2 g of medication in 100 mL of solution. A further breakdown of this concept would be 2 g equals 2000 mg; therefore, each 100 mL of solution contains 2000 mg of lidocaine. Breaking it down further, 1 mL contains 20 mg of lidocaine. A quick calculation is to move the decimal point one place to the right as this will determine mg/mL of local anesthetic. Examples are:

2.0% = 20 mg/mL
1.0% = 10 mg/mL
0.25% = 2.5 mg/mL

Table A Maximum Dosages of Commonly Used Local Anesthetic Agents*

Agent	Concentration	Maximum Dosage Guidelines (Total cumulative adult dose per procedure)	Onset	Duration
Esters				
Procaine (Novocain)	0.25%-0.5%	7 mg/kg, not to exceed 350-600 mg (infiltrative)	2-5 min	15-60 min
Chloroprocaine (Nesacaine)	1%-2%	w/o epinephrine: 11 mg/kg, not to exceed 800 mg; w/epinephrine: 14 mg/kg, not to exceed 1000 mg (infiltrative)	6-12 min	15-30 min
Tetracaine (Pontocaine)	0.5%	Not to exceed 20 mg (topical application)	3-8 min	30-60 min
Amides				
Lidocaine (Xylocaine)	1%-2%	w/o epinephrine: 4.5-5 mg/kg, not to exceed 300 mg; w/epinephrine: 7 mg/kg, not to exceed 500 mg (infiltrative)	< 2 min < 2 min	w/o epinephrine: 60-120 min; w/epinephrine: 60-400 min
Mepivacaine (Carbocaine)	1%	7 mg/kg, not to exceed 400 mg (infiltrative)	3-5 min	w/o epinephrine: 45-90 min; w/epinephrine 120-360 min
Bupivacaine (Marcaine)	0.25%	w/o epinephrine: 2.5 mg/kg, not to exceed 175 mg; w/epinephrine: not to exceed 225 mg (infiltrative)	5 min	w/o epinephrine 120-240 min; w/epinephrine: 240-420 min
Ropivacaine (Naropin)	0.5%	5 mg. not to exceed 200 mg (for minor nerve block)	15-30 min	120-360 min

**It should be noted that sources vary slightly in onset and duration times.*

Local anesthetics are typically in lower concentrations when used for infiltration anesthesia. Infiltration anesthesia involves administration of the anesthetic intradermally, subcutaneously, or submucosally across the nerve paths that supply the involved body areas. The dose depends upon the type of procedure, the degree of anesthesia required, and the patient's condition.

A reduced dosage of local anesthetic is indicated for patients who are debilitated, acutely ill, very young, very old, and have liver disease, arteriosclerosis, or occlusive arterial disease.

EPINEPHRINE ADDITIVE TO LOCAL ANESTHETICS

Epinephrine acts as a vasoconstrictor that not only decreases bleeding but also slows the rate of systemic absorption of the anesthetic. This allows the body more time to metabolize the anesthetic and prolongs the anesthetic effects. Given the slower absorption rate, a larger volume of anesthetic with epinephrine can be injected without causing toxicity. Epinephrine can be used in a variety of surgical procedures. An example of this would be septoplasty with inferior turbinectomies. A local anesthetic with epinephrine is beneficial because of the vascularity of the nasal mucosa and the confined space within the nasal cavity.

Concentrations of epinephrine are described as a ratio (for example, 1:100,000 or 1:200,000) and are calculated as the number of grams of the agent in a given volume of solution. The previous examples show 1 g of epinephrine in 100,000 mL of solution and 1 g of epinephrine in 200,000 mL of solution, respectively. If the number of grams is always 1, then the greater the number on the other side of the ratio, the less concentrated the solution becomes. A 1:100,000 solution of epinephrine is stronger than a 1:200,000 solution.

CAUTION

Local anesthetics containing epinephrine should never be used in an area where vascular supply is minimal. For example: fingers, tip of nose, penis, and toes.

POSTOPERATIVE PAIN MANAGEMENT WITH LOCAL AND REGIONAL ANESTHETICS

Traditionally oral or intramuscular anesthetics or opioids have been used for postoperative pain management. The patient's reaction to pain is subjective and depends upon the individual's perception of pain, **pain threshold**, and **tolerance**; as well as the physiologic changes due to an operative procedure. Despite the belief that opioids provide optimal pain relief, studies have shown that more than half of the surgical patients receiving opioids remain in moderate to severe pain. The surgical first assistant should also recognize that narcotics such as the opioids can cause respiratory depression to the point of respiratory arrest if the dose is too great. The recognition that unrelieved pain contributes to perioperative morbidity and mortality has inspired preemptive analgesic techniques to control postoperative pain. The surgical first assistant may be involved with implementing various techniques for pain control during the procedure.

Local anesthetics can be administered into the incision sites or intra-articularly. An example is bupivacaine (Marcaine), which can provide up to approximately 6 hours of pain control. The maximum dose of bupivacaine for infiltration is 175 mg (70 mL of 0.25% solution). Another alternative is continuous local infusion therapy (site specific infusion) when a catheter is placed in the incision site or intra-articularly and a continuous infusion or boluses of local anesthetic can be administered with patient-controlled pumps. This is known as patient-controlled analgesia or PCA. The pump dispenses 2 mL or 4 mL of local anesthetic to the surgical site per hour. Depending on the type of pump a 4-mL bolus chamber can be squeezed providing additional medication to the site. These pumps are disposable and have 2-day or 4-day duration.

ASSISTANT *ADVICE*

Local anesthetics containing epinephrine will have red labels and/or red printing noting the concentration of epinephrine.

Advanced Practices Bibliography

Fulcher E, Fulcher R, Soto C: *Pharmacology principles and applications*, ed 2, St. Louis, 2009, Saunders/Elsevier.

Fuller JK: *Surgical technology: principles and practice*, ed 5, St. Louis, 2010, Saunders/Elsevier.

Jensen SC, Peppers MP: *Pharmacology and drug administration for imaging technologists*, ed 2, St. Louis, 2006, Mosby/Elsevier.

Moscou K, Snipe K: *Pharmacology for pharmacy technicians*, St. Louis, 2009, Mosby/Elsevier.

Rothrock J: *Alexander's care of the patient in surgery*, ed 13, St. Louis, 2007, Mosby/Elsevier.

Advanced Practices Internet Resources

eMedicine from WebMD: *Local Anesthetic Agents, Infiltrative Administration by Mary L Windle, PharmD.* http://emedicine.medscape.com/article/149178-overview.

eMedicine from WebMD: *Toxicity, Local Anesthetics by Raffi Kapitanyan, MD and Mark Su, MD.* http://emedicine.medscape.com/article/819628-overview.

eMedicine from WebMD: *Regional Anesthesia for Postoperative Pain Control by Raymond Graber, MD and Matthew Kraay, MD.* http://emedicine.com/orthoped/topic581.htm.

McKinley Medical: *ACCUFUSER Post-Op Pain Control Pump.* www.drmele.com/_pdf/AccufuserPatientGuide.pdf.

RxList: *Naropin.* www.rxlist.com/naropin-drug.htm.

RxMed: *PONTOCAINE.* www.rxmed.com/b.main/b2.pharmaceutical/b2.1.monographs/CPS-%20Monographs/CPS-%20(General%20Monographs-%20P)/PONTOCAINE.html.

Savoie FH, Field LD, Jenkins RN, et al: The pain control infusion pump for postoperative pain control in shoulder surgery, *Arthroscopy* 16(4):339–342, 2000. Available at www.ncbi.nlm.nih.gov/pubmed/10802469. Accessed July 28, 2010.

http://www.moog.com/products/medical-pump-systems/post-operative-pain-management-systems/accufuser/.

Virtual Anaesthesia Textbook. www.virtual-anaesthesia-textbook.com/index.shtml.

WebMD: *Pain Management: Patient-Controlled Analgesia (PCA).* www.webmd.com/pain-management/guide/pca.

Advanced Practices: Learning the Language (Key Terms)

Using your textbook or a standard medical dictionary, look up and write the definitions of each term.

- circumoral
- erythema
- para-aminobenzoic acid (PABA)
- pain threshold
- pain tolerance
- tinnitus
- urticaria

Advanced Practices: Review Questions

1. Explain the difference between aminoesters and aminoamides.
2. Why should patients with hepatitis be closely monitored while on amides?
3. Name the two principal adverse effects upon the patient from local anesthetics.
4. What is the difference between a local and a systemic allergic reaction? Give clinical signs of each.
5. What causes systemic toxicity of local anesthetics? Give two symptoms.
6. Why can a larger volume of local anesthetic with epinephrine be injected into tissues without causing toxicity?

KEY CONCEPTS

- The vital signs of all patients undergoing surgical intervention must be closely monitored.
- Vital signs monitored on all patients include heart rate and rhythm, oxygen saturation, BP, and respirations.
- Additional parameters measured under general anesthesia include temperature, expired CO_2, consciousness level, and neuromuscular function.
- Certain patient conditions and surgical procedures may require additional invasive monitoring such as arterial pressure, central venous pressure, or pulmonary artery pressure.
- When basic monitoring parameters are established, the appropriate anesthesia method is administered. More invasive monitors may be placed after the patient is under anesthesia.
- Four major classifications of anesthesia techniques are local, regional, sedation/MAC, and general anesthesia.
- Several agents are used to produce local anesthesia and the surgical technologist handles these agents on a daily basis.
- Several techniques are used to accomplish regional anesthesia, and there are many applications for these techniques.

Bibliography

Aronson J: *Meyler's side effects of drugs used in anesthesia,* Amsterdam, 2009, Elsevier.

Evers A, Maze M: *Anesthetic pharmacology: physiologic principles and clinical practice,* St. Louis, 2004, Churchill Livingstone/Elsevier.

Karlet M: *Nurse Anesthesia Secrets,* St. Louis, 2005, Mosby/Elsevier.

Kost M: *Moderate sedation/analgesia,* ed 2, St Louis, 2004, Saunders/Elsevier.

Nagelhout J, Plaus K: *Nurse anesthesia,* ed 4, St. Louis, 2010, Saunders/Elsevier.

Rathmell JP: *Regional anesthesia: the requisites in anesthesiology,* Philadelphia, 2004, Mosby/Elsevier.

Stoelting R, Miller R: *Basics of anesthesia,* ed 5, St. Louis, 2007, Churchill Livingstone/Elsevier.

Internet Resources

American Association of Nurse Anesthetists: *Scope and Standards for Nurse Anesthesia Practice,* © 2007. www.aana.com/uploadedFiles/Resources/Practice_Documents/scope_ stds_nap07_2007.pdf.

American Society of Anesthesiologists: *ASA House of Delegates, Standards for Basic Anesthetic, Monitoring.* www.asahq.org/publicationsAndServices/standards/02.pdf.

American Society of Anesthesiologists: *ASA Position on Monitored Anesthesia Care.* www.asahq.org/publicationsAndServices/standards/23.pdf.

American Society of Anesthesiologists: *ASA Statement on Continuum of Depth of Sedation.* www.asahq.org/publicationsAndServices/standards/20.pdf.

American Society of Anesthesiologists: *ASA Statement on Distinguishing MAC from Conscious Sedation.* www.asahq.org/publicationsAndServices/standards/35.pdf.

American Society of Anesthesiologists: Updated Report by the ASA Task Force on Sedation and Analgesia by Non-Anesthesiologists, *Anesthesiology* 96:1004–1017, 2002. Available at www.asahq.org/publicationsAndServices/sedation1017.pdf.

APP Pharmaceuticals, LLC: *NAROPIN.* www.naropin-us.com/.

Drugs.com: *Bupivacaine.* www.drugs.com/pro/bupivacaine.html.

Naropin Feb 2010 FDA: Council on Surgical and Perioperative Safety: *Patient Monitoring. www.cspsteam.org/patientmonitoring/patientmonitoring.html.*

Qualified Providers of Sedation and Analgesia. www.aana.com/qualifiedproviders_sedation.aspx.

www.accessdata.fda.gov/drugsatfda_docs/label/2010/020533s020s021lbl.pdf.

LEARNING THE LANGUAGE (KEY TERMS)

Using your textbook or a standard medical dictionary, look up and write the definitions of each term.

auscultation
blood pressure
capnometry
electrocardiography
epidural
exsanguination
intrathecally
local anesthesia
monitored anesthesia care (MAC)
pulse oximetry
regional anesthesia

REVIEW QUESTIONS

1. How is each physiologic vital sign monitored in surgery?
2. Which types of monitoring are considered invasive?
3. What are the four major types of anesthesia?
4. What kinds of surgical procedures may be performed under local or regional anesthesia?
5. Which agents are used to accomplish local and/or regional anesthesia?
6. What should you know about the use of epinephrine with local anesthetic agents?
7. Can you list some types of regional anesthesia? What types of procedures may be performed under each?

CRITICAL THINKING

Scenario 1

Ms. Ortiz is a 78-year-old woman with emphysema. She has recently undergone a hysterectomy for uterine cancer. The pelvic lymph nodes were positive for cancer. She has been admitted to surgery for placement of a venous access port for chemotherapy.

1. Would you select local anesthesia or monitored anesthesia care? Justify your answer.
2. How would her medical condition affect the pulse oximetry measurements? Why?

Scenario 2

Mr. Delano is a 69-year-old man admitted to surgery for placement of a transvenous pacemaker. The surgeon's preference card indicates that you should have 50 mL of 1% lidocaine with epinephrine 1:100,000 on the back table for injection.

1. Would you select local anesthesia or monitored anesthesia care? Justify your answer.
2. Is the agent indicated on the preference card acceptable for this procedure? Why or why not?

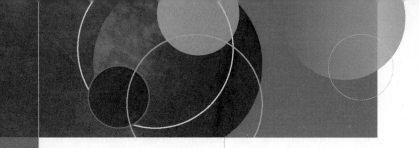

CHAPTER 15 General Anesthesia

OBJECTIVES *After completing this chapter, you should be able to:*

1. Define terminology related to anesthesia.
2. Discuss indications for general anesthesia.
3. Identify anesthesia equipment.
4. Explain the basic components of a general anesthetic.
5. List methods of inducing general anesthesia.
6. Define the phases of general anesthesia.
7. Discuss options for airway management.
8. Describe the process of endotracheal intubation.
9. Discuss the concept of awareness under anesthesia.
10. Identify categories and purposes of agents used in general anesthesia.
11. List agents used to accomplish general anesthesia in each category.
12. Identify generic and trade names of common agents used in anesthesia.
13. State the phase of anesthesia in which various agents are administered.
14. Compare and contrast depolarizing and nondepolarizing muscle relaxants.

KEY TERMS

anesthesia
emergence phase
emulsion
endotracheal (ET) tube
extubation
fasciculation
induction phase
intubation
lacrimation
laryngeal masked airway (LMA)
maintenance phase
minimum alveolar concentration (MAC)
opioid
post-anesthesia care unit (PACU)
preinduction phase
rapid sequence induction (RSI)

General **anesthesia** is a systemic state of anesthesia, rather than anesthesia in a large area (regional) or a specific site (local). The term *anesthesia* is literally defined as an absence of sensation, but in the context of general anesthesia it is more correctly defined as a drug-induced temporary loss of consciousness during which patients are not arousable, even by painful stimulation.

The decision to use a general anesthetic is based both on the requirements of the surgical procedure to be performed and on the individual patient. For instance, a general anesthetic is used when there are multiple operative sites or for a procedure on an area that is difficult to block regionally, such as the thoracic or abdominal cavities. Examples of surgical procedures on multiple locations include skin grafts, breast reconstruction, and autologous bone grafts. Surgical procedures that require an absolutely motionless field, such as retinal surgery, are also performed under general anesthesia. In addition, the expected duration of the surgical procedure may influence the choice of general anesthesia because of patient discomfort when the patient is required to lie flat on the operating room bed for a long period of time.

Patient factors that influence the selection of general anesthesia include patient age, cognitive ability, mental or emotional state, and (when possible) patient preference. Patient age is a primary consideration in that children are almost never candidates for regional or local anesthesia, regardless of the surgical procedure being performed. General anesthesia is usually indicated when the patient's cognitive ability is impaired, causing an inability to understand, communicate, or cooperate with directions required in regional or local anesthesia. For example, mentally disabled patients or those with Alzheimer disease may not be capable of understanding what is happening to them, so general anesthesia is the method of choice. Patient preference is taken into account when possible; for example, if a patient is very frightened at the idea of a spinal needle being inserted into the back and is in otherwise good health, general anesthesia may be a more appropriate choice than a regional.

Historically, early agents used to produce general anesthesia had unwanted side effects—they were extremely toxic to the patient or they were explosive (Insight 15-1). However, modern advances in the pharmacology of anesthesia have produced many agents that accomplish general anesthesia with a high degree of

INSIGHT 15-1 Yesterday and Today: Anesthesia

In today's world, surgery and anesthesia are inseparable concepts. However, this was not always true. Surgery can actually be divided into two eras: preanesthesia and postanesthesia. In the preanesthesia era, surgery was based on speed, because the patient would often die from hemorrhage, shock, or the trauma of the operation. Ironically, shock may have helped to relieve some of the pain before death occurred. The postanesthesia era began in the 19th century when discoveries were finally published, accepted, and used.

Attempts to alleviate pain probably date back as far as humankind has experienced suffering. These first attempts treated pain as an evil spirit or demon, and the idea was to frighten it away. Thus, early anesthesia involved tattoos, jewelry, talismans, amulets, and charms. Pain relievers existed and were used in ancient times, but they were impure, unsafe, and unreliable. Ancient pain remedies documented include a Babylonian clay tablet from approximately 2250 BC that gives the remedy for a toothache. Early Egyptian surgeons applied pressure to nerves or blood vessels, which caused insensibility to a specific part of the body for an operation.

Many early methods of pain control used drugs. Alcohol was often used in the form of spirits or wines. Along with opium and marijuana, ancient literature contains many references to the mandragora (mandrake, or mandragon) plant as a pain reliever that produced a confused mental state. Dioscorides, a first-century Greek physician, administered the mandragora root boiled in wine to his patients before they went under his knife. Mandragora was also known as the "potion of the condemned," because it was given to criminals to decrease the agonies of crucifixion.

Besides drugs, other pain-control methods were used in the preanesthesia era. One method was to produce unconsciousness by compressing the carotid arteries to decrease heart rate; another was to place a wooden bowl over the patient's head and strike the bowl to cause a concussion. Another method came from China in the form of acupuncture, which decreased pain sensations. A third method was cryothermia. This was documented in England in 1050 in an Anglo-Saxon manuscript that instructed the surgeon to wait a while before making the incision as the patient sat in cold water "until it can become deadened."

The word *anesthesia* comes from the Greek word *anaisthesis,* which means "no sensation." *Anesthesia* appeared in *Bailey's English Dictionary* in 1721.

IN SIGHT 15-1 Yesterday and Today: Anesthesia—Cont'd

However, the term itself was reportedly coined by Oliver Wendell Holmes in a letter in 1846.

Unfortunately, many agents with anesthetic properties were known for generations but were not applied in surgery. The great alchemist Paracelsus (1493?-1541) mixed sulfuric acid with alcohol and distilled his concoction. He believed this mixture, called sweet vitriol, could quiet suffering and relieve pain. We know this mixture today as ether. Nitrous oxide was discovered by Joseph Priestly in 1772. However, both nitrous oxide and ether were popularized by traveling "professors" as entertainment tools. Volunteers would inhale the gases and become intoxicated. This fad produced "laughing gas parties" and "ether frolics." Little known to the public at the time was the fact that in 1800 a man named Humphrey Davy had described the use of nitrous oxide to relieve pain produced by a wisdom tooth.

It was after one of these public demonstrations of ether that a young physician named Crawford W. Long contemplated its use as an anesthetic during surgery. He was inspired when he saw friends receive injuries without pain while under the vapor's influence. So, on March 30, 1842, Dr. Long administered ether to James M. Venable and successfully removed a tumor from the patient's neck. A dentist named Horace Wells observed a similar demonstration of nitrous oxide in 1844 and used it in his dental practice for many years to relieve pain from tooth extractions. Unfortunately, Wells's demonstration to Harvard Medical School was not a success, possibly because of incomplete administration of the gas, and nitrous oxide was not accepted. Wells's partner, Dr. William T.G. Morton, realized that although nitrous oxide was unreliable, an alternative could be found in ether vapor. After numerous experiments, Morton contacted Dr. John Warren, a senior surgeon of the Massachusetts General Hospital. A demonstration was arranged for October 16, 1846. This demonstration was a success as a tumor was removed from the jaw of a 20-year-old male, who remained insensible throughout the procedure. Thus the postanesthesia era was officially begun with Dr. Warren's famous remark, "Gentlemen, this is no humbug."

The widespread use of anesthesia began in England on April 7, 1853, when Queen Victoria accepted the use of chloroform during childbirth. Her physician was Dr. Sir James Young Simpson. Chloroform had been discovered in 1831; however, its use by the queen led to its acceptance by the medical community. From these beginnings, anesthesia has developed into the vital branch of medicine we know today.

safety. Several classes of drugs are used to achieve general anesthesia, often in combination. The desired result is a patient who (1) remains unconscious, (2) is pain free, (3) retains no memory of the event, (4) is immobile, and (5) maintains normal cardiovascular function. Although several theories have been suggested, the exact mechanism of agents used to induce and maintain general anesthesia is still not clearly understood. Different categories of agents affect different parts of the body at the cellular level; for example:

- Drugs used to produce an unconscious state affect the reticular activating system in the brain stem.
- Agents used to produce analgesia (opioids) bind with receptors on cell membranes in the brain and spinal cord, altering the transmission of pain signals.
- Muscle relaxants work at the neuromuscular junction of skeletal muscles.

The ability to safely provide general anesthesia is an art as well as a science. The anesthesia provider manages a delicate balance of agents to achieve the necessary components of general anesthesia while maintaining the patient in a stable physiologic state. Additionally, the anesthesia provider manages the timing of these agents so that the anesthetic effect is wearing off as the surgical procedure is concluding. In most situations, the goal is to have patients awake, alert, and breathing on their own before transport to the **post-anesthesia care unit (PACU)**.

In addition to pharmacologic agents, various pieces of equipment that assist in the process of administering general anesthesia are used by the anesthesia provider. Much of this equipment is integrated into the anesthesia workstation (Fig. 15-1). Components of an anesthesia workstation include manual and automatic ventilation systems, breathing circuits, oxygen and nitrous oxide

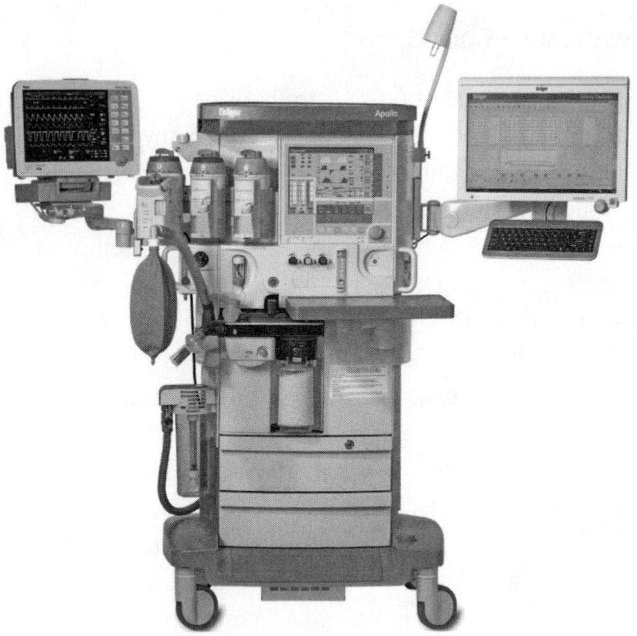

Figure 15-1 An anesthesia workstation. © *Drager Medical GmbH, Lubek-Germany (All rights reserved. Not to be reproduced without written permission.)*

(N_2O) central pipeline hoses and backup tanks, vaporizers (for volatile gases), pressure regulators and gas-mixing components, and gas-scavenging systems. Exhaled gases are routed through a CO_2 absorbent (soda lime) canister. A number of respiratory and physiologic monitors are used, including electrocardiogram (ECG), pulse oximeter, blood pressure (BP) monitor, level of consciousness monitor, and instruments to measure inhaled and exhaled oxygen, carbon dioxide, and anesthetic agent levels. Physiologic and respiratory monitors are equipped with audible alarm systems for additional safety. Alarms are set to emit a signal when readings occur outside of preset parameters. Each component is checked for proper function prior to admitting the patient to the operating room. Additional equipment used to assist the delivery of anesthesia and provide physiologic support to the patient includes infusion control devices (see Chapter 11, Fig. 11-5), thermoregulatory devices, fluid warmers (see Chapter 11, Fig. 11-9), and fluid pumps.

COMPONENTS OF GENERAL ANESTHESIA

General anesthesia is accomplished by administering agents to achieve four major goals. These goals, or components, of general anesthesia are unconsciousness (a state of being unaware), analgesia (painlessness), amnesia (memory impairment), and immobility (skeletal muscle relaxation) (Box 15-1). That is, the patient must remain unconscious, pain free, and immobile while retaining no explicit memory of the event. Different agents are used to accomplish each of these required components. The anesthesia provider monitors the effects of the agents administered and works to maintain the patient's cardiovascular stability throughout the course of anesthesia.

ADMINISTRATION METHODS

Two methods, or routes, are used to administer general anesthetic agents: inhalation and intravenous injection. An inhalation anesthetic is administered as a gas the patient breathes, whereas intravenous agents are administered directly into the bloodstream through a small catheter placed in a vein (Fig. 15-2). No intravenous agent in current use can provide all the required effects and only those effects, so a combination of administration methods is used. The term *balanced anesthesia* refers to the technique that uses a combination of inhalation and intravenous agents to accomplish general anesthesia. Another (but much less common) anesthesia technique uses a combination of a regional block, such as an epidural, and a light general anesthetic. This technique is useful for select patients undergoing major vascular procedures because it decreases the amount of general anesthetic agents required, helping to maintain cardiovascular stability, and provides an effective means of postoperative pain control. This technique is also valuable for use in selected orthopedic, thoracic, and other surgical specialty procedures. In the 1990s, the rectal route was used to induce anesthesia in children but results were inconsistent. This method of administration of anesthesia is rarely used in current practice.

Box 15-1 COMPONENTS OF GENERAL ANESTHESIA

Amnesia	Muscle relaxation
Analgesia	Unconsciousness

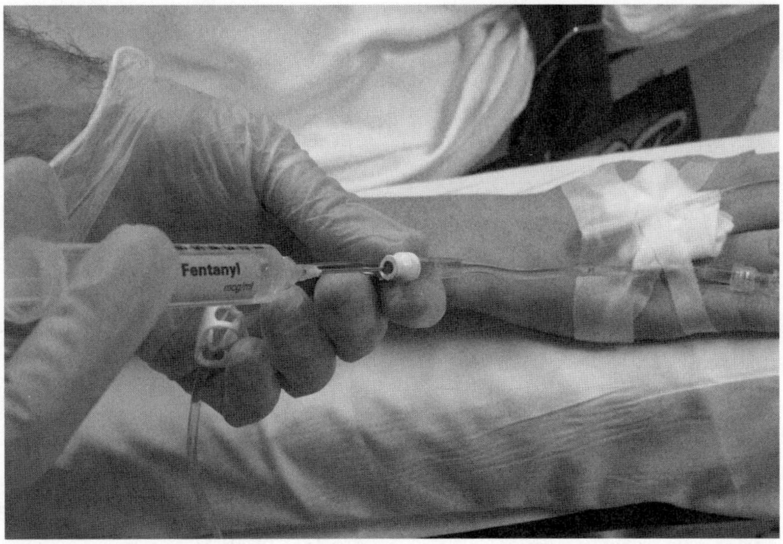

Figure 15-2 Some anesthetic agents are administered intravenously.

PHASES OF GENERAL ANESTHESIA

There are five phases of general anesthesia: preinduction, induction, maintenance, emergence, and recovery (Box 15-2). Preinduction includes preoperative assessment and preparation of the patient, both physically and psychologically (see Chapter 13). The intraoperative phases of general anesthesia are induction, maintenance, and emergence. Recovery is the postoperative phase. Phases of general anesthesia are not to be confused with the concept of stages of anesthesia (Insight 15-2), which was based on the effects of ether.

PREINDUCTION PHASE

The **preinduction phase** begins as the patient is admitted to the preoperative holding area and continues up to the point of administration of anesthetic agents. In this phase, the patient is assessed and prepared for anesthesia and surgery. Part of the history and physical exam specific to anesthesia includes assessment of the patient's airway—even for patients not scheduled to undergo general anesthesia. A history is obtained regarding airway issues and a physical examination is conducted to determine neck mobility and assess other factors that might indicate potential for a difficult airway. Classification systems such as Mallampati score and Cormack-Lehane score are used to categorize the patient's risk for difficult airway management. Appropriate medications are administered during this phase as ordered by the anesthesia provider (see Chapter 13). One goal of the preinduction phase is to have the patient arrive in the operating room calm, physiologically stable, and fully prepared for anesthesia.

The preinduction phase continues as the patient is transported to the operating room and transferred to the operating room bed. The circulator secures the safety belt over the patient's thighs and obtains warm blankets for patient comfort. The anesthesia provider begins by attaching monitoring devices to the patient and obtaining baseline vital signs. The vital functions of all patients receiving a general anesthetic are continuously monitored (see Chapter 14). Heart rate and ECG, BP, respirations, oxygen saturation, expired gases

Box 15-2 PHASES OF GENERAL ANESTHESIA

Preinduction
Induction
Maintenance
Emergence
Recovery

INSIGHT 15-2 Stages of Anesthesia

Classic texts describe four stages of anesthesia. These stages are based on the physiologic effects of ether, one of the first anesthetic agents. Each stage was based on observations of body movement, respiratory rhythm, oculomotor reflexes, and muscle tone.

Stage 1. *Amnesia:* Induction to loss of consciousness.

Stage 2. *Delirium* (or excitement): Patient is unconscious but still responding reflexively and unpredictably to certain stimuli.

Stage 3. *Surgical anesthesia:* Adequate depth of anesthesia is reached so that an incision can be made and procedure performed without negative patient response (such as hypertension or tachycardia).

Stage 4. *Overdose* (or medullary depression): Level of anesthesia is so deep that cardiovascular and respiratory function is compromised to the point of collapse due to depression of those centers in the brain.

It is important to note that the stages as traditionally described are no longer as useful in anesthesia practice. Current anesthetic agents are able to bring the patient more quickly through stages 1 and 2, and so may exhibit different signs during induction and make the early stages more difficult to identify. These signs, based on muscular responses, are also invalidated with the current frequent practice of administration of muscle relaxants. Additionally, modern anesthetic agents are much more predictable than ether, so stage 4 is less likely to occur.

(end-tidal CO_2, O_2, and anesthetic gases), and temperature are closely observed to constantly assess the physiologic status of the patient. An anesthesia mask is usually placed over the patient's nose and mouth and 100% oxygen is administered, a process known as preoxygenation. This practice is performed to bring the oxygen saturation of the patient's blood to the highest possible level prior to induction.

INDUCTION PHASE

The **induction phase** begins when medications are administered to initiate general anesthesia and concludes when an adequate depth of anesthesia is reached and the patient's airway is secured.

CAUTION

The patient may experience a period of agitation or excitement during induction. Hearing sensitivity is also heightened (hyperacusis) during induction of anesthesia. The effect of loud noises and sudden movement may be intensified during this time, inducing a stress reaction in the patient. The stress response may be characterized by unstable cardiovascular functions, which is potentially harmful to the patient. In addition, moving the patient suddenly at this time can trigger laryngospasm. Thus, the surgical technologist and all members of the surgical team must make every effort to minimize unnecessary operating room noise and movement of the patient during induction.

Induction agents are usually administered by intravenous injection. The option of masked induction with an inhalation anesthetic may be chosen for children to avoid the emotional trauma of placing an intravenous catheter. Various induction agents are used to produce an unconscious state, amnesia, and analgesia. A variation of standard induction technique called neuroleptanesthesia (Insight 15-3) was used in specific situations but is rarely used in current practice. When the patient becomes unconscious, the anesthesia provider ensures that an adequate airway is maintained.

Airway Management

The exchange of oxygen and carbon dioxide (respiration) is a vital function that must be sustained throughout any surgical procedure. An unconscious patient requires additional support to ensure optimal respiratory function and various methods of airway management are used to provide that support. The patient's airway may be managed with a mask for surgical procedures of short duration when muscle relaxation is not required, such as myringotomy with placement of pressure equalization (PE) tubes. When the patient becomes unconscious, a nasal or a pharyngeal (oral) airway may be placed as needed to displace the tongue and facilitate air exchange through the mask. The mask is held in position with straps and the anesthesia provider supports the airway by maintaining the patient's head in a chin-lift position.

In select patients, the airway may be managed with a **laryngeal masked airway (LMA)** (Fig. 15-3), also known as a supraglottic airway. An LMA consists of a flexible shaft attached to a silicone mask that is inflated

INSIGHT 15-3 Neuroleptanesthesia

Occasionally, you may hear the term *neuroleptanesthesia* used in surgery. This strange-sounding term is used to indicate an anesthetic state that produces sedation and analgesia while allowing the patient to breathe on his or her own and move on command. Also called a dissociative anesthetic state, its effects are similar to those of ketamine. Fentanyl, droperidol, and nitrous oxide are the agents used to produce neuroleptanesthesia. When indicated, this technique was used for induction of anesthesia in high-risk patients undergoing vascular procedures because of the minimal negative impact on cardiovascular and hemodynamic stability. A variation of this technique is called neuroleptic analgesia, in which pain relief is provided through the use of fentanyl and droperidol without nitrous oxide. Recently, however, the FDA has required a "Black Box" warning on droperidol because of an associated increased risk of fatal cardiac arrhythmias. Thus, the use of droperidol is significantly limited, and as a result, the techniques of neuroleptanesthesia and neuroleptic analgesia are used rarely if at all in current practice.

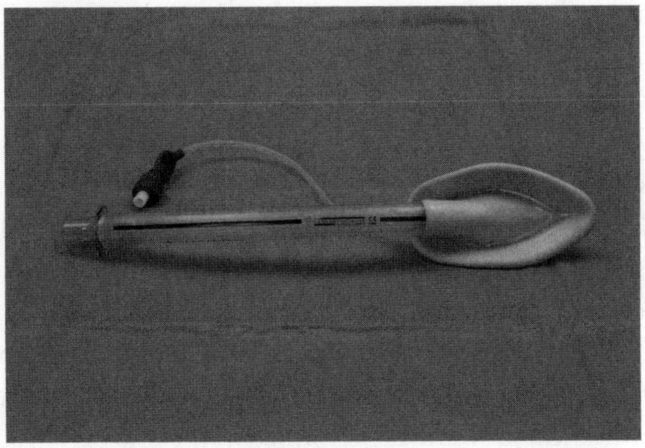

Figure 15-3 Laryngeal masked airway.

to seal the airway. Sizes range from 1 to 5 and the proper size is selected based on the patient's weight. After induction of anesthesia, an LMA is inserted and positioned in the laryngopharynx to cover the epiglottis and larynx. The LMA cuff is inflated to provide a seal, and the tube is connected to the breathing circuit. The patient may continue to breathe on his or her own (if no muscle relaxant is needed for the surgical procedure), or respirations may be controlled with the use of a ventilator or by manual ventilation (if muscle relaxants are administered). The LMA, which does not require laryngoscopy or muscle relaxation, is particularly useful for ambulatory surgical procedures. Contraindications to LMA include procedures on the oral cavity, obesity, hiatal hernia, gastroesophageal reflux disease (GERD), and low pulmonary compliance. Several variations of the LMA are available including an Intubating LMA (ILMA), LMA Ctrach, and LMA ProSeal, allowing for expanded applications in select patients.

Many patients are not appropriate candidates for masked or laryngeal masked airway and require more precise control of the airway. In addition, many surgical procedures are of longer duration, require deep muscle relaxation, or are performed in a lateral or prone position, all of which require a more highly controlled airway. Deep muscle relaxation is achieved by the administration of neuromuscular blockers, which cause temporary relaxation of skeletal muscles including the muscles of respiration. During a surgical procedure requiring deep muscle relaxation, the patient will not be breathing on his or her own, so respirations are controlled by mechanical ventilation through a tube placed into the patient's trachea called an **endotracheal (ET) tube** (Fig. 15-4). Endotracheal tubes are made of clear, flexible polyvinyl chloride (PVC) and are sized by internal diameter in 0.5-mm increments. External markings on the tube are in centimeters and are used to determine the length of tube insertion.

An ET tube is placed through the patient's mouth into the trachea to establish the most direct and precisely controlled airway. The placement of an endotracheal tube, called **intubation**, begins after induction agents and muscle relaxants are administered to render the patient unconscious and immobile.

TECH TIP

The circulator assists the anesthesia provider during intubation and should be present at the patient's head as soon as induction begins.

When the patient's airway is adequately managed with masked ventilation, a short-acting muscle relaxant

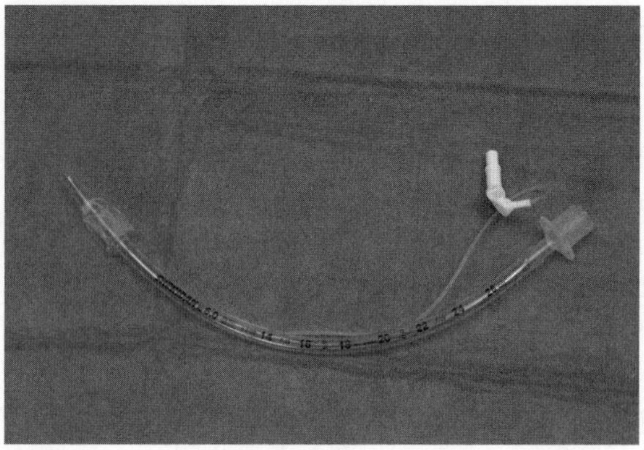

Figure 15-4 An endotracheal tube.

(neuromuscular blocker) is administered to relax the vocal cords and facilitate placement of the ET tube. When the patient is adequately relaxed to suppress the laryngeal reflex, an ET tube is inserted past the epiglottis, through the vocal cords, and into the trachea under direct visualization with a laryngoscope (Fig. 15-5). An intubating laryngoscope is somewhat similar to an operating laryngoscope and is used to retract the tongue and lift the jaw to visualize the larynx and vocal cords. Detachable laryngoscope blades such as a Macintosh (curved) or a Miller (straight) of various sizes are used to retract the patient's tongue. A flexible stylet may be placed inside the ET tube to guide the tube along the correct path, and the circulator may be asked to remove the stylet when the tube is in position. The end of the tube is placed midway between the vocal cords and the carina of the trachea (the carina is the place where the trachea bifurcates into right and left main stem bronchi). Correct placement of the ET tube is verified by clinical assessment, measurement of exhaled CO_2, and auscultation of bilateral breath sounds.

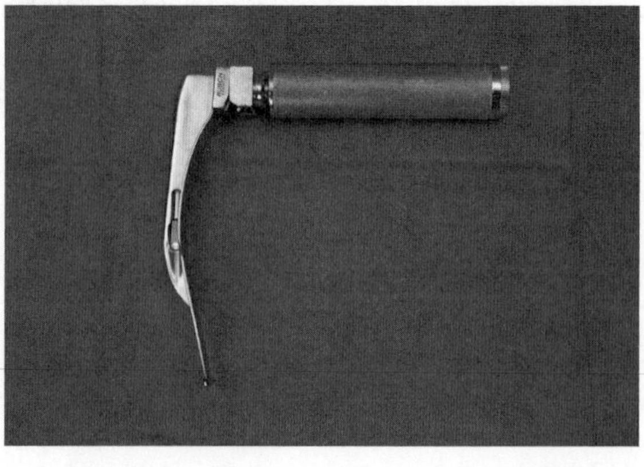

Figure 15-5 A laryngoscope.

A variation on standard induction technique called **rapid sequence induction (RSI)** may be used for patients who are at an increased risk for gastric reflux and pulmonary aspiration. RSI is used for patients who have not been NPO (especially trauma patients), and those with a history of hiatal hernia, GERD, previous gastrointestinal surgery, diabetes, or obesity. Rapid sequence induction is used to secure and control the airway quickly. The patient is preoxygenated and an induction agent is administered. Fentanyl may be given 1 to 3 minutes prior to the induction agent to minimize reaction to laryngoscopy and intubation. A non-paralyzing dose of a non-depolarizing neuromuscular blocker (such as pancuronium) and a dose of 1 to 2 mg/kg of succinylcholine (a depolarizing neuromuscular blocker) are administered. Cricoid pressure (also known as the Sellick maneuver, Fig. 15-6) is applied with the thumb and index finger to the cricoid cartilage, gently compressing the esophagus downward against the cervical vertebrae, in an effort to prevent gastric contents from entering the trachea and lungs. Cricoid pressure is maintained until the ET tube is in correct position. Placement is verified as described previously and a nasogastric tube may be placed through the mouth to empty stomach contents.

In certain circumstances, other intubation techniques may be indicated. Nasal intubation may be used for particular surgical procedures performed in the oral cavity, such as repair of mandibular fractures, when the presence of the ET tube in the mouth may not be desirable. The ET tube is inserted through the nose to the oropharynx, a laryngoscope is used to visualize the vocal cords, and a Magill forceps may be used to guide the ET tube into place.

If the preoperative evaluation indicates a potential significant problem for ventilation and intubation (difficult airway), the patient may be intubated prior to induction using fiberoptic endotracheal intubation. This technique is reserved for patients with specific conditions such as morbid obesity, a history of difficult intubation, facial deformities, laryngeal cancer, unstable cervical spine fractures, or other conditions that may compromise the airway. Preparation for intubation prior to induction begins with administration of an antisialagogue (an agent to dry salivary secretions) such as glycopyrrolate (Robinul) 0.2 mg IV approximately 30 minutes before intubation. The patient's gag reflex may be suppressed with the use of a topical anesthetic agent such as Cetacaine (a combination of benzocaine, tetracaine, and butamben) spray. Sedation is administered so that the patient can tolerate the intubation and yet continue to

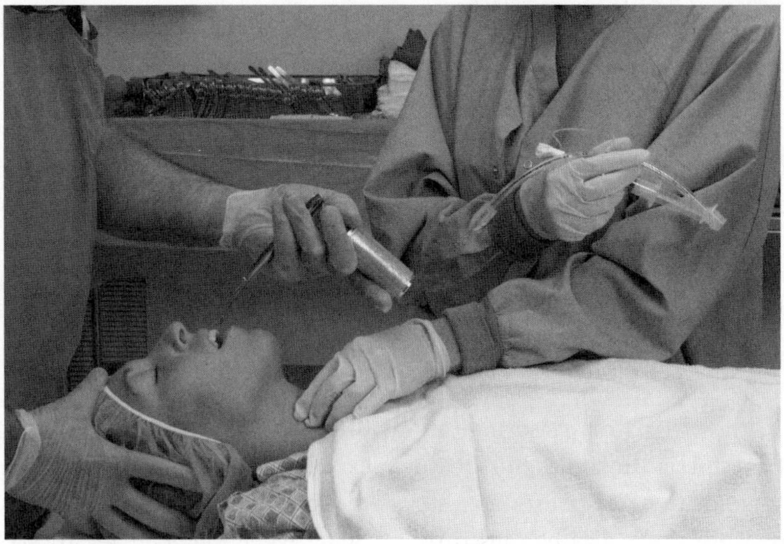

Figure 15-6 Application of cricoid pressure prior to endotracheal intubation.

breathe and protect his or her own airway. Intubation may be accomplished by nasal or oral route, depending on the situation. If a nasal intubation is selected, topical vasoconstrictors such as cocaine, oxymetazoline (Afrin), or phenylephrine may be used intranasally to prevent bleeding (epistaxis). The ET tube is loaded over a flexible fiberoptic bronchoscope, and the scope is gently guided into the trachea. The ET tube is placed in position and the bronchoscope removed.

Regardless of the method, once intubation is accomplished the ET tube is connected to a breathing circuit leading to the ventilator (Fig. 15-7). The ET tube position is verified by auscultation during the delivery of manual ventilations. When proper ET tube position is confirmed, respirations are controlled with mechanical ventilation set to the appropriate volume and rate. The ET tube is secured in position, and an adequate depth of anesthesia is achieved to begin the surgical procedure, concluding the induction phase of anesthesia.

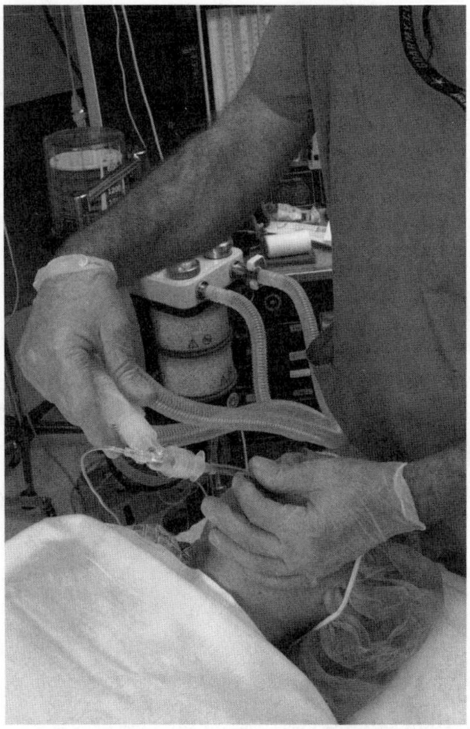

Figure 15-7 The endotracheal tube is connected to the ventilator.

MAINTENANCE PHASE

The **maintenance phase** begins as the patient's airway is established and secured and continues until the surgical procedure has been completed. Additional anesthetic agents are administered during the maintenance phase as needed to maintain a depth of anesthesia appropriate to the surgical procedure. Abdominal and thoracic procedures require a much deeper level of anesthesia than superficial procedures, for example. The patient is maintained in an unconscious state by using a combination of intravenous and inhalation agents, some of which also produce amnesia and analgesia. Muscle relaxants are administered as needed to keep the patient immobile and facilitate retraction and visualization of the surgical site. Opioids are administered as needed for analgesia. The anesthesia provider maintains the delicate balance of administering the appropriate agents in the appropriate amounts at the appropriate times to achieve a level of anesthesia neither too deep nor too light for the surgical procedure while maintaining a stable cardiovascular state in the patient.

The anesthesia provider uses direct measurements of vital signs and clinical observation to continually assess the patient's status and need for additional anesthetic agents. For example, if the analgesic agents are wearing off most surgical patients demonstrate a measurable physiologic response to pain such as an increase in blood pressure or heart rate. Indirect measures (clinical observations) such as sweating and **lacrimation** (the production of tears) are also considered reliable indicators of pain response. However, these signs may also indicate an insufficient depth of anesthesia. In addition, specific conditions may cause some of these responses as well. For example, an increased heart rate may be caused by hypovolemia rather than a painful stimulus. Some medications, for example, β-blockers and calcium channel blockers (agents administered for specific heart conditions), can prevent the normal heart rate increase in response to pain. Each patient and each surgical situation present unique challenges in assessing and responding to patient needs under anesthesia.

Awareness Under Anesthesia

A disturbing phenomenon known as awareness under anesthesia has emerged as one of the most challenging problems in current anesthesia practice. It is important to note that dreams and/or fleeting perceptions on induction or emergence are *not* considered true awareness under anesthesia. For reasons that remain unclear, some patients do not demonstrate characteristic (measurable or observable) physiologic responses to pain or have inadequate depth of anesthesia during surgery. The result is that the patient may have direct recall, or explicit memory (Insight 15-4), of intraoperative events. When muscle relaxants are used, the patient is unable to move or speak and therefore is unable to communicate this awareness to the anesthesia provider. An average of 0.1% to 0.2% of all patients undergoing general anesthesia experience some sort of awareness (1-2 per 1000 anesthetics). Because about 21 million patients in the United States receive general anesthesia each year, an estimated 20,000 to 40,000 cases of awareness under anesthesia may be occurring yearly. The risk of awareness appears to be greater when it is necessary to use the lowest possible dose of anesthesia medications to avoid undesirable side effects. Patients who are hemodynamically unstable (such as trauma patients) are also at greater risk for awareness under anesthesia, as well as those undergoing cardiac and emergency obstetric procedures. Patients with a history of substance abuse and patients with chronic pain are also at greater risk. Although the extent of awareness is highly variable, about half of these patients report auditory recall, half report a sensation of being unable to breathe,

INSIGHT 15-4 Explicit and Implicit Memory Under Anesthesia

The term *explicit memory* refers to the ability to recall events—that is, conscious recollection. When a patient has explicit memory of events during surgery, it may be quite traumatic. Although explicit memory may be somewhat vague, some patients have been able to recall specific comments and conversations that took place during their surgical procedure. Much effort is being directed at preventing such occurrences.

But what is *implicit* memory? *Implicit memory* is the term used to describe subconscious processing of information by the brain, demonstrated by changes in the performance of tasks. For example, you know how to tie your shoelaces, but you may not remember exactly how or when you learned to do so. Another example of implicit memory is posthypnotic suggestion. Popular nightclub acts offer hypnosis to audience volunteers. The volunteer is hypnotized and asked to perform some particular behavior when a cue is given. The volunteer is awakened from the hypnotic state and the cue is given, causing the volunteer to display the suggested behavior. The experience occurred, and the behavior was displayed, but the volunteer has no conscious recollection (explicit memory) of why he or she is doing so.

A few experiments have shown that some learning (similar to hypnotic suggestion) is possible while under anesthesia, indicating that implicit memory during anesthesia exists in some form. Surgical patients who agreed to participate in these studies were routinely anesthetized for surgery. During the surgical procedure, verbal instructions were given asking the patient to perform a simple task (such as scratching the nose) on cue during the postoperative interview.

INSIGHT 15-4 Explicit and Implicit Memory Under Anesthesia—Cont'd

On the prearranged cue, a surprising number of patients displayed the suggested behavior, yet without remembering why they were doing so. These studies seem to indicate that a significant number of surgical patients hear and remember what is said (implicit memory), but without conscious recall (explicit memory). The potential impact of implicit memory and the surgical patient is enormous and much remains unknown. Could pessimistic comments made by the surgeon and other surgical team members during surgery have a negative effect on the patient's recovery? Could positive suggestions given under anesthesia actually speed recovery? Until the impact of implicit memory is clearly identified, all surgical team members should consider making only positive, affirming comments and keeping conversations on an encouraging and professional level during surgery. After all, it appears that our patients may be hearing and implicitly remembering everything we say throughout their operations.

and one third recall pain. A number of these patients reportedly go on to develop post-traumatic stress disorder as a result.

TECH TIP

Previously, the surgical team was periodically reminded that the patient's hearing is the last sense to go and the first to return. Inherent in that statement is a belief that what was said during a patient's surgical procedure did not affect the patient. What we now understand about explicit and implicit memory and the number of patients who experience auditory recall (explicit memory) should motivate us to try to effect significant change in surgical team behaviors. We can no longer assume that the patient is unaffected by our conversations and comments during surgery. As surgical technologists, we can support the anesthesia providers in their efforts to bring this understanding to the attention of all surgical team members.

Prevention measures include administration of midazolam for amnesia (provides anterograde amnesia only) and avoidance of the use of neuromuscular blocking agents whenever possible.

Additional methods of patient monitoring have been developed in an effort to predict and prevent awareness under anesthesia. Rather than measure physiologic responses, these devices monitor brain activity and are modified types of electroencephalography. These devices may be known as level-of-consciousness or anesthesia-depth monitors (see Chapter 14). Brain function monitoring is not indicated for all patients, but may be used for select patients based on procedural and physiologic risk factors. It is important to note, however, that although these monitors may provide additional information on patient consciousness, there is not yet a perfect system for preventing awareness under anesthesia.

Muscle Relaxation

Whereas a short-acting muscle relaxant is administered to allow intubation, a long-acting muscle relaxant is often given during the maintenance phase to facilitate exposure of the surgical site. The amount of muscle relaxation required depends on the surgical procedure, with abdominal procedures requiring the deepest relaxation. In addition to depth, timing of relaxation is a crucial factor. The duration of a long-acting muscle relaxant and the anticipated length of the surgical procedure are taken into consideration when selecting and administering the appropriate agent.

The depth of neuromuscular blockade is monitored with the use of a peripheral nerve stimulator. The peripheral nerve stimulator administers an electrical stimulus to a nerve-muscle group and the motor response is assessed, indicating the extent of muscle blockade. Electrodes are placed at the desired location, usually the wrist, and connected to the unit. Alternatively, the unit may be placed directly over a branch of the facial nerve. Different stimuli patterns may be used as indicated, but one of the most common is the train-of-four (TOF) pattern, a series of four electrical stimuli delivered approximately 0.5 seconds apart. Recall from Chapter 14 that the presence of four of the four twitches indicates no muscle relaxation, and zero of the four twitches indicates complete muscle relaxation. The patient's motor response is assessed and used to determine when and how much additional muscle relaxant is necessary to maintain optimal surgical exposure. Ideally, muscle relaxation is present through closure of the deep wound layers and wears off as the superficial layers are closed.

EMERGENCE PHASE

As the procedure is completed, the **emergence phase** begins, during which anesthetic agents are discontinued and allowed to wear off. If indicated, the duration of certain anesthetic agents may be shortened by the administration of reversal agents to permit the patient to gradually awaken. The emergence phase ends when the patient is transported to the PACU.

CAUTION

The emergence phase of anesthesia is another time when the patient is hypersensitive to loud noises and movement. Because the surgical procedure has concluded and pressure exists to minimize the operating room turnover time, surgical technologists in the scrub role are busy with various tasks to break down the sterile back table. These tasks involve manipulation of instruments and metal pans and basins, which can produce loud noises. In addition, the surgical technologist in the circulating role may be performing various duties around the patient, such as dressing application, replacement of blankets, and preparation for patient transfer. Each of these activities may cause a sudden movement of the patient, which in turn may cause laryngospasm. The surgical technologist must always maintain an awareness of the surgical patient's status and make every effort to minimize movement of the patient and noise during the emergence phase of anesthesia.

As the patient awakens and becomes able to maintain his or her own airway, the items used to provide airway support are removed. In masked airway, the pharyngeal airway is removed (if present), but the mask may be left in place to administer oxygen. If an LMA was used, it is removed and replaced with a regular mask for oxygen administration as needed. If the patient has been intubated, particular care is used to assess the appropriate timing for removal of the endotracheal tube, a process called **extubation**. The patient must be breathing on his or her own, with airway reflexes present, and must demonstrate sufficient muscle strength to be able to maintain the airway independently. A mask may be used to administer oxygen if necessary. When vital signs are stable, the patient is carefully moved to a transport stretcher and taken to PACU for the recovery phase. The anesthesia provider gives a detailed report to the PACU staff nurses, who closely monitor the patient during the recovery phase. When it is deemed safe, the patient is discharged from PACU to the appropriate care location.

AGENTS USED FOR GENERAL ANESTHESIA

Several different classes of drugs have been used to achieve general anesthesia. Multiple agents are used to provide an unconscious state, analgesia, amnesia, and muscle relaxation. These medications are presented by category, and the phases of general anesthesia in which they are administered are indicated. The broad categories covered are intravenous induction agents, analgesics, inhalation agents, neuromuscular blocking agents, and reversal agents (Box 15-3).

INTRAVENOUS INDUCTION AGENTS

Intravenous induction agents are administered to produce a rapid loss of consciousness. Agents used to induce unconsciousness are classified as either sedatives or hypnotics. Benzodiazepines are sedatives (see Chapter 13) that may be used for induction. Hypnotic agents used for induction include barbiturates (thiopental and methohexital), ketamine (Ketalar), etomidate (Amidate), and propofol (Diprivan). These agents may also be used during maintenance of general anesthesia.

Benzodiazepines, which have both sedative and amnestic effects, are used preoperatively and occasionally as induction agents in combination with other agents. Benzodiazepines are not commonly used for induction because of the high doses required to induce an unconscious state. Recall that the benzodiazepines include midazolam (Versed), diazepam (Valium), and lorazepam (Ativan). Lorazepam is used to treat anxiety but not for induction and/or maintenance of anesthesia. Midazolam may be

Box 15-3 MAJOR CATEGORIES OF ANESTHESIA MEDICATIONS

Intravenous induction agents
Analgesics
Inhalation agents
Neuromuscular blocking agents
Reversal agents

administered for induction in a dose of 0.1 to 0.3 mg/kg IV, but it causes a greater drop in blood pressure than diazepam. Fentanyl 50 to 100 mcg IV may be given 3 minutes prior to midazolam to speed the onset of unconsciousness. Benzodiazepines do not provide analgesia.

Barbiturates are ultra–short-acting hypnotic agents derived from barbituric acid. Prior to the development of propofol (Diprivan), the most frequently used induction agents were barbiturates—2.5% thiopental (Pentothal) and 1% methohexital (Brevital). Thiopental, for instance, takes only seconds to travel from the injection site to the brain; thus, it is rapidly taken up by the brain, but it is also rapidly eliminated. Methohexital is ultra–short-acting and is more often used for procedures that take place outside the operating room such as cardioversion. Both agents are alkaline (pH greater than 10) and will cause precipitation when administered with acidic agents such as some neuromuscular blocking drugs. Barbiturates induce anesthesia, but have no analgesic effect; patients may therefore be agitated and disoriented during the emergence phase because of the pain they experience.

Ketamine (Ketalar) is a dissociative hypnotic agent used for induction of general anesthesia. Chemically related to the drug phencyclidine (PCP) or "angel dust", ketamine is a powerful amnestic and analgesic—the only hypnotic agent with this property. Induction dose is 1 to 2 mg/kg and the onset of action is 30 to 60 seconds after intravenous injection. When ketamine is used, patients appear to be awake and their eyes may be open; however, they are dissociated from their environment and they do not consciously recall surgical events. Ketamine can cause hallucinations and distorted visual, auditory, and tactile sensations. It also exaggerates the effect of sudden loud noises. Involuntary movements may be present and the dissociative state may make patients difficult to handle. It may be combined with a benzodiazepine to increase amnesia and reduce emergence reactions. Ketamine is not commonly used for maintenance of anesthesia but may be used for superficial procedures of short duration, such as painful dressing changes, débridements, or skin grafts. Ketamine does not produce skeletal muscle relaxation.

Etomidate (Amidate) is a hypnotic agent that produces an unconscious state in less than a minute but provides no analgesia and no muscle relaxation. The induction dose is typically 0.2 to 0.3 mg/kg. This agent is often used for patients with compromised myocardial contractility who cannot tolerate the myocardial depression often seen with other induction agents. Rapid onset and a minimal effect on BP make etomidate an excellent alternative to propofol and the barbiturates. Etomidate is also ideal for brief procedures such as cardioversion. It is particularly useful for induction in trauma patients, who may be hypovolemic and hence unable to tolerate any additional hypotension.

Propofol is a hypnotic agent chemically unrelated to any other anesthetic agent. The active drug is 2, 6-diisopropylphenol suspended in an **emulsion** (a mixture of two liquids not mutually soluble) of 10% soybean oil, 2.25% glycerol, and 1.2% lecithin (a protein found in egg yolk). The most commonly used agent for induction, it is injected intravenously in doses of 1 to 2.5 mg/kg. Propofol produces an unconscious state within a minute, but does not provide analgesia or muscle relaxation. Propofol has a characteristic milky white appearance (Fig. 15-8). Strict aseptic technique must be maintained when handling propofol because it contains no antimicrobial preservatives and can support rapid growth of microorganisms. Unused portions of propofol, as well as intravenous lines, or solutions containing propofol injection, must be discarded at the end of the procedure or within 12 hours (6 hours if propofol was transferred from the original container).

Potential adverse effects include hypotension, bradycardia, and apnea. Many patients (40% to 90%) report a stinging sensation at the injection site. A continuous propofol infusion of 100 to 200 mcg/kg/minute may be used for maintenance of general anesthesia. Because of its brief

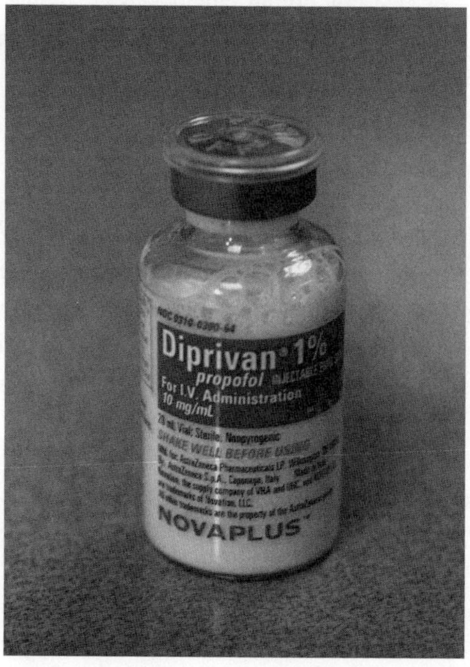

Figure 15-8 Propofol (Diprivan) is an intravenous induction agent.

Box 15-4 INTRAVENOUS INDUCTION AGENTS USED IN GENERAL ANESTHESIA

Sedatives (benzodiazepines)
midazolam (Versed)
diazepam (Valium)
Hypnotics (barbiturates)
thiopental (Pentothal)
methohexital (Brevital)
Hypnotics (various chemical categories)
propofol (Diprivan)
ketamine (Ketalar)
etomidate (Amidate)

duration (4 to 6 minutes), patients recover alert and free of the usual side effects of an anesthetic agent.

See Box 15-4 for a summary of intravenous induction agents used in general anesthesia.

ANALGESICS

Analgesic agents are given during maintenance of general anesthesia to prevent pain during surgery. If adequate pain control is achieved, the amount of other anesthetic agents required may be reduced.

MAKE IT SIMPLE

Apply what you already know to assist you in learning pharmacology. The term *analgesia* literally means "without pain." An analgesic, then, is an agent given to prevent or treat pain. You are already familiar with many examples of analgesics available over the counter, such as aspirin (Bayer, Excedrin, etc.) and acetaminophen (Tylenol). Remember, just as you take aspirin or acetaminophen (analgesics) to relieve the pain of a headache (e.g., that caused by studying so hard to learn all this pharmacology information), we give analgesics (different ones, however) to our patients to relieve the pain of surgery.

The most common analgesic agents administered for anesthesia are classified as opioids. The term ***opioid*** refers to drugs (natural and synthetic) that produce morphine-like effects. The brain has its own natural pain suppression system, in part consisting of neurochemicals called endorphins (or endogenous opioids) and specific receptors sites for these chemicals. Opioids used in anesthesia are able to bind with the brain's natural receptor sites, initiating pain suppression. These agents are most effective when administered prior to a painful event.

{NOTE} *Previously, the term narcotic was used to describe analgesics used for anesthesia and was associated with the production of a state of stupor. In current use, however, the word narcotic is used to indicate any drug that can cause dependence. Thus the term narcotic analgesic is no longer used in reference to anesthesia.*

Opioids are available from several drug sources:

- Plants (also known as a natural source; from the opium poppy, *Papaver somniferum*)
- Semi-synthetic (modified from the natural alkaloids found in the poppy)
- Synthetic (manufactured from chemicals)

Natural opioids are morphine and codeine. Morphine will have an onset of action in 15 to 30 minutes, reach a peak in 45 to 90 minutes, and has a duration of action lasting approximately 4 hours. Codeine is available in Tylenol 3, a combination of acetaminophen and codeine, which may be prescribed for postoperative pain relief.

{NOTE} *Although* NOT *an analgesic, another natural derivative of the opium poppy is papaverine (Insight 15-5), a smooth muscle relaxant that may be administered from the sterile back table.*

Synthetic opioids used for anesthesia are fentanyl (Sublimaze), alfentanil (Alfenta), sufentanil (Sufenta), and remifentanil (Ultiva). These drugs are useful in anesthesia because of their relatively short action and intense analgesic effect. Synthetic opioids are more potent analgesics than morphine, but at equivalent analgesic doses, they cause the same degree of respiratory depression.

Fentanyl is 100 times more potent than morphine. This drug has a rapid onset, about 30 seconds, with a duration of 20 to 40 minutes. Fentanyl provides analgesia plus some sedation. When used as the sole induction agent, the dose is 50 to 150 mcg/kg of body weight. When used in addition to other agents, the dose is 2 to 20 mcg/kg. Alfentanil has one fourth the potency of

INSIGHT 15-5 Papaverine

Papaverine is a chemical derived from the opium poppy *(Papaver somniferum)* that is used as a smooth-muscle relaxant during surgery. Papaverine may be administered from the sterile field during procedures on small blood vessels (such as coronary artery bypass grafts). It is injected at the vessel wall to prevent vasoconstriction from vascular muscle spasms caused by surgical manipulation.

fentanyl and its onset of action is rapid. Lasting just 10 to 15 minutes, alfentanil is classified as an ultra–short-acting opioid. Sufentanil is five to ten times more potent than fentanyl, but it is more rapidly cleared from the body, providing a very rapid recovery. Onset is rapid, with effects lasting 20 to 45 minutes. Remifentanil (Ultiva) is the newest ultra–short-acting opioid and is 20 to 40 times more potent than alfentanil. Onset of effects occurs in 1 to 3 minutes, but duration is only 5 to 10 minutes. An induction dose is typically 1 mcg/kg IV administered over 60 to 90 seconds. If used for maintenance of the analgesia component of general anesthesia, remifentanil is given as a continuous infusion of 0.05 to 2 mcg/kg/minute.

See Table 15-1 for a comparison of opioids used for analgesia during general anesthesia.

INHALATION AGENTS

Inhalation agents are gases or vaporized liquids that induce anesthesia when administered in the air the patient breathes. The first inhalation anesthetics used were ether, chloroform, nitrous oxide, and cyclopropane. Of these, only nitrous oxide gas is in use currently. Ether and cyclopropane are explosive and chloroform is toxic to the liver, so use of these agents was discontinued as new agents were developed. Halothane (Fluothane), introduced in 1956, was the first nonexplosive inhalation agent. Additional inhalation agents have been developed, each generation of new agents improving on previous agents.

Inhalation anesthetics (also called volatile anesthetics) are distributed in liquid form packaged in bottles. The liquid agent is poured into the appropriate vaporizer on an anesthesia machine, and the administration rate is adjusted as needed (Fig. 15-9). The vaporizer turns the liquid agent into a gas that is relatively easy to administer via breathing mask, LMA, or ET. Inhalation agents, which are measured by the percentage of vapor present in the mixture the patient inhales, diffuse into the blood from the air in the alveoli, then rapidly diffuse out of the blood and into the brain—the site of action. Inhalation anesthetics are eliminated from the body quickly, most via the pulmonary, hepatic, and renal systems. The potency of inhalation agents is compared using a measurement called **minimum alveolar concentration (MAC).** The MAC is the concentration that, at one atmosphere of pressure, stops the motor response to incision in 50% of patients.

TECH TIP

Don't confuse the concept of monitored anesthesia care (MAC) discussed in Chapter 14 with minimum alveolar concentration (MAC). If the abbreviation MAC is used in reference to an anesthesia method involving administration of sedation, anxiolysis, and/or analgesia and patient assessment provided by an anesthesia professional, it stands for "monitored anesthesia care." If the abbreviation MAC is used in reference to an inhalation agent (used in general, not local, anesthesia), it stands for "minimum alveolar concentration."

Table 15-1 COMPARISON OF OPIOIDS USED FOR ANALGESIA DURING GENERAL ANESTHESIA

Generic Name	Trade Name	Onset	Duration (min)
fentanyl	Sublimaze	30 seconds	45-60
alfentanil	Alfenta	30 seconds	10-15
sufentanil	Sufenta	30 seconds	20-45
remifentanil	Ultiva	1-3 minutes	5-10

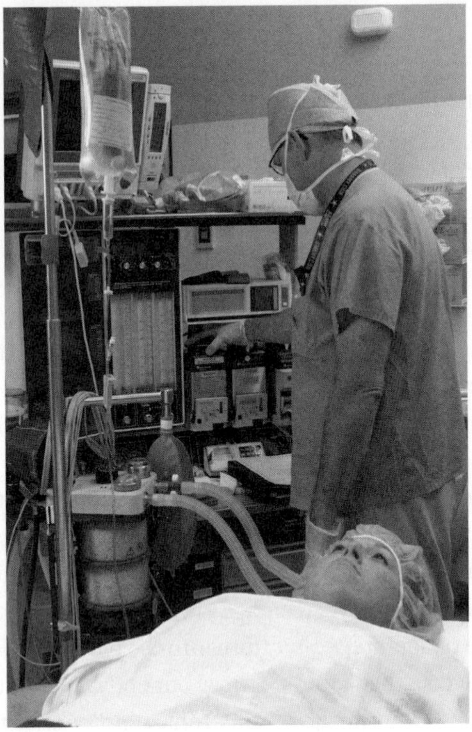

Figure 15-9 Concentration of inhalation anesthetics is controlled in an anesthesia machine.

The disadvantages of inhalation agents include an increased potential for cardiovascular depression and lack of postoperative analgesia. The selection of an inhalation agent is influenced by factors such as solubility of the gas and the patient's cardiac output. The most common inhalation agents in use today include the gas nitrous oxide and three volatile liquid anesthetics, isoflurane (Forane), desflurane (Suprane), and sevoflurane (Ultane).

Nitrous oxide (N_2O)—a colorless, odorless, tasteless gas—is one of the most widely used inhalation anesthetics in clinical practice. Nitrous oxide provides rapid onset and emergence and is completely eliminated by the lungs. Its mild analgesic and amnestic characteristics make it an excellent adjunct to volatile liquid inhalation anesthetic agents. Nitrous oxide is often used in conjunction with volatile anesthetics to reduce the amount of the latter needed. A muscle relaxant must also be given if needed. An interesting characteristic of nitrous oxide is that it will rapidly diffuse out of the circulatory system and into a closed, air-filled cavity such as the middle ear. The resulting increase in pressure can push against a newly placed tympanic membrane graft, so the surgeon may request that nitrous oxide be turned off prior to graft placement during tympanoplasty.

MAKE IT SIMPLE

To help identify the category of an agent, use common word parts as hints. For example, if the name of an agent ends in "-ane," it is probably an inhalation anesthetic. Similarly, the names of local anesthetic agents usually end in "-caine."

The three most common volatile liquid anesthetics are isoflurane (Forane), desflurane (Suprane), and sevoflurane (Ultane). These agents are quite similar to previous volatile liquid anesthetic agents, except that they provide more precise control of maintenance and more rapid induction and emergence. Volatile agents are highly potent and doses can be adjusted to provide some muscle relaxation and rapid emergence. Cardiac depression may be seen with higher doses, so the volatile agents are often used in combination with nitrous oxide. See Table 15-2 for a list of inhalation anesthetic agents.

CAUTION

Inhalation anesthetic agents (except for nitrous oxide), either alone or in combination with succinylcholine (Anectine, Quelicin), have been identified as triggering agents of a rare but life-threatening condition called malignant hyperthermia (see Chapter 16).

NEUROMUSCULAR BLOCKING AGENTS

Agents categorized as neuromuscular blockers are administered to relax skeletal muscles for intubation and surgery. Patients under general anesthesia may be unconscious, pain free, and memory free, but their skeletal muscles continue to respond to stimuli. To receive an endotracheal tube, the patient must be adequately relaxed; that is, the muscles must be relaxed. During some surgical procedures, especially in the abdomen, the patient's muscles must be relaxed to facilitate exposure of the surgical site.

Muscle Physiology Review

There are three types of muscle tissue: cardiac, smooth, and skeletal. Muscles function in circulation, labor and delivery, and intestinal movements, as well as in body movement. For a muscle to contract, it must be stimulated by a motor nerve. The neuromuscular junction is an area where the motor nerve axon is very near the muscle fiber. The space between an axon and a muscle fiber is called a synapse. The neurotransmitter at the neuromuscular junction is acetylcholine (ACh). When

Table 15-2 INHALATION ANESTHETICS

Generic Name	Trade Name
GAS	
nitrous oxide (N_2O)	N/A
VOLATILE LIQUID (VAPOR)	
isoflurane	Forane
desflurane	Suprane
sevoflurane	Ultane

ACh is released from the axon, it diffuses across the synapse (synaptic cleft) and binds to receptor sites on the cell membrane of the muscle fiber (the sarcolemma). ACh causes a wave of depolarization to spread across the muscle fiber to T-tubules, which conduct the wave of depolarization deep into the muscle fibers. As a result of the spreading wave of depolarization, calcium is released from its storage sites within the sarcoplasmic reticulum. The presence of calcium ions allows the contractile elements of the muscle, actin and myosin, to engage, resulting in muscle contraction. For muscle fibers to return to a resting state, ACh must diffuse away from the receptor sites at the neuromuscular junction and be broken down, or recycled, by an enzyme called acetylcholinesterase. This enzyme, which is present abundantly in extracellular fluid, breaks down ACh and terminates the contraction. Calcium ions are then transported back into the sarcoplasmic reticulum for storage and later release. Depolarizing muscle relaxants act like ACh; they bind with receptor sites and initiate a contraction (depolarization). Such contractions are observed as **fasciculations**, small involuntary muscle twitches just under the skin. Subsequent contractions are prevented as long as the depolarizing muscle relaxant stays on the binding sites. Nondepolarizing muscle relaxants act as ACh antagonists; they competitively block receptor sites and prevent ACh binding, thus preventing a contraction (see Fig. 1-11 in Chapter 1).

{NOTE} *Students should consult an anatomy and physiology text to review the physiology of muscle contraction in more depth.*

There are two basic types of muscle relaxants classified according to their action on the motor end-plate: depolarizing and nondepolarizing. Examples of each type are listed with a brief description.

Succinylcholine (Anectine, Quelicin) is the only depolarizing muscle relaxant in use. Succinylcholine acts similarly to the neurotransmitter ACh, but its duration is longer. It causes persistent depolarization and produces fasciculations followed by flaccidity. Succinylcholine is administered in a dose of 0.5 to 1.5 mg/kg IV and effects are seen in 30 to 60 seconds. Duration of effects is also short, usually only 5 to 10 minutes; but because no antagonist or reversal agent is currently available, succinylcholine must be allowed to wear off. Some adverse effects associated with administration of succinylcholine include increased intracranial pressure, increased intraocular pressure, increased intragastric pressure (which increases the potential for regurgitation), and muscle soreness postoperatively. Elevated serum potassium levels have been noted in burn patients receiving succinylcholine. Patients with pseudocholinesterase deficiency may experience prolonged neuromuscular blockade and respiratory paralysis because succinylcholine is not eliminated effectively without that enzyme. The U.S. Food and Drug Administration (FDA) warns against using succinylcholine in children because of cases of unrecognized muscular dystrophy that may lead to hyperkalemia and cardiac arrest. Succinylcholine may be used in children when emergency airway control is necessary (see Chapter 16).

CAUTION

Succinylcholine has been identified as a triggering agent for malignant hyperthermia. See Chapter 16 for additional information.

There are several nondepolarizing muscle relaxants, categorized as long, intermediate, and short-acting. These agents include pancuronium bromide (Pavulon), atracurium besylate (Tracrium), vecuronium bromide (Norcuron), cisatracurium (Nimbex), rocuronium bromide (Zemuron), and mivacurium chloride (Mivacron). The first muscle relaxant, tubocurarine chloride (Curare), is also nondepolarizing (Insight 15-6). Nondepolarizing muscle relaxants prevent muscle contractions by binding to cholinergic receptors, preventing ACh from binding to the receptor sites. Nondepolarizing muscle relaxants do not cause fasciculations and may be used prior to administration of succinylcholine to prevent fasciculations. The selection of a particular nondepolarizing muscle relaxant depends on its pharmacologic properties, such as onset and duration of effects, and side effects, such as those seen in the cardiovascular

IN SIGHT 15-6 The First Muscle Relaxant

The earliest known muscle relaxant was curare. It is a toxin that is extracted from plants found in the rain forest. Indigenous peoples on three separate continents—South America, Africa, and Southeast Asia—used curare on the tips of darts to immobilize monkeys and other tree-dwelling animals. Once discovered by Western culture, curare was used in the experimental laboratory for various purposes. A German report in 1912 described the use of curare on humans as an adjunct to anesthesia; however, the report was generally ignored. Not until 1942 was curare first used in surgery; it was used to relax abdominal muscles of a patient undergoing an appendectomy. Discovery of the benefits of curare radically changed anesthesia practice. Patients could now be routinely intubated, a sporadic practice prior to the use of curare. Since the introduction of curare, many agents have been developed to provide muscle relaxation.

Table 15-3 COMPARISON OF DURATION OF NEUROMUSCULAR BLOCKING AGENTS

Category	Generic Name	Trade Name	Duration (min)
Depolarizing	succinylcholine	Anectine	4-6
Nondepolarizing	mivacurium chloride	Mivacron	6-10
	atracurium besylate	Tracrium	20-35
	vecuronium bromide	Norcuron	25-30
	cisatracurium besylate	Nimbex	45-75
	rocuronium bromide	Zemuron	15-85
	pancuronium bromide	Pavulon	40-65

system. See Table 15-3 for a comparison of the duration of effects of neuromuscular blocking agents. Adverse effects of nondepolarizing muscle relaxants on the cardiovascular system include hypotension or hypertension, tachycardia, bradycardia, and arrhythmias. Dosage is variable, depending on onset time and depth of block required. Nondepolarizing muscle relaxants may be reversed if necessary with an antagonist such as neostigmine (Prostigmine). Neostigmine works by competing with ACh for attachment to acetylcholinesterase. This competition causes a buildup of ACh, which facilitates transmission of impulses across the neuromuscular junction. In addition, some reversal agents, for example edrophonium, stimulate the presynaptic release of ACh as well as binding to acetylcholinesterase.

REVERSAL AGENTS

Occasionally, the surgical procedure may be completed sooner than expected. An example of this situation is a radical hysterectomy. This procedure is expected to take several hours, and so several different long-acting anesthetic agents are administered. If unexpected metastases are discovered in the liver or scattered over the intestines, the procedure may be terminated without resection. This situation may require the administration of reversal agents to counteract specific anesthetic agents. Naloxone (Narcan), nalmefene (Revex), and naltrexone (ReVia, Trexan) are used to reverse opioid analgesics if necessary. Naloxone may be given in a dose of 1 to 4 mcg/kg IV to reverse respiratory depression caused by opioids. It has a short duration of action, 30 to 45 minutes. Nalmefene is a long acting opioid antagonist. Benzodiazepines may be reversed with flumazenil (Mazicon), 8 to 15 mcg/kg IV. When indicated, nondepolarizing muscle relaxants may be reversed with neostigmine (Prostigmin) or edrophonium (Tensilon). Neostigmine is an acetylcholinesterase inhibitor and may be given in doses up to a maximum of 60 to 70 mcg/kg. See Table 15-4 for a list of reversal agents for various anesthetics.

Table 15-4 REVERSAL AGENTS FOR ANESTHETICS

Reversal Agent	Used to Reverse
naloxone (Narcan)	Opioid analgesics
nalmefene (Revex)	Opioid analgesics
naltrexone (ReVia, Trexan)	Opioid analgesics
flumazenil (Mazicon)	Benzodiazepines
neostigmine (Prostigmin)	Nondepolarizing muscle relaxants
edrophonium (Tensilon)	Nondepolarizing muscle relaxants

ADVANCED PRACTICES FOR THE SURGICAL FIRST ASSISTANT

CHAPTER 15—General Anesthesia

Key Terms

acupuncture
biomedicine
cryoanesthesia
hypnoanalgesia
methods to achieve lack of sensation

According to its definition, the term *anesthesia* means "lack of sensation." How this effect is achieved may employ many methods. In addition to the ones mentioned in the previous two chapters, the surgical first assistant should be familiar with some of these alternate anesthesia methodologies. **Cryoanesthesia**, or cryoanalgesia, is also known as frost or refrigeration anesthesia. It is defined as a local anesthesia produced by chilling a part of the body or peripheral nerves to near-freezing temperature to numb the area against pain. The application of cold to tissues creates a conduction block that is similar to a local anesthetic's effect. This technique uses an applicator (cryoprobe) or sprays such as Frigiderm (dichlorotetrafluoroethane). Cryotherapy is used in surgical specialties such as dermatology for dermabrasion or removal of skin lesions, and gynecology for endometrial cryoablation. In these procedures, the extreme cold freezes and destroys the targeted tissues.

Hypnosis has long been associated with entertainment; however, there is a therapeutic hypnosis used in medical applications as well. Called **hypnoanalgesia**, it was approved by the American Medical Association in 1958 as an alternative form of medicine and has been used by dentists, obstetricians, and midwives in place of local anesthesia for many years. In a hypnotized state, a part of the central nervous system shows greater activity and influence on the patient's senses (as feeling and thoughts) and on the sensation of pain. However, this form of therapy can be unpredictable, because its effect depends upon the patient's willingness and acceptance of the method, and the fact that not everyone can be hypnotized.

Acupuncture originated in China more than 2000 years ago and is one of the oldest and most commonly used medical procedures worldwide. This group of procedures involves the stimulation of anatomic points of the body by varying methods. The most studied scientifically is the penetration of the skin with thin, metallic needles that are manipulated by hand or by an electrical stimulation (electroacupuncture). Acupuncture became better known to the American public after James Reston wrote an article for *The New York Times* about his experience in China in the 1970s. He had an emergency appendectomy while visiting there and acupuncture was used to help with his postoperative pain control. The first acupuncture clinic in the United States is claimed to have been opened by Dr. Yao Wu Lee in Washington, D.C., on July 9, 1972. The FDA approved acupuncture needles for use by licensed practitioners in 1996. According to acupuncture theory, pain signals travel from the area of the injury to the spinal cord and brain. Acupuncture generates a stimulus that travels faster and crowds out the pain signals to effectively block and prevent them from reaching the brain. The result is that the patient never experiences the pain.

ALTERNATIVE HEALING THERAPIES

Alternative healing therapies, in addition to those mentioned earlier, are now being accepted into the concepts of Western medicine. They may be defined as treatments for which scientific evidence of safety and usefulness are lacking. The current medical system is based on the conventional approach of theory, knowledge, and research. This is termed ***biomedicine*** or theoretical medicine. However, in the 1990s, consumers began to look outside of the traditional approach toward alternative medicines. In 1992, the U.S. Congress established the Office of Alternative Medicine (OAM) within the National Institutes of Health. In 1998, this office became the National Center for Complementary and Alternative Medicine (NCCAM). Now more funding and research projects for information are possible. The NCCAM has categorized alternative healing and complementary medicines into five main areas: alternative medical systems, mind-body interventions, biologically based therapies, manipulative and body-based methods, and energy therapies.

Alternative medical systems include Asian systems, folk health care, herbal medicines, massage, energy therapy, acupressure, acupuncture, and qigong. A traditional system from India is known as Ayurveda, which aspires to restore the individual's harmony of body, mind, and spirit. Native American, Middle Eastern, Tibetan, Central and South American, and African cultures also have developed traditional alternative medical systems. Other examples include naturopathic and homeopathic medicine. Naturopathic practices are based on the belief that the human body has an innate healing ability. These practices use diet, exercise, lifestyle changes, and natural therapies to enhance the body's ability to ward off and combat disease. Homeopathic medicine is based on the concept that "like cures like." Patients are treated with heavily diluted preparations that practitioners claim cause effects similar to the symptoms presented. Homeopaths also use aspects of the patient's physical and psychological state in recommending remedies.

Mind-body explores the concept that the mind has an ability to affect the body (mental healing). These interventions include meditation, some types of hypnosis, music and art therapy, dance, and prayer. Biologically based therapies include dietary supplements such as herbs and orthomolecular therapies. Herbs are considered as dietary supplements and so are regulated by the Department of Agriculture and the FDA. However, in this category, herbs are not subject to the strict regulations that apply to medications. Orthomolecular therapies use different chemical concentrations to treat disease. These include magnesium, melatonin, and megadoses of vitamins. Manipulative and body-based methods include chiropractic methods, osteopathy, and massage. And finally, energy therapies include biofield and electromagnetic field therapies. Biofield therapies are those that focus on fields that come from the body and include acupuncture, Reiki, qigong, and therapeutic touch. Electromagnetic fields come from sources other than the body and include magnetic fields, alternating current fields, or direct current fields. While these fields have yet to be proven, the therapies are used with patients who have arthritis, cancer, or pain.

Advanced Practices Bibliography

Fulcher E, Fulcher R, Soto C: *Pharmacology principles and applications*, ed 2, St. Louis, 2009, Saunders/Elsevier.

Fuller JK: *Surgical technology: principles and practice*, ed 5, St. Louis, 2010, Saunders/Elsevier.

Mosby's medical dictionary, ed 8, St. Louis, 2009, Mosby/Elsevier.

Rothrock J: *Alexander's care of the patient in surgery*, ed 13, St. Louis, 2007, Mosby/Elsevier.

Advanced Practices Internet Resources

American Association of Acupuncture and Oriental Medicine: www.aaaomonline.org/.

The American Association of Naturopathic Physicians: www.naturopathic.org/content.asp?contentid=59.

Baumann L, Frankel S, Welsh E, et al: Cryoanalgesia with dichlorotetrafluoroethane lessens the pain of botulinum toxin injections for the treatment of palmar hyperhidrosis, *Dermatol Surg* 29(10):1057–1060, Published Online: 17 Sep 2003, © 2010 American Society of Dermatologic Surgery. Available at www3.interscience.wiley.com/journal/118893512/abstract. Accessed August 2, 2010.

Dermabrasion and Chemical Peels, Grand Rounds of the UTMB Department of Otolaryngology. www.utmb.edu/otoref/grnds/chempeel.htm.

Lewis DO: Hypnoanalgesia for chronic pain: the response to multiple inductions at one session and to separate single inductions, *J R Soc Med* 85(10):620–624, 1992. Available at www.ncbi.nlm.nih.gov/pmc/articles/PMC1293691/. Accessed August 2, 2010.

National Acupuncture Foundation: www.nationalacupuncturefoundation.org/pages/about.html.

RxList: *Ethyl Chloride*. www.rxlist.com/ethyl-chloride-drug.htm.

Song S: Health: Mind over Medicine, *Time*, March 19, 2006. Available at www.time.com/time/magazine/article/0,9171,1174707-2,00.html. Accessed August 2, 2010.

Trescot AM: Cryoanalgesia in interventional pain management, *Pain Physician* 6(3):345–360, 2003. Available at www.ncbi.nlm.nih.gov/pubmed/16880882. Accessed August 2, 2010.

Washington Acupuncture Center: www.acupunctureflorida.com/lee.html.

WebMD Feature: *Hypnosis, Meditation, and Relaxation for Pain Treatment*. www.webmd.com/balance/features/hypnosis-for-pain.

Advanced Practices: Learning the Language (Key Terms)

Using your textbook or a standard medical dictionary, look up and write the definitions of each term.

- acupuncture
- biomedicine
- cryoanesthesia
- hypnoanalgesia

Advanced Practices: Review Questions

1. Describe how cryoanesthesia produces a local anesthetic effect.
2. Who has used hypnosis in the past to achieve an anesthetic effect?
3. How does hypnosis produce a local anesthetic effect?
4. Which alternative medical practice to achieve anesthesia is among the oldest and most widely used?
5. Describe how acupuncture produces an anesthetic effect.

KEY CONCEPTS

- Safely providing anesthesia is an art as well as a science. Various drugs and techniques have been used to achieve a state of anesthesia. Although several theories have been proposed, in some cases the exact mechanism of action of anesthetic drugs remains unclear.
- For some procedures, it is important that the patient be under general anesthesia, that is, unconscious, pain free, and immobile. General anesthesia may be necessary because of patient factors or the nature of the surgical procedure.
- Four major components must be accomplished in general anesthesia: hypnosis, analgesia, amnesia, and muscle relaxation.
- There are five phases of administration of a general anesthetic: preinduction, induction, maintenance, emergence, and recovery.
- The two methods or routes used to deliver general anesthetics are intravenous and inhalation.
- Intravenous induction agents include barbiturates, benzodiazepines, ketamine, etomidate, and propofol.
- Analgesics administered as an adjunct to general anesthesia are fentanyl, alfentanil, sufentanil, and remifentanil.
- Common inhalation agents include the gas nitrous oxide and volatile liquid anesthetics such as isoflurane, desflurane, and sevoflurane.
- Muscle relaxants, given as an adjunct to general anesthesia, are categorized as depolarizing and nondepolarizing neuromuscular blockers.
- Agents that may be administered during emergence include naloxone, nalmefene, naltrexone, flumazenil, neostigmine, and edrophonium.
- Anesthesia is a complex physiologic state, often taken for granted by operating room personnel. To function effectively on the surgical team, the surgical technologist must understand the basic concepts of anesthesia and the names of common agents used.

Bibliography

Aronson J: *Meyler's side effects of drugs used in anesthesia,* Amsterdam, 2009, Elsevier.

Evers A, Maze M: *Anesthetic pharmacology: physiologic principles and clinical practice,* St. Louis, 2004, Churchill Livingstone/Elsevier.

Nagelhout J, Plaus K: *Nurse anesthesia,* ed 4, St. Louis, 2010, Saunders/Elsevier.

Stoelting R, Miller R: *Basics of anesthesia,* ed 5, St. Louis, 2007, Churchill Livingstone/Elsevier.

Internet Resources

Anesthesia Awareness Campaign: www.anesthesiaawareness.com/.

Diprivan 1% Injectable Emulsion (propofol). www1.astrazeneca-us.com/pi/diprivan.pdf.

Laryngeal Mask Airway. www.airwaycarnival.com/LMA.htm.

LMA Airway Management. www.lmana.com/index.php.

LMA ProSeal. www.lmaco.com/proseal.php.

Preventing, and Managing the Impact of Anesthesia Awareness, *Sentinel Event Alert* The Joint Commission: Issue 32 - October 6, 2004. www.jointcommission.org/sentinelevents/sentineleventalert/sea_32.htm.

LEARNING THE LANGUAGE (KEY TERMS)

Using your textbook or a standard medical dictionary, look up and write the definitions of each term.

anesthesia
emergence phase
emulsion
endotracheal (ET) tube
extubation
fasciculation
induction phase
intubation
lacrimation
laryngeal masked airway (LMA)
maintenance phase
minimum alveolar concentration (MAC)
opioid
post-anesthesia care unit (PACU)
preinduction phase
rapid sequence induction (RSI)

REVIEW QUESTIONS

1. What does the term *anesthesia* mean?
2. What are the indications for general anesthesia?
3. What is the surgical technologist in the scrub role doing during each phase of general anesthesia? What is the circulating surgical technologist doing?
4. What are the components of a general anesthetic?
5. Which categories of agents are used to accomplish general anesthesia?
6. Can you name an agent in each category?
7. How are depolarizing and nondepolarizing muscle relaxants alike? How are they different?
8. How should the potential for awareness under anesthesia impact the surgical technologist's practice?

CRITICAL THINKING

Scenario 1

Mrs. Diaz is a 45-year-old woman. She sustained a fractured wrist when she slipped on an icy sidewalk exiting a restaurant. She has been admitted to surgery for closed reduction and cast application.

1. Which method of airway control do you think the anesthesia provider will select for Mrs. Diaz? Justify your answer.

Scenario 2

Johnny Duncan is a 5-year-old boy. He sustained a greenstick fracture of the forearm when he fell from a park swing set. He has been admitted to surgery for a closed reduction and cast application.

1. Which method of administration do you think the anesthesia provider will select for Johnny? Justify your answer.

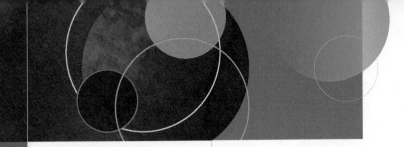

CHAPTER 16 Emergency Situations

OBJECTIVES *After completing this chapter, you should be able to:*

1. Define terminology related to emergency situations.
2. Identify emergency situations associated with anesthesia.
3. Identify medications used in emergency situations.
4. State the purpose of drugs used in emergency situations.
5. Identify the category of specified emergency medications.
6. Discuss the role of the surgical technologist during a cardiac emergency in surgery.
7. List clinical signs of malignant hyperthermia.
8. Outline the basic course of treatment for malignant hyperthermia.
9. Discuss the role of the surgical technologist in a malignant hyperthermia crisis.

KEY TERMS

anaphylaxis
asystole
bradycardia
bronchospasm
diaphoresis
hemoglobinuria
pyrexia
tachycardia
tachypnea
urticaria

One goal of anesthesia is to maintain the patient in a stable physiologic state throughout the course of anesthesia and surgery. However, surgery and anesthesia are complex processes that significantly impact the human physiologic state. Additionally, many patients requiring surgery are critically ill and some may have multiple organ system failure. The most common anesthesia emergency situations, which vary from mild to life-threatening, merit careful study by the surgical technologist. Emergency situations in the operating room may be due to existing disease, trauma, the surgical procedure, anesthesia, or may be of unknown origin and may occur at any point during the patient's care. This chapter is specifically focused on anesthesia-associated emergencies that require pharmacologic treatment. Two of the most pertinent to the surgical technologist—cardiac arrest and malignant hyperthermia (MH)—are discussed at length. The surgical technologist should be able to respond appropriately as a surgical team member to any patient emergency. To function in a competent manner, the surgical technologist must have a thorough knowledge of the medications frequently used in emergency situations.

RESPIRATORY EMERGENCIES

Intraoperative respiratory impairment or obstruction may be caused by a number of factors including swelling from trauma or inflammation, bronchospasm, or laryngospasm. In rare cases, surgical intervention (tracheotomy) may be indicated.

BRONCHOSPASM

Bronchospasm is defined as impaired breathing from constriction and inflammation of the bronchi. Severe bronchospasm could result in brain injury or death. When bronchospasm occurs in surgery, it is not usually due to an acute asthma event—especially when the asthma patient is asymptomatic at the time of surgery. Acute bronchospasm can be triggered by chemical or mechanical irritation, the most common of which is tracheal irritation caused during intubation (also known as reflex bronchospasm). Placement of a laryngeal masked airway (LMA) does not trigger bronchospasm. Other factors that place patients at greater risk for bronchospasm may include mucosal edema, increased mucus production, and inflammation of the airway.

If indicated, patients with symptomatic asthma may be treated preoperatively with oral or inhaled steroids. Preoperative breathing treatments may also include β-adrenergic agonists (see Insight 16-1 later in this chapter) such as albuterol (Proventil, Ventolin).

Signs of bronchospasm may include wheezing, prolonged exhalation, decreased breath sounds, decreased oxygen saturation (called desaturation), increased airway pressures during positive pressure ventilation, and hypotension. When presented with these signs, the anesthesia provider will look for mechanical causes such as blockage of the endotracheal tube. The anesthesia provider will also assess the depth of anesthesia, which is critical to prevention of bronchospasm before and during airway management and intubation.

When intraoperative bronchospasm is diagnosed, 100% oxygen is administered and the patient is ventilated manually. The underlying condition, such as a foreign body or secretions in the airway, incorrect endotracheal (ET) tube placement, or inadequate depth of anesthesia is identified and corrected. Several different categories of medications may be used to treat bronchospasm. A group of drugs called β-adrenergic agonists (classified by physiologic action, see Chapter 1) are particularly effective. Albuterol may be aerosolized (nebulized) and administered via the ET tube. Another β-agonist, terbutaline (Brethine), may be administered subcutaneously. Epinephrine (Adrenalin) is a hormone (see Chapter 8) that may be aerosolized through the ET tube or given subcutaneously (0.1 to 0.5 mL of a 0.1% solution) for bronchospasm. Anticholinergics (see Chapter 13) such as atropine and ipratropium (Atrovent) may also be administered aerosolized through the ET tube to treat bronchospasm. If bronchospasm persists, corticosteroids (see Chapter 8) such as hydrocortisone, methylprednisolone, or dexamethasone may be delivered in aerosolized form, but are usually given intravenously.

ANAPHYLAXIS

Anaphylaxis is a severe, systemic allergic reaction in a susceptible person caused by a second exposure to a triggering agent. It is the most severe type of hypersensitivity reaction to medications, anesthetics, latex, or blood administered in surgery. All patients receiving parenteral medications are at risk, especially those with a history of allergic reactions. Anaphylaxis is estimated to occur in 1 of every 4,000 to 25,000 administrations of anesthetic agents. The most common cause of allergic reactions during anesthesia are the neuromuscular blocking agents (see Chapter 15), responsible for approximately 65% of allergic reactions. Latex allergy is the second most common cause, followed by antibiotic agents. Other items implicated in allergic reactions include bone cement, chlorhexidine, and vascular grafts.

{NOTE} *Medications that cause the most frequent allergic reactions include neuromuscular blockers such as atracurium, antibiotics such as penicillin, contrast media, codeine, morphine, meperidine, and thiopental.*

Signs of allergic reactions can occur in 2 to 20 minutes and persist for up to 36 hours. Allergic reactions range from mild signs such as **urticaria** (hives or raised skin patches) to severe cardiovascular and respiratory problems indicating anaphylaxis. Respiratory symptoms include bronchospasm, dyspnea (labored breathing), **tachypnea** (rapid breathing), respiratory obstruction, and laryngeal edema. Anaphylactic shock is a complete cardiovascular collapse, which occurs rapidly and may include cardiac and respiratory arrest.

Under general anesthesia, however, the first sign of anaphylaxis usually noted is hypotension. Hypotension is treated with intravenous fluids, and medications used to raise blood pressure (vasopressor or inotropic agents) are administered as needed. Vasopressor agents include dopamine (Intropin) and dobutamine (Dobutrex). Agents such as ephedrine or phenylephrine (Neo-Synephrine) may also be used to treat hypotension associated with allergic reaction.

Treatment for anaphylaxis differs from treatment for a mild allergic reaction. If early signs of a mild allergic reaction appear, potentially triggering medications being administered are discontinued and a 0.5 to 0.7 mg/kg dose of diphenhydramine (Benadryl) may be given intravenously. Diphenhydramine (Benadryl, Allergan 50) is an antihistamine; it is used to treat allergic reactions or as an adjunct in treatment of anaphylaxis. Steroids such as methylprednisolone (15-25 mg/kg) or hydrocortisone (4-15 mg/kg) may be administered. If this treatment is effective, surgery may continue, but without the use of the suspected agent. If conservative treatment is not effective, the allergic reaction may quickly progress to anaphylaxis. An IV bolus of epinephrine (0.2-1 mcg/kg) may be administered for moderate cases and a repeat dose may be necessary. If circulatory collapse occurs, 3 to 15 mcg/kg of epinephrine IV may be administered.

Transfusion (Hemolytic) Reaction

Blood transfusion reaction is an infrequent, but important, type of intraoperative allergic reaction. Any adverse reaction to the administration of blood or blood products in surgery is a condition treated and managed by the anesthesia provider. Transfusion reactions may be one of three types: febrile nonhemolytic, allergic, or hemolytic. Febrile nonhemolytic reaction is caused by antibodies binding to donor white blood cells (WBCs) or platelets and is rarely seen during surgery. It is characterized by a temperature increase of 1° C and is usually treated with antipyretic agents, such as acetaminophen. Allergic transfusion reaction is usually mild and caused by medications taken by the blood donor or additives used in blood product preparation. Mild allergic transfusion reaction is treated as any mild allergic reaction previously discussed.

Hemolytic transfusion reaction occurs when ABO-type–incompatible blood or blood products are administered (see Chapter 11). Mixing of incompatible donor red blood cell (RBC) antigens and recipient antibodies causes hemolysis. Numerous safety precautions are taken during all phases of blood replacement to ensure that the patient receives only compatible blood, but errors can occur. Hemolytic transfusion reaction may be characterized by hypotension, **hemoglobinuria** (hemoglobin in urine), anuria or oliguria, fever, and disseminated intravascular coagulopathy (DIC). Hemolytic transfusion reactions are first treated by discontinuation of blood products, followed by control of hypotension as described previously. Diuretics such as mannitol (Osmitrol) may be administered to maintain kidney function.

LARYNGOSPASM

Laryngospasm is an involuntary constriction of the vocal cords that may result in partial or complete closure. It may occur during intubation or shortly after extubation as a reaction to the endotracheal tube. Patients are most at risk for laryngospasm if they are lightly anesthetized at the time of extubation. Laryngospasm is seen more frequently in children and infants, and is characterized by a high-pitched "crowing" sound (called stridor) on inspiration. The risk is increased for infants 0 to 3 months of age and significantly increased for those with asthma or upper respiratory infection.

Positive airway pressure is administered by masked ventilation with chin-lift in an effort to break a partial spasm, but may actually make a complete spasm worse. If the spasm does not respond to positive pressure ventilation, and pulse oximetry shows oxygen desaturation, a 0.1 to 2 mg/kg dose of the depolarizing muscle relaxant succinylcholine (Anectine) will be administered intravenously. (For further discussion of succinylcholine, see Chapter 15.) Generally, small doses of succinylcholine (5-10 mg) will achieve reasonable vocal cord relaxation and allow adequate mask ventilation. Larger doses of succinylcholine can be used to relax muscles to allow reintubation, which may be necessary to achieve adequate ventilation and oxygenation. Atropine may be administered in pediatric patients to treat bradycardia caused by hypoxemia.

CARDIAC ARREST

Cardiac arrest is the sudden, unexpected loss of cardiac function, breathing, and consciousness. Cardiac arrest may occur at any time before, during, or after an anesthetic. Cardiac arrest may be attributed to several causes. For example, some anesthetic agents can cause cardiac irritability or arrhythmias; in other cases, the patient may have an existing condition, such as cardiac disease, low serum potassium, or hypovolemia that might precipitate a cardiac arrest. Cardiac or respiratory arrest in surgery may be called a "code blue" or "code 99." When cardiac arrest occurs in other departments of the hospital, an announcement is usually made throughout the hospital over the public address system to notify members of the code blue team (including an emergency physician and designated members of the anesthesia and respiratory care departments) to report to the location of the arrest. Most surgery departments do not announce the code blue to the entire hospital, however, because the surgical team is its own code blue team.

All surgical technologists should be certified in basic cardiac life support at the healthcare provider level by the American Heart Association. Surgical technologists should know exactly what must be done to treat cardiac arrest in the operating room. Cardiac arrest in surgery could occur in any number of possible scenarios, so it is helpful to use critical thinking techniques to analyze each situation. The surgical technologist must be familiar with the roles of various team members and understand the functions performed by each team member during cardiac resuscitation.

Usually, it is the anesthesia provider who makes the diagnosis, officially calls the code blue, and initiates treatment. The ABCDs of cardiopulmonary resuscitation techniques (airway, breathing, circulation, and defibrillation) are followed. The anesthesia provider manages the airway and breathing. If the ET tube has not been placed when the cardiac arrest occurs, an immediate laryngoscopy is performed, the ET tube is placed, and mechanical ventilation is initiated. If the patient has been intubated prior to the arrest, mechanical ventilation continues. Cardiac compressions may be administered by any member of the surgical team trained in cardiopulmonary resuscitation, depending on the situation. For example, if the operation has not yet begun, any member of the team may begin compressions. If the operation is in progress, the surgeon may administer cardiac compressions from the sterile field. Alternately, the circulator may perform cardiac compressions under the sterile drapes. A designated team member calls for, or goes to get, the crash cart, which contains emergency medications and a cardiac defibrillator (Fig. 16-1). The defibrillator is brought into the operating room and prepared for

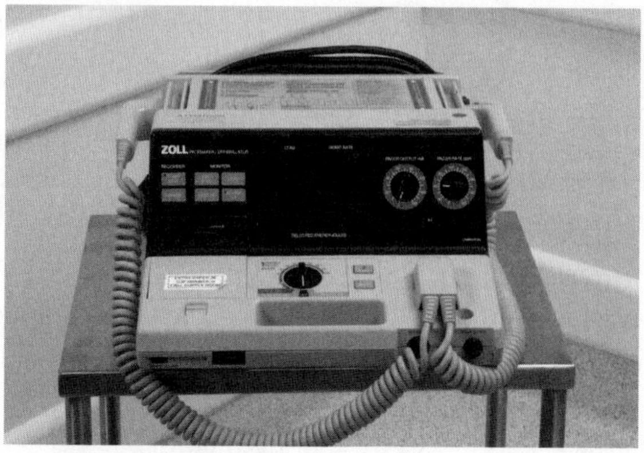

Figure 16-1 Cardiac defibrillator.

use. Defibrillator paddles are placed on the patient's chest by a physician, physician's assistant, surgical first assistant, or registered nurse and used to deliver electric shocks to the patient's heart in an effort to reinstate normal cardiac rhythm. If the thoracic cavity is open, sterile internal defibrillator paddles are opened and placed by the surgeon into direct contact with the heart muscle.

Several factors influence the tasks the surgical technologist performs in resuscitation efforts, including the time of day (how much help is available) and whether or not an incision has been made (need to protect sterility of the surgical site). In addition, the tasks may vary depending on the role the surgical technologist is performing on the surgical team: scrub role, second assistant, surgical first assistant, or circulator. In the scrub role, the surgical technologist may remain sterile to cover the wound if necessary or prepare the internal defibrillator paddles for use. If an additional surgical technologist is scrubbed in as a second assistant, he or she may be asked to break scrub to obtain the crash cart. If necessary, the second assistant may be designated as the official record keeper, documenting all medications given, dosages, and times of events on a special cardiac resuscitation form provided on the crash cart. A surgical technologist in the surgical first assistant role may perform cardiac compressions, close the surgical incision if needed, or serve as record keeper. In the circulating role, the surgical technologist may notify appropriate personnel of the situation, bring in or call for the crash cart, assist the anesthesia provider, perform cardiac compressions, or serve as record keeper.

Regardless of the role, it is vital that the surgical technologist be familiar with medications given during a cardiac emergency, their usual dosages, and their purposes. The following is a brief synopsis of drugs

Table 16-1 SUMMARY OF CARDIAC RESUSCITATION DRUGS

Generic Name	Purpose
epinephrine	Raise blood pressure to perfuse heart muscle
vasopressin	Raise blood pressure to perfuse heart muscle
amiodarone	Treat ventricular dysrhythmias
lidocaine	Treat ventricular dysrhythmias
magnesium sulfate	Treat hypomagnesemia
sodium bicarbonate	Treat metabolic acidosis

frequently used in treatment of a cardiac arrest (Table 16-1).

Epinephrine (Adrenalin) is a hormone (see Chapter 8) that acts as a vasopressor (causes vasoconstriction and raises blood pressure), to improve coronary perfusion pressure and myocardial blood flow. During cardiac arrest, epinephrine may be administered intravenously in an effort to restore both force and rate of myocardial contractions. Intravenous dosage of epinephrine for cardiac arrest is usually 1 mg bolus (depending on patient's weight), which may be repeated every 3 to 5 minutes as needed. One dose of the anti-diuretic hormone vasopressin (Pitressin), 40 units IV, may be given to replace the first or second dose of epinephrine in adults. Vasopressin causes intense peripheral vasoconstriction to support myocardial blood flow during a cardiac event.

Additional medications that may be administered during cardiac arrest include anti-dysrhythmic agents amiodarone (Cordarone) and lidocaine (Xylocaine). These agents are used in an effort to restore normal cardiac rhythm in cases of ventricular tachycardia or ventricular fibrillation. Amiodarone is administered IV in a dose of 300 mg and an additional dose of 150 mg may be administered if the condition persists. Lidocaine may be given in an initial dose of 1 to 1.5 mg/kg IV, followed by 0.5 to 0.75 mg/kg IV for a maximum dose of 3 mg/kg if necessary. If ventricular fibrillation leads to **asystole**—failure of ventricles to contract—then atropine 1 mg may be administered IV and repeated every 3 to 5 minutes up to 3 doses.

Magnesium sulfate (1 to 2 mg bolus intravenously) may be administered to correct hypomagnesemia if present. Sodium bicarbonate is used to treat metabolic acidosis, which is frequently seen in cardiac arrest. Hyperventilation and effective cardiac compressions usually correct acidosis, so sodium bicarbonate is indicated only when blood gas analysis demonstrates significant acidosis. Sodium bicarbonate neutralizes excess hydrogen ion concentration in the blood, thus raising blood pH. When administered during cardiac arrest, the dose of sodium bicarbonate is 1 mEq/kg intravenously, repeated 0.5 mEq/kg every 10 minutes.

TECH TIP

Many different drugs may be used during a cardiac emergency, and only the most common are introduced here. It is strongly suggested that the surgical technology student review an actual crash cart at a local clinical facility to further study the medications used to treat cardiac arrest.

MISCELLANEOUS CARDIOVASCULAR DRUGS

There are a huge number of cardiovascular drugs, only a few of which are of concern to the routine practice of surgical technology. The surgical patient may be taking various cardiovascular medications to manage chronic heart problems such as angina or congestive heart failure. In addition, some cardiovascular medications may be administered during the course of anesthesia and surgery. These agents are classified in several categories (see Insight 16-1), and only the most common agents are discussed in this chapter.

Adrenergic Agonists

Adrenergic agonists, also called sympathomimetics, are agents that mimic the effect of epinephrine and norepinephrine. Dopamine (Intropin) is an adrenergic agonist and anti-arrhythmic agent used to increase blood pressure and cardiac output. It may be given in a dose of 2 to 10 mcg/kg/minute to treat **bradycardia** (slow heart rate, usually fewer than 60 beats per minute).

Phenylephrine (Neo-Synephrine) and methoxamine (Vasoxyl) are α-adrenergic agonists used to treat cardiac arrhythmias and to treat hypotension by causing peripheral vasoconstriction.

Dobutamine (Dobutrex) is a β-adrenergic agonist and positive inotropic agent used to treat cardiac failure (medically, for chronic conditions) and hypotension (intraoperatively, for acute situations).

IN SIGHT 16-1 Cardiovascular Medications and the Autonomic Nervous System

The majority of cardiovascular drugs are agonists or antagonists (see Chapter 1). Recall that agonists are drugs that bind to or have an affinity (attraction) for a receptor, causing a particular response. Antagonists, then, are drugs that bind to a receptor and prevent a response, also called receptor blockers. Cardiovascular drugs affect the autonomic nervous system, adrenergic agents affect the sympathetic system, and cholinergic agents affect the parasympathetic system. Recall from physiology class that neurotransmitters are the natural chemicals that cause responses in the autonomic nervous system. The sympathetic neurotransmitters are epinephrine and norepinephrine, and the major cholinergic neurotransmitter is acetylcholine. Adrenergic agonists, therefore, are agents that mimic the effect of epinephrine and norepinephrine (sympathomimetics). Cholinergic agonists mimic the effects of acetylcholine (parasympathomimetics). Adrenergic antagonists block the effects of epinephrine and norepinephrine (sympatholytics). Cholinergic antagonists (called anticholinergics) block the effects of acetylcholine (parasympatholytics).

Adrenergic receptors are further divided into alpha (α)-receptors and beta (β)-receptors, and each subtype is divided into two further subtypes: α-1 and α-2, and β-1 and β-2. α-Adrenergic receptors respond to norepinephrine and β-adrenergic receptors respond to epinephrine. An additional type of adrenergic receptor responds to the neurotransmitter dopamine (called dopaminergic receptors).

Adrenergic agonists include the catecholamines epinephrine (α-1, β-1, β-2), norepinephrine, dopamine, dobutamine, and isoproterenol (β-1 and β-2). Other adrenergic agonists are ephedrine, phenylephrine, and methoxamine. Selective β-2 adrenergic agonists are albuterol and terbutaline, used as bronchodilators.

Adrenergic antagonists (blockers) include the α-blocker prazosin (Minipress), used to treat hypertension; the β-blockers metoprolol (Lopressor) used to treat hypertension, angina, and heart failure; propranolol (Inderal) used to treat hypertension, angina, and arrhythmias; and a nonselective adrenergic antagonist, labetalol (Normodyne), used to manage hypertension.

Cholinergic agonists include pilocarpine (used in ophthalmology for miosis and treatment of open-angle glaucoma) and neostigmine (used to reverse nondepolarizing muscle relaxants).

Cholinergic antagonists (anticholinergics) include atropine, glycopyrrolate (Robinul), and scopolamine (preoperative medications; see Chapter 13). Atropine in low doses slows the heart rate, but in high doses increases the heart rate by blocking the vagus nerve's ability to inhibit the SA and atrioventricular (AV) nodes of the intrinsic rate mechanism of the heart. Ipratropium (Atrovent) is an anticholinergic used to reverse bronchoconstriction associated with chronic obstructive pulmonary disease (COPD).

In addition to the classification as agonists or antagonists, several other medical terms are used to classify cardiac drugs by their action on the heart. Inotropic agents change the force of cardiac muscle contractions. Dromotropic agents increase the conductivity of nerve or muscle fibers. Chronotropic agents influence the rate of cardiac contractions.

Isoproterenol hydrochloride (Isuprel) is a β-adrenergic agonist and positive inotropic agent administered to increase the rate and force of myocardial contractions. It is also used to treat bradyarrhythmias and serves as a bronchodilator.

Norepinephrine bitartrate (Levophed) is a β-1 agonist and potent peripheral vasoconstrictor used to raise blood pressure, subsequently increasing coronary artery blood flow.

Albuterol (Proventil, Ventolin) and terbutaline (Brethine) are selective β-2 adrenergic agonists used to treat bronchospasm as earlier described for respiratory emergencies.

Adrenergic Antagonists

Adrenergic antagonists, also called sympatholytics, are agents that block the effects of epinephrine and norepinephrine. Labetalol (Normodyne) and atenolol (Tenormin) are β-adrenergic antagonists, or β-blockers, that slow the heart rate and are used to treat cardiac arrhythmias and hypertension. β-Blockers are also classified as Class II anti-arrhythmic drugs.

CHOLINERGIC AGENTS

Cholinergic agonists, also called parasympathomimetics, are agents that mimic the effects of acetylcholine (ACh). Cholinergic antagonists, also called anticholinergics or parasympatholytics, are agents that block the effects of ACh.

Cholinergic agonists are not used in the treatment of cardiac conditions, but cholinergic antagonists (anticholinergics) may be used in certain instances. Atropine sulfate is a cholinergic antagonist used to block the effects of the vagus nerve on the sinoatrial (SA) node of the heart. Recall that atropine or a similar drug, glycopyrrolate (Robinul), may be given preoperatively (see Chapter 13) to dry oral secretions (antisialagogue). Blocking the effects of the vagus nerve also prevents bradycardia resulting from a stimulus such as stretching the peritoneum or placing traction on eye muscles. If asystole (absence of heartbeat) occurs as a response to such actions, cardiac resuscitation is initiated. Additional amounts of atropine (up to a maximum of 3 mg) may be injected during the resuscitation process.

Anti-arrhythmics

Anti-arrhythmics are agents used to prevent or treat irregularities in the force or rhythm of the heart. Lidocaine (Xylocaine) is a local anesthetic that also has anti-arrhythmic effects. As a cardiac anti-arrhythmic agent, lidocaine is administered intravenously to treat ventricular arrhythmias such as premature ventricular contractions (PVCs). Lidocaine in a 1% or 2% solution is administered slowly in doses of 1 to 1.5 mg/kg IV. This may be repeated 0.5 to 0.75 mg/kg every 2 to 5 minutes as needed, not to exceed 3 mg/kg. Additional anti-arrhythmic agents include amiodarone (Cordarone) and procainamide (Pronestyl) to treat atrial fibrillation, lidocaine-resistant ventricular arrhythmias, and paroxysmal atrial tachycardia (PAT). Digoxin (Lanoxin) is an anti-arrhythmic agent and positive inotropic drug used to treat atrial arrhythmias because it helps to slow signals originating in the SA node of the heart.

Anti-arrhythmic agents are classified in four categories. Class I drugs are sodium channel blockers such as procainamide (Procanbid, Pronestyl). Class II anti-arrhythmics are β-blockers such as metoprolol (Lopressor) and propranolol (Inderal). Class III agents are potassium channel blockers such as sotalol (Betapace) and Class IV drugs are calcium channel blockers such as verapamil (Isoptin).

Calcium Channel Blockers

Calcium channel blockers are agents that reduce the flow of calcium into cells of the heart and blood vessels, resulting in relaxation of the blood vessels (vasodilation). These medications are also categorized as Class IV anti-arrhythmic agents. Nicardipine (Cardene) and nifedipine (Procardia) are arterial vasodilators used to treat hypertension and stable angina. Verapamil hydrochloride (Isoptin) is a calcium channel blocker also used to treat hypertension and angina, and is helpful in treating tachyarrhythmias.

Vasodilators

Vasodilators are agents that relax smooth muscle cells in blood vessel walls, reducing blood pressure and enabling less restricted blood flow to vital tissues. Nitroglycerine (Transderm-Nitro, Nitrodisc) and nitroprusside (Nipride) are nitrovasodilators used to treat hypertension, angina, and cardiogenic shock.

Inotropic Agents

Inotropic agents are drugs that alter the force of cardiac muscle contraction. Positive inotropic agents increase the force of muscle contraction and negative inotropic agents weaken contractions. Positive inotropic agents include digoxin (Lanoxin), dopamine, dobutamine (Dobutrex), epinephrine, and norepinephrine. Negative inotropic agents include β-blockers, calcium channel blockers, and procainamide (Pronestyl), all of which are also classified as anti-arrhythmic agents. Digoxin is a positive inotropic agent used to treat congestive heart failure (CHF), atrial fibrillation and flutter, and PAT. Digoxin is administered intravenously, 0.5 to 1.0 mg in divided doses.

MALIGNANT HYPERTHERMIA

Malignant hyperthermia (MH) is a rare but life-threatening reaction triggered in susceptible individuals by administration of certain anesthetic agents. MH is an inherited muscle condition that causes a hypermetabolic state in patients exposed to those specific trigger agents. It is estimated to occur in 1 in 15,000 children and 1 in 50,000 adults. When trigger agents are administered, massive amounts of calcium accumulate in muscle cells causing sustained contractions. At first, the patient's metabolism is aerobic, causing increased oxygen consumption, an increase in end-tidal carbon dioxide (hypercarbia), respiratory acidosis, and heat production. As adenosine triphosphate (ATP) is used up, metabolism becomes anaerobic resulting in lactic acid production, metabolic acidosis, and more heat production. Muscle cell membranes become stressed and break down (rhabdomyolysis), releasing potassium, myoglobin (a muscle cell protein), and creatine kinase.

If untreated, mortality is nearly 80%. Agents known to trigger this disease are succinylcholine (Anectine) and all inhalation anesthetics except nitrous oxide. Although the condition is rare, it is crucial that the surgical technologist understand the signs, treatment, and pharmacology involved in such a crisis in order to provide competent assistance to the anesthesia team. It is important to realize that patients who are identified preoperatively as positive for malignant hyperthermia should ***not*** be at risk for an intraoperative MH episode because trigger agents should *not* be administered to those patients during the course of general anesthesia.

CAUTION

Once MH has been triggered, the patient can die in as short a time as 15 minutes, so prompt diagnosis and treatment are vital.

CLINICAL SIGNS OF MALIGNANT HYPERTHERMIA

Contrary to popular belief, **pyrexia** (rapid increase in body temperature) is *not* an early indicator of MH (Box 16-1). A rise in patient temperature indicates that a full crisis is in effect. The earliest sign presented is an increase in end-tidal carbon dioxide. An increase of even 5 mm Hg could be significant. End-tidal CO_2 can increase for several reasons other than MH; but when other possibilities have been ruled out, the anesthesia provider may begin to alert the operating room staff that potential exists for an MH crisis.

Additional early signs include **tachycardia** and **tachypnea** (rapid breathing). These conditions may have other causes, but in combination with the signs described here, tachycardia and tachypnea are classic symptoms of MH. Both tachycardia and tachypnea are means the body uses to eliminate the excess carbon dioxide that is accumulating because of the hypermetabolic crisis.

Muscle rigidity, especially masseter muscle rigidity (MMR), can be an early warning of MH; but there are other, benign causes of MMR. Opinions vary on the correlation here; but if MMR is present, the patient should be closely monitored for MH. In combination with signs described previously, MMR is considered a classic sign of MH. In addition, the patient may exhibit an unstable blood pressure, arrhythmias, cyanosis, **diaphoresis** (profuse sweating), and a rapid increase in body temperature (pyrexia). Temperatures of higher than 42° C have been reported. Other late signs include skin mottling, myoglobinuria, and hyperkalemia.

MALIGNANT HYPERTHERMIA TREATMENT PROTOCOL

Once MH has been identified, the surgical procedure is stopped if possible and all triggering agents are discontinued. The patient is hyperventilated with 100% oxygen to help eliminate the excess CO_2 that accumulates in the blood. Dantrolene sodium (Dantrium), a skeletal muscle relaxant developed specifically to treat MH, is administered intravenously (Fig. 16-2). Initial dosage is a bolus of 2.5 mg/kg. Dantrolene is packaged, freeze-dried, in vials of 20 mg with 3 g of mannitol, and must be reconstituted with 60 mL of sterile water. In an adult patient weighing 80 kg (176 lb), 200 mg of dantrolene (10 vials) is required to begin treatment. Dosages may reach 10 mg/kg, so in this case, 800 mg (40 vials) of dantrolene might need to be reconstituted. If additional help is not available (as seen when doing emergency on-call procedures), it may become necessary for the scrubbed surgical technologist to break scrub and help reconstitute dantrolene as directed by the anesthesia provider. Once sterile water has been injected into the vial, the mixture must be shaken vigorously until the solution becomes clear yellow, indicating complete reconstitution. Dantrolene may be repeated in a dose of 2 mg/kg every 5 minutes, then 1 to 2 mg/kg/hr, and is administered until symptoms disappear. MH may also be seen in children, so

Box 16-1 CLINICAL SIGNS OF MALIGNANT HYPERTHERMIA

Increase in end-tidal CO_2
Tachycardia
Tachypnea
Masseter muscle rigidity (MMR)
Unstable blood pressure
Arrhythmias
Cyanosis
Diaphoresis
Pyrexia

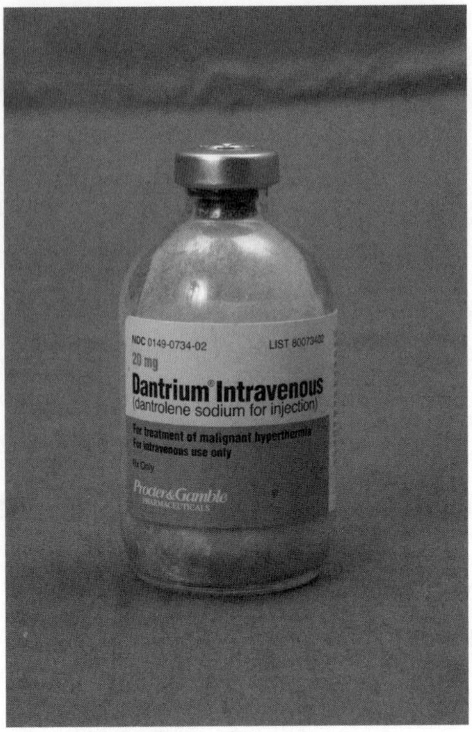

Figure 16-2 Vial of dantrolene (Dantrium) used to treat malignant hyperthermia.

the number of vials reconstituted is adjusted accordingly by patient weight.

Sodium bicarbonate is given intravenously in doses of 1 to 2 mEq/kg to treat the metabolic acidosis resulting from high concentrations of lactate in the blood. Blood gases are monitored frequently. The patient must be rapidly cooled to prevent brain damage. Ice packs are applied to groin, neck, and axilla in an effort to lower the temperature. Iced lavage of stomach, rectum, or bladder may be performed to cool the patient's core temperature.

Muscle cells are destroyed during an MH crisis, and the myoglobin that is released in this process tends to accumulate in the kidneys, obstructing flow. To keep the kidneys functioning properly, diuretics such as 20% mannitol (Osmitrol) or furosemide (Lasix) are given intravenously. Each 20 mg vial of dantrolene contains 3 mg of mannitol.

Procainamide or lidocaine is given intravenously to treat arrhythmias secondary to electrolyte imbalances. Procainamide (Procan SR, Pronestyl) and lidocaine (Xylocaine) are anti-arrhythmic agents used to control cardiac arrhythmias seen in MH. Glucose and insulin are administered to treat hyperkalemia, frequently seen because potassium (K^+) is released as muscle cells are destroyed. All these treatment steps are taken virtually simultaneously and are arranged to help remember key points. All patient vital functions are monitored closely to determine response to treatment. Continuous monitoring of expired CO_2 (capnography) is crucial, as are establishment of arterial lines, frequent blood gas assessment, and accurate temperature measurement. A Foley catheter should be in place to measure urine output. Basic treatment steps for an MH crisis are summarized in Box 16-2.

MAKE IT SIMPLE

The treatment steps for MH are easier to learn if you formulate an easy-to-remember acronym such as "How do surgical technologists do it?" or HDSTDI. "H" stands for hyperventilate, "D" for dantrolene, "S" for sodium bicarbonate, "T" for temperature management, "D" for diuretics, and "I" for insulin.

For additional information, visit the Malignant Hyperthermia Association of the United States website at www.mhaus.org.

A 24-hour hotline staffed by volunteer physicians has been established to assist with information to treat an MH crisis: 1-800-MH HYPER (1-800-644-9737).

Treatment can be considered successful when vital signs and blood gases return to within normal limits. Elective surgery is discontinued. Life-threatening surgery is resumed, but with different anesthetic agents and a different anesthesia machine to prevent residual inhalation agent from triggering a second crisis. On cancellation or completion of the surgical procedure, the patient is transported to the intensive care unit (ICU) or post-anesthesia intensive unit (PACU) accompanied with the replenished MH cart, because another episode could yet occur. Always consult

Box 16-2 MALIGNANT HYPERTHERMIA TREATMENT STEPS

Hyperventilate—with 100% oxygen
Dantrolene—administer 2.5 to 10 mg/kg intravenously
Sodium bicarbonate—administer intravenously to treat metabolic acidosis
Temperature management—treat with ice packs and lavage
Diuretics—administer mannitol or furosemide intravenously
Insulin—treat hyperkalemia

and follow individual institution policies covering an MH crisis. The surgical technologist should become familiar with all institutional policies covering any emergency situation, including MH. In addition, the surgical technologist should be familiar with signs, treatment, and pharmacology of MH to provide competent assistance during an MH crisis as directed by the anesthesia provider.

KEY CONCEPTS

- A number of emergency situations arise associated with anesthesia, including respiratory conditions, cardiac arrest, and MH.
- Although not common in surgery, these situations merit careful study and continuing education. As an allied health professional, the surgical technologist must attain and maintain the proficiency required to function effectively in these emergency situations.
- Drugs used to treat cardiac arrest include epinephrine, vasopressin, amiodarone, lidocaine, procainamide, magnesium sulfate, and sodium bicarbonate.
- Numerous miscellaneous cardiovascular drugs are also administered in surgery to treat various conditions.
- MH is a hypermetabolic crisis triggered by some anesthetic agents. Signs of an MH crisis include tachycardia, tachypnea, masseter muscle rigidity, unstable blood pressure, arrhythmias, cyanosis, diaphoresis, and pyrexia. Basic treatment steps for MH include hyperventilation with 100% oxygen, intravenous injection of dantrolene and sodium bicarbonate, temperature management, and administration of diuretics.

Bibliography

Atlee JL: *Complications in anesthesia*, Philadelphia, 2007, Saunders/Elsevier.

Nagelhout J, Plaus K: *Nurse anesthesia*, ed 4, St. Louis, 2010, Saunders/Elsevier.

Stoelting R, Miller R: *Basics of anesthesia*, ed 5, St. Louis, 2007, Churchill Livingstone/Elsevier.

Internet Resources

American Association of Nurse Anesthetists (search for "malignant hyperthermia"): www.aana.com/.

American Heart Association: www.americanheart.org.

American Society of Anesthesiologists: www.asahq.org/.

Malignant Hyperthermia Association of the United States: www.mhaus.org/.

Texas Heart Institute Heart Information Center (topics about medicines for cardiovascular disease): www.texasheartinstitute.org/HIC/Topics/Meds/index.cfm.

LEARNING THE LANGUAGE (KEY TERMS)

Using your textbook or a standard medical dictionary, look up and write the definitions of each term.

anaphylaxis
asystole
bradycardia
bronchospasm
diaphoresis
hemoglobinuria
pyrexia
tachycardia
tachypnea
urticaria

REVIEW QUESTIONS

1. What are some complications that can occur during anesthesia?
2. Which medications may be used to treat those complications?
3. Can you name some drugs used to treat cardiac arrest? What is the purpose of each of those agents?
4. What are the signs of malignant hyperthermia?
5. What are the basic treatment steps for MH?

6. What would the surgical technologist do during a cardiac emergency in the scrub role? In the assistant circulating role?
7. What would the surgical technologist do during a malignant hyperthermia crisis in the scrub role? In the assistant circulating role?

CRITICAL THINKING

Scenario 1

You have just finished first scrubbing for a tonsillectomy. While you are cleaning up, the patient is extubated and begins emitting a high-pitched "crowing" sound indicating that the patient is experiencing laryngospasm.

1. What steps do you take?
2. What steps does the anesthesia provider take?

Scenario 2

You are scheduled to scrub an abdominal aortic aneurysm repair on a 63-year-old man who has tested positive for malignant hyperthermia.

1. What additional preparations must be made for this patient and why?

Scenario 3

It is 8 AM, and you have just scrubbed in to retract (second scrub role, not first scrub) on a gastric resection procedure. The patient is draped, but no incision has been made when anesthesia calls a code blue. The patient is in cardiac arrest.

1. Which basic duties will be performed by each team member?
2. What duties might you be required to perform?

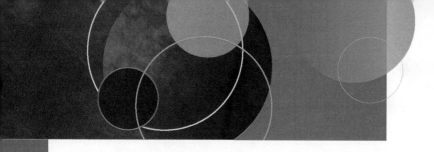

Drug Category Index

Medication Categories Commonly used from the Sterile Back Table by Surgical Specialty

Category	Chapter
General Surgery	
Antibiotics	Chapter 5
Contrast Media	Chapter 6
Fluids and Irrigation Solutions	Chapter 11
Hemostatic Agents	Chapter 9
Local Anesthetics	Chapter 14
Obstetrics and Gynecology	
Dyes	Chapter 6
Fluids and Irrigation Solutions	Chapter 11
Hemostatics, Chemical	Chapter 9
Hormones	Chapter 8
Staining Agents	Chapter 6
Genitourinary	
Contrast Media	Chapter 6
Dyes	Chapter 6
Fluids and Irrigation Solutions	Chapter 11
Orthopedic Surgery	
Antibiotics	Chapter 5
Fluids and Irrigation Solutions	Chapter 11
Hemostatic Agents	Chapter 9

Category	Chapter
Hormones, Anti-inflammatory agents	Chapter 8
Local Anesthetics	Chapter 14
Otorhinolaryngology	
Antibiotic Ointments and Suspensions	Chapter 5
Epinephrine	Chapter 8
Fluids and Irrigation Solutions	Chapter 11
Hemostatic Agents	Chapter 9
Local Anesthetics	Chapter 14
Ophthalmology	
Antibiotics, ophthalmic	Chapter 10
Anti-glaucoma Agents	Chapter 10
Anti-inflammatory Agents	Chapter 10
Dyes, ophthalmic	Chapter 10
Enzymes	Chapter 10
Irrigation Solutions	Chapter 10
Local Anesthetics	Chapter 10
Miotics	Chapter 10
Mydriatics and Cycloplegics	Chapter 10
Viscoelastic Agents	Chapter 10

Category	Chapter
Plastic and Reconstructive Surgery	
Antibiotics	Chapter 5
Dyes	Chapter 6
Hemostatic Agents	Chapter 9
Hormones, Anti-inflammatory Agents	Chapter 8
Local Anesthetics	Chapter 14
Peripheral Vascular Surgery	
Antibiotics	Chapter 5
Anti-coagulants, systemic	Chapter 9
Contrast Media	Chapter 6
Hemostatic Agents	Chapter 9
Local Anesthetics	Chapter 14
Cardiovascular Surgery	
Antibiotics	Chapter 5
Anti-coagulants, systemic	Chapter 9

Category	Chapter
Contrast Media	Chapter 6
Hemostatic Agents	Chapter 9
Local Anesthetics	Chapter 14
Papaverine	Chapter 15 (Insight 15-5)
Thoracic Surgery	
Dyes	Chapter 6
Hemostatic Agents	Chapter 9
Local Anesthetics	Chapter 14
Neurosurgery	
Antibiotics	Chapter 5
Dyes	Chapter 6
Fluids and Irrigation Solutions	Chapter 11
Hemostatic Agents	Chapter 9
Hormones, Anti-inflammatory agents	Chapter 8
Local Anesthetics	Chapter 14

Index

Note: Page numbers followed by *b* indicate boxes, *f* indicate figures and *t* indicate tables.

A

D

E

I

Q

R

S

T

U

V

W

X

Z